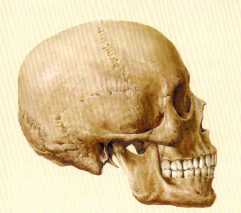

主审 ■ 钟世镇　柏树令

主编 ■ 徐国成　韩秋生　霍　琨

人体解剖学

彩色图谱

HUMAN ANATOMY

第二版

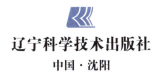

辽宁科学技术出版社

中国·沈阳

《人体解剖学彩色图谱》编委会名单

主　　审　钟世镇　柏树令

主　　编　徐国成　韩秋生　霍　琨

副主编　王效杰　陈永春　刘海兴　李德华　周播江　戈　果　张玉和　滕诚毅　秦　毅　雍刘军

编绘人员　（按姓氏笔画为序）

丁银秀　马全瑞　马江波　王正东　王剑华　令狐艳　冯利强　卢　辰　司马学琴　宁志丰
田　伟　任占川　刘文庆　刘　兵　刘　富　孙慧哲　扬　畅　朱颖飞　许本柯　邢雪松
齐金萍　何红云　余资江　余修贵　张本斯　张　杰　张　晔　张莲香　李永涛　李军平
李寿田　李斯宁　李立新　杜赵康　邹卫东　陈拥彬　单　伟　孟　健　金春峰　金海峰
姚立杰　赵　海　唐　莹　聂　政　曹小明　崔　勇　康朝胜　梁栋阳　曾　亮　蒋彦军
谢立平　焦旭文　颜　玲

标本制作　刘铁生　刘瑞昌　佟玉章　姜振林

图书在版编目（CIP）数据

人体解剖学彩色图谱（第二版）/ 徐国成，韩秋生，霍琨主编. —2 版. —沈阳：辽宁科学技术出版社，2010.9（2020.9 重印）

ISBN 978-7-5381-6653-8

I. ①人… II. ①徐… ②韩… ③霍… III. ①人体解剖学–图谱 IV. ①R322-64

中国版本图书馆 CIP 数据核字（2010）第 167694 号

人　体　解　剖　学　彩　色　图　谱

出版发行　辽宁科学技术出版社
　　　　　地址：沈阳市和平区十一纬路 29 号
　　　　　邮编：110003
　　　　　联系电话：024-23284360
　　　　　邮购热线：024-23284502　23284357
　　　　　E-mail：lkzzb@mail.lnpgc.com.cn
　　　　　http://www.lnkj.com.cn
印 刷 者　辽宁新华印务有限公司
经 销 者　各地新华书店
幅面尺寸：190mm×260mm
印　　张：16
字　　数：350 千字

插　　页：4
印　　数：96001-102000
出版时间：2003 年 8 月第 1 版
　　　　　2010 年 9 月第 2 版
印刷时间：2020 年 9 月第 17 次印刷
责任编辑：宋纯智
封面设计：刘　枫
版式设计：于　浪
责任校对：东　戈　淑　敏
书　　号：ISBN 978-7-5381-6653-8
定　　价：75.00 元

序

PREFACE

解剖学是每个临床医生必须掌握的基本知识，特别是系统解剖学更为重要。举例来说，一支动脉起自何处，其行走途径和终末支进入何处，在手术时是否可以结扎，或在行介入治疗时应如何调控导管的插入方向，都要有系统解剖学的知识，才能进行检查或治疗。同样，对一条神经也必须知道它起自何处、行走途径及其分支的分布情况。总之，人体各部分是不可分割的，任何一个体内病变多会涉及到人的整体；临床医生切不可局限地、孤立地来考虑临床问题。因此，掌握系统解剖学知识对临床医生的重要性也就不言而喻了。

记得70年前我在同济大学医学院上医学的第一课，就是系统解剖学的运动系统，包括骨骼、关节和肌肉。当时是上午上课，下午在尸体上自己动手解剖，每周六老师必来考问，所以我们老一辈的系统解剖学知识还是很牢固的，到今天还很熟悉这门重要课程。现在的情况不同了，缺少尸体供医学生自己动手解剖，只能以大体标本来示教，或仅仅从教材的线条图上学习，这当然是远远不够的。那么，补救的最好办法就是阅读一本实用的系统解剖学彩色图谱了。

人体的形态结构和层次毗邻关系复杂，要清晰逼真地显示出来，必须用彩色来表达，使读者阅读时一目了然。迄今为止我国还缺少一部人工绘制的按人体系统编绘的中国人自己的《人体解剖学彩色图谱》。今天，这部精美的图谱终于问世了，这是医学界的一件大喜事。编绘者历时6年，共编绘彩图近500幅，由运动系统、内脏学、脉管系统、感觉器官和神经内分泌系统五个部分组成。编绘中，作者首次将水彩绘画技巧融入到医学图谱的绘制中，使图谱本身不仅具有科学性、严谨性、实用性，更显示了其艺术性。特别要提出的，这本图谱是根据中国人自己的人体结构绘画的，清晰明了，是当今不可多得的一部好书。相信这部《人体解剖学彩色图谱》的问世将对解剖学科的建设起到促进作用，对临床多科医生在工作中起到辅助作用。

我乐于为此书作序，并热忱地把这本巨著推荐给广大的医学生、研究生，特别是临床多科医生。

裘法祖

中国科学院院士
全国高等医药院校临床医学专业
教材评审委员会名誉主任委员

前言
INTRODUCTION

人体解剖学图谱是高等医学院校学生学习、认识人体结构和功能的工具书。近年来，国内有很多解剖学图谱相继问世，但还缺乏一部人工绘制的较系统和全面的适合医学生和临床医生使用的人体解剖学彩色图谱。为此我们编绘了这部按系统排列的《人体解剖学彩色图谱》。彩图不仅能清晰、逼真地表现人体复杂的形态、结构关系，而且能更好地指导医学生和医务工作者的学习和临床实践。

这部《人体解剖学彩色图谱》遵循国内高、中等医学院校教学大纲的要求，系统地展示了正常人体的形态、结构。在参阅了大量的国内外图谱资料的基础上，又编绘了一些特殊剖面的彩图，画龙点睛，突出了大纲的重点、难点内容。

本书共编绘了近500幅彩图，是一本采用水彩绘画语言表现人体结构的医学图谱。这种写实的绘画风格使本书更具特色，不仅具有内容的科学性、严谨性，而且具有审美价值。这是将水彩绘画技巧引入到医学图谱绘制上的一种创新尝试。为了准确地表现中国人体的结构特点，大部分彩图都以标本写生为主，并尽力还原器官结构的本来色彩，使彩图更具真实性和艺术性。

本书共分五大部分，包括运动系统、内脏学（消化系统、呼吸系统、泌尿系统和生殖系统）、脉管系统、感觉器官和神经内分泌系统。这部图谱除系统地展示人体的形态结构外，还详细地揭示了人体重要部位结构间的毗邻关系，使人体的复杂结构一目了然。全书名词以全国自然科学名词审定委员会公布的"人体解剖学名词"（1991）为准。

本书在编绘过程中，得到了中国医科大学各级领导的关心和支持；得到了国内兄弟院校的大力协助；还荣幸地得到了国内著名的医学界前辈裘法祖院士和钟世镇院士的勘误、斧正以及人民卫生出版社具有丰富医学图谱编辑经验的张之生编审的鼎力支持，在此深表谢意。

本书自第一版出版以来，已近八年时间，受到了广大读者的欢迎，此次修订为第二版，改正了书中的差错和疏漏。由于编者水平所限，虽经第二版修订，缺点和错误在所难免，敬请同行不吝赐教，以便进一步完善。

编 者

2010 年 8 月于中国医科大学

目录
CONTENTS

运动系统 LOCOMOTOR SYSTEM

1. 人体骨骼（前面观）The human skeleton（anterior aspect）-------------------------- 2
2. 人体骨骼（后面观）The human skeleton（posterior aspect）------------------------ 3
3. 骨的构造 Structure of the bones -- 4
4. 骨的连结 The osseous joint --- 4
5. 脊柱（前面观）The spinal column（anterior aspect）--------------------------------- 5
6. 脊柱（后面观）The spinal column（posterior aspect）-------------------------------- 5
7. 脊柱（外侧面观）The spinal column（lateral aspect）-------------------------------- 5
8. 各部椎骨的形态 Features of the individual vertebrae ------------------------------ 6
9. 骶骨（前面观）The sacrum（anterior aspect）------------------------------------- 7
10. 尾骨（前面观）The coccyx（anterior aspect）------------------------------------ 7
11. 骶骨（后面观）The sacrum（posterior aspect）----------------------------------- 7
12. 尾骨（后面观）The coccyx（posterior aspect）----------------------------------- 7
13. 椎骨的连结（正中矢状切面）The intervertebral joints（median sagittal section）------------ 8
14. 椎骨的连结（前面观）The intervertebral joints（anterior aspect）--------------------- 8
15. 椎间关节和椎间盘（水平切面）The intervertebral joint and disc（horizontal section）--------- 8
16. 项韧带（外侧面观）Ligamentum nuchae（lateral aspect）------------------------- 9
17. 寰枕和寰枢关节（后面观）The atlantooccipital joint and atlantoaxial joint（posterior aspect）-------- 9
18. 骨性胸廓（前面观）The osseous thorax（anterior aspect）------------------------ 9
19. 胸骨（前面观）The sternum（anterior aspect）---------------------------------- 10
20. 胸骨（侧面观）The sternum（lateral aspect）---------------------------------- 10
21. 胸肋关节（前面观）Sternocostal joint（anterior aspect）------------------------- 10
22. 肋椎关节（前面观）Costovertebral joint（anterior aspect）----------------------- 10
23. 第一肋骨 First rib -- 10
24. 第七肋骨 Seventh rib --- 10
25. 颅（前面观）The skull（anterior aspect）-------------------------------------- 11
26. 颅（外侧面观）The skull（lateral aspect）------------------------------------- 12
27. 颅底（内面观）The base of the skull（internal aspect）------------------------- 13
28. 颅底（外面观）The base of the skull（external aspect）------------------------- 14
29. 颅骨（正中矢状切面）The skull（median sagittal section）----------------------- 15
30. 颅（上面观）The skull（superior aspect）-------------------------------------- 15
31. 颅（后面观）The skull（posterior aspect）------------------------------------- 15
32. 新生儿颅（前面观）The skull of a newborn infant（anterior aspect）-------------- 16
33. 新生儿颅（外侧面观）The skull of a newborn infant（lateral aspect）------------- 16
34. 新生儿颅（上面观）The skull of a newborn infant（superior aspect）------------- 16
35. 新生儿颅底（下面观）The base of skull of a newborn infant（inferior aspect）------- 16
36. 骨性鼻腔外侧壁 The lateral wall of the bony nasal cavity ----------------------- 17
37. 骨性鼻腔外侧壁（示鼻旁窦的开口）The lateral wall of the bony nasal cavity
    （showing the apertures of the paranasal sinuses）-------------------------------- 17

38. 颅冠状切面（前面观）Coronary section of the skull（anterior aspect）---------------- 17

39. 下颌骨（外侧面观）The mandible（lateral aspect）---------------- 17

40. 舌骨 The hyoid bone ---------------- 17

41. 额骨（前面观）The frontal bone（anterior aspect）---------------- 18

42. 额骨（下面观）The frontal bone（inferior aspect）---------------- 18

43. 筛骨（上面观）The ethmoid bone（superior aspect）---------------- 18

44. 筛骨（后面观）The ethmoid bone（posterior aspect）---------------- 18

45. 上颌骨（外面观）The maxilla（external aspect）---------------- 19

46. 上颌骨（内面观）The maxilla（internal aspect）---------------- 19

47. 颞骨（外面观）The temporal bone（external aspect）---------------- 19

48. 颞骨（内面观）The temporal bone（internal aspect）---------------- 19

49. 颞骨（下面观）The temporal bone（inferior aspect）---------------- 20

50. 腭骨（后面观）The palatine bone（posterior aspect）---------------- 20

51. 腭骨（内面观）The palatine bone（internal aspect）---------------- 20

52. 蝶骨（前面观）The sphenoid bone（anterior aspect）---------------- 21

53. 蝶骨（后面观）The sphenoid bone（posterior aspect）---------------- 21

54. 枕骨和蝶骨（上面观）The occipital bone and sphenoid bone（superior aspect）---------------- 22

55. 颞下颌关节（外面观）The temporomandibular joint（external aspect）---------------- 22

56. 颞下颌关节（矢状切面）The temporomandibular joint（sagittal section）---------------- 22

57. 锁骨（上面观）The clavicle（superior aspect）---------------- 23

58. 肩胛骨（前面观）The scapula（anterior aspect）---------------- 23

59. 锁骨（下面观）The clavicle（inferior aspect）---------------- 23

60. 肩胛骨（后面观）The scapula（posterior aspect）---------------- 23

61. 肱骨（前面观）The humerus（anterior aspect）---------------- 24

62. 肱骨（后面观）The humerus（posterior aspect）---------------- 24

63. 桡骨和尺骨（前面观）The radius and ulna（anterior aspect）---------------- 24

64. 桡骨和尺骨（后面观）The radius and ulna（posterior aspect）---------------- 24

65. 手骨（掌侧面）The bones of the hand（palmar aspect）---------------- 25

66. 手骨（背侧面）The bones of the hand（dorsal aspect）---------------- 25

67. 肩关节（前面观）The shoulder joint（anterior aspect）---------------- 26

68. 肩关节（内面观，去掉肱骨）The shoulder joint（internal aspect, without humerus）---------------- 26

69. 肩关节（冠状切面）The shoulder joint（coronal section）---------------- 26

70. 肘关节（前面观）The elbow joint（anterior aspect）---------------- 26

71. 肘关节矢状切面（示肱尺关节）Sagittal section of the elbow joint（showing the humeroulnar joint）---------------- 27

72. 前臂骨的连结（前面观）The radioulnar syndesmosis（anterior aspect）---------------- 27

73. 手关节（掌面观）The joints of the hand（palmar aspect）---------------- 28

74. 腕关节（冠状切面）The joints of the wrist（coronal section）---------------- 28

75. 髋骨（内面观）The hip bone（internal aspect）---------------- 29

76. 髋骨（外面观）The hip bone（external aspect）---------------- 29

77. 小儿髋骨（外面观）The hip bone of a child（external aspect）---------------- 29

78. 股骨（前面观）The femur（anterior aspect）---------------- 30

79. 股骨（后面观）The femur（posterior aspect）---------------- 30

80. 髌骨（前面观）The patella（anterior aspect）---------------- 30

81. 髌骨（后面观）The patella（posterior aspect）---------------- 30

82. 胫骨和腓骨（前面观）The tibia and fibula（anterior aspect）---------------- 30

83. 胫骨和腓骨（后面观）The tibia and fibula（posterior aspect）---------------- 30

84. 足骨（背面观）Bones of the foot（dorsal aspect）---------------- 31

85. 足骨（跖面观）Bones of the foot（plantar aspect）---------------- 31

86. 骨盆的韧带（前面观和后面观）The ligaments of the pelvis（anterior aspect and posterior aspect）---------------- 32

87. 骨盆（上面观）The pelvis（superior aspect）---------------- 32

88. 骨盆（正中矢状切面）The pelvis（median sagittal section）---------------- 33

89. 髋关节（前面观）The hip joint（anterior aspect）---------------- 33

90. 髋关节（后面观）The hip joint（posterior aspect）-- 33
91. 切开关节囊（示髋关节腔内面）The opened articular capsule
　　（showing the internal surface of the hip joint cavity）--- 34
92. 髋关节（冠状切面）The hip joint（coronal section）-- 34
93. 膝关节（前面观）The knee joint（anterior aspect）-- 34
94. 膝关节（后面观）The knee joint（posterior aspect）--- 34
95. 切开关节囊前部（示膝关节腔内面）The anterior aspect of the opened articular capsule
　　（showing the internal surface of the knee joint cavity）--- 35
96. 膝关节半月板和交叉韧带（上面观）The articular meniscus and cruciate ligament of the knee joint
　　（superior aspect）--- 35
97. 膝关节前面观（切除关节囊）The anterior aspect of the knee joint（without the articular capsule）
98. 膝关节后面观（切除关节囊）The posterior aspect of the knee joint（without the articular capsule）--------------------- 35
99. 足关节（切面）The joints of foot（section）-- 36
100. 小腿骨连结（前面观）The tibiofibular syndesmosis（anterior aspect）-------------------------------- 36
101. 距小腿关节和足关节（外侧面观）The talocrural joint and the joints of foot（lateral aspect）----------- 37
102. 足关节（下面观）The joints of foot（inferior aspect）-- 37
103. 全身肌肉（前面观）Muscles of the whole body（anterior aspect）-------------------------------------- 38
104. 全身肌肉（后面观）Muscles of the whole body（posterior aspect）------------------------------------- 39
105. 头颈肌（前面观）Muscles of the head and neck（anterior aspect）------------------------------------- 40
106. 头颈肌的浅层（外侧面观）Superficial layer of the muscles of the head and neck（lateral aspect）------------------- 41
107. 头颈肌的深层（外侧面观）Deep layer of muscles of the head and neck（lateral aspect）------------------ 41
108. 颈深肌群（前面观）Deep cervical muscle group（anterior aspect）------------------------------------- 42
109. 胸部肌深层（前面观）Muscles of the deep layer of the thorax（anterior aspect）---------------------- 42
110. 胸前壁（内面观）The anterior thoracic wall（internal aspect）-- 43
111. 胸后壁（内面观）The posterior thoracic wall（internal aspect）--------------------------------------- 43
112. 腹前外侧壁肌（前面观）Muscles of the anterolateral abdominal wall（anterior aspect）-------------- 44
113. 腹后壁肌及膈（前面观）Muscles of the posterior abdominal wall and the diaphragm（anterior aspect）-------------- 44
114. 腹壁的层次 The layers of the abdominal wall --- 45
115. 腹前壁的内面 The internal aspect of the anterior abdominal wall------------------------------------- 46
116. 腹股沟区（1）Inguinal region（1）--- 47
117. 腹股沟区（2）Inguinal region（2）--- 47
118. 腹股沟区（3）Inguinal region（3）--- 48
119. 腹股沟区（4）Inguinal region（4）--- 48
120. 腹股沟三角（内面观）Inguinal triangle（internal aspect）--- 48
121. 背部肌肉(1) Muscles of the back(1) -- 49
122. 背部肌肉(2) Muscles of the back(2) -- 49
123. 膈（上面观）The diaphragm（superior aspect）-- 50
124. 膈（下面观）The diaphragm（inferior aspect）-- 50
125. 上肢肌（前面观）（1）Muscles of the upper limb（anterior aspect）（1）----------------------------- 51
126. 上肢肌（前面观）（2）Muscles of the upper limb（anterior aspect）（2）----------------------------- 51
127. 上肢肌（外侧面观）Muscles of the upper limb（lateral aspect）-------------------------------------- 52
128. 上肢肌（后面观）（1）Muscles of the upper limb（posterior aspect）（1）--------------------------- 52
129. 上肢肌（后面观）（2）Muscles of the upper limb（posterior aspect）（2）--------------------------- 52
130. 手掌侧肌（1）Palmar muscles of the hand（1）-- 53
131. 手掌侧肌（2）Palmar muscles of the hand（2）-- 53
132. 手掌侧肌（3）Palmar muscles of the hand（3）-- 54
133. 手背侧肌（1）Dorsal muscles of the hand（1）-- 54
134. 手背侧肌（2）Dorsal muscles of the hand（2）-- 54
135. 手掌侧腱鞘 The tendinous sheaths of the palmar side of the hand ----------------------------------- 55
136. 手背侧腱鞘 The tendinous sheaths of the dorsal side of the hand ----------------------------------- 55
137. 下肢肌深层（前面观）Deep layer of the muscles of the lower limb（anterior aspect）--------------- 56
138. 下肢肌深层（后面观）Deep layer of the muscles of the lower limb（posterior aspect）-------------- 56

139. 下肢肌（外侧面观）Muscles of the lower limb（lateral aspect）--- 57

140. 足底肌（1）Plantar muscles（1）--- 58

141. 足底肌（2）Plantar muscles（2）--- 58

142. 足腱鞘（内侧面观）The tendinous sheaths of the foot（medial aspect）--- 59

143. 足腱鞘（外侧面观）The tendinous sheaths of the foot（lateral aspect）--- 59

144. 男性会阴肌 Male perineal muscles --- 60

145. 女性会阴肌 Female perineal muscles --- 60

内脏学 SPLANCHNOLOGY

146. 消化系统全貌 General arrangement of the alimentary system --- 62

147. 口腔的结构（1）Structure of the oral cavity（1）--- 63

148. 口腔的结构（2）Structure of the oral cavity（2）--- 63

149. 牙的构造（模式图）The structure of tooth（schema chart）-- 64

150. 上颌恒牙的排列（下面观）Arrangement of the permanent teeth of maxilla（inferior aspect）-------------- 64

151. 下颌恒牙的排列（上面观）Arrangement of the permanent teeth of mandible（superior aspect）---------- 64

152. 恒牙（外面观）The permanent teeth（external aspect）--- 65

153. 乳牙（外面观）The deciduous teeth（external aspect）--- 65

154. 舌（冠状切面）The tongue（coronal section）-- 65

155. 舌（正中矢状切面）The tongue（median sagittal section）--- 65

156. 腮腺、下颌下腺和舌下腺 The parotid gland, submandibular gland and sublingual gland ------------------- 66

157. 腮腺、下颌下腺和舌下腺（内面观）The parotid gland, submandibular gland and sublingual gland
（internal aspect）--- 66

158. 咽与鼻、口、喉的交通 Connection of the pharynx and nose, mouth, larynx --------------------------------- 67

159. 咽腔（后面观）The pharyngeal cavity（posterior aspect）-- 68

160. 咽肌（内面观）The pharyngeal muscles（internal aspect）--- 68

161. 咽肌（外侧面观）The pharyngeal muscles（lateral aspect）--- 69

162. 咽肌（后面观）The pharyngeal muscles（posterior aspect）--- 69

163. 食管的位置及毗邻 Position and relations of the esophagus --- 70

164. 胃的肌肉 The gastric muscles --- 70

165. 胃腔 The gastric lumen --- 70

166. 十二指肠及毗邻（前面观）The duodenum and its relations（anterior aspect）------------------------------ 71

167. 空肠 The jejunum --- 71

168. 回肠 The ileum -- 71

169. 小肠和大肠（前面观）The small intestine and the large intestine（anterior aspect）----------------------- 72

170. 盲肠和阑尾 The cecum and vermiform appendix --- 72

171. 回盲部（内面观）The ileocecal part（internal aspect）-- 72

172. 直肠（冠状切面）The rectum（coronal section）-- 73

173. 直肠和肛管的肌肉 Muscles of the rectum and the anal canal --- 73

174. 肛门括约肌（冠状切面）The anal sphincter（coronal section）--- 73

175. 肝（前面观）The liver（anterior aspect）--- 74

176. 肝（后面观）The liver（posterior aspect）--- 74

177. 肝（上面观）The liver（superior aspect）--- 75

178. 肝（下面观）The liver（inferior aspect）-- 75

179. 输胆管道及开口（前面观）The bile passage and its openings（anterior aspect）--------------------------- 76

180. 呼吸系全貌 General arrangement of respiratory system -- 77

181. 鼻旁窦的开口 The openings of paranasal sinuses --- 78

182. 甲状软骨（侧面观）The thyroid cartilage（lateral aspect）--- 78

183. 杓状软骨和小角软骨（前面观）The arytenoid and corniculate（anterior aspect）--------------------------- 78

184. 环状软骨（侧面观）The cricoid cartilage（lateral aspect）--- 78

185. 喉软骨和韧带（前面观）The cartilages and ligaments of larynx（anterior aspect）----------------------- 79

186. 喉软骨和韧带（后面观）The cartilages and ligaments of larynx（posterior aspect）--------------------- 79

187. 喉软骨和韧带（外侧面观）The cartilages and ligaments of larynx（lateral aspect）-------------------- 80

188. 喉肌（外侧面观）Muscles of the larynx（lateral aspect）-------------------------- 80

189. 喉腔（后面观）The laryngeal cavity（posterior aspect）------------------------- 81

190. 喉腔冠状切面（后面观）Coronal section through the laryngeal cavity（posterior aspect）--------------------------- 81

191. 气管和肺段支气管 The trachea and segmental bronchi---------------------------- 82

192. 右肺（前面观）Right lung（anterior aspect）------------------------------------ 83

193. 右肺（内侧面观）Right lung（medial aspect）------------------------------------ 83

194. 左肺（前面观）Left lung（anterior aspect）------------------------------------- 83

195. 左肺（内侧面观）Left lung（medial aspect）------------------------------------- 83

196. 支气管肺段（前面观）The bronchopulmonary segments（anterior aspect）---------------------- 84

197. 支气管肺段（后面观）The bronchopulmonary segments（posterior aspect）---------------------- 84

198. 支气管肺段（左外侧面观）The bronchopulmonary segments（left lateral aspect）------------------ 85

199. 支气管肺段（右外侧面观）The bronchopulmonary segments（right lateral aspect）----------------- 85

200. 支气管肺段（左内侧面观）The bronchopulmonary segments（left medial aspect）------------------ 85

201. 支气管肺段（右内侧面观）The bronchopulmonary segments（right medial aspect）---------------- 85

202. 肺和胸膜（前面观）The lungs and the pleura（anterior aspect）---------------------- 86

203. 纵隔（左外侧面观）The mediastinum（left lateral aspect）--------------------------- 87

204. 纵隔（右外侧面观）The mediastinum（right lateral aspect）------------------------- 88

205. 男性泌尿生殖系统全貌 General arrangement of the male urogenital system----------------- 89

206. 腹后壁（示肾和输尿管）Posterior abdominal wall（showing the kidneys and the ureters）-------------- 90

207. 右肾（前面观）The right kidney（anterior aspect）--------------------------------- 91

208. 右肾（后面观）The right kidney（posterior aspect）-------------------------------- 91

209. 肾窦及其结构 The renal sinus and its structures--------------------------------- 91

210. 肾的冠状切面（后面观）The coronal section of the kidney（posterior aspect）-------------- 91

211. 肾段和肾段动脉（前面观）The renal segments and the segmental arteries（anterior aspect）----------- 92

212. 肾段和肾段动脉（后面观）The renal segments and the segmental arteries（posterior aspect）--------- 92

213. 肾的位置和毗邻（前面观）The position of the kidneys and their relations（anterior aspect）--------- 92

214. 肾的位置和毗邻（后面观）The position of kidneys and their relations（posterior aspect）---------- 93

215. 肾和输尿管的体表投影 The surface projection of the kidneys and ureters----------------- 93

216. 睾丸、附睾及其被膜（外侧面观）The testis, epididymis and their capsule（lateral aspect）-------- 94

217. 睾丸、附睾的内部结构 Internal structures of the testis and the epididymis------------------ 94

218. 膀胱、前列腺及精囊腺（后面观）The urinary bladder, prostate and seminal vesicles（posterior aspect）-------------- 95

219. 膀胱底及男性尿道前列腺部（内面观）The fundus of bladder and the prostatic part of the male urethra（internal aspect）-------------------------- 95

220. 阴茎的海绵体（1）Cavernous bodies of the penis（1）---------------------------- 96

221. 阴茎的海绵体（2）Cavernous bodies of the penis（2）---------------------------- 96

222. 阴茎体横切面 Transverse section through body of the penis----------------------- 96

223. 男性盆腔（正中矢状切面）Male pelvic cavity（median sagittal section）------------------ 97

224. 女性盆腔（正中矢状切面）Female pelvic cavity（median sagittal section）--------------- 97

225. 女性盆腔器官（上面观）Female pelvic organs（superior aspect）---------------------- 98

226. 女性内生殖器（冠状切面）Female internal genital organs（coronal section）--------------- 98

227. 女性外生殖器 Female external genital organs-------------------------------- 99

228. 前庭球和前庭大腺 The bulb of vestibule and the greater vestibular gland---------------- 99

229. 男性会阴分区 The divisions of the male perineum-------------------------------- 99

230. 女性会阴分区 The divisions of the female perineum------------------------------- 99

231. 女性乳房（前面观）Female mamma（anterior aspect）---------------------------- 100

232. 女性乳房（矢状切面）Female mamma（sagittal section）-------------------------- 100

233. 男性盆腔（冠状切面）Male pelvic cavity（coronal section）------------------------- 101

234. 女性盆腔（冠状切面）Female pelvic cavity（coronal section）----------------------- 101

235. 小网膜和大网膜 Lesser omentum and greater omentum----------------------------- 102

236. 小网膜和胃 The lesser omentum and stomach----------------------------------- 103

237. 网膜囊（1）The omental bursa（1）--- 103

238. 网膜囊（2）The omental bursa（2）--- 104

239. 网膜囊（3）The omental bursa（3）-- 104

240. 大肠及腹后壁腹膜的配布 The large intestine and distribution of the peritoneum on the posterior abdominal wall ---- 105

241. 腹后壁腹膜的配布（示系膜根）Distribution of the peritoneum on the posterior abdominal wall
(showing the radix of mesentery) --- 105

242. 女性腹腔（正中矢状切面）Female abdominal cavity（median sagittal section）------------------------------------- 106

脉管系统 VASCULAR SYSTEM

243. 心包及毗邻器官 Pericardium and its adjacent organs -- 108

244. 心脏的位置和毗邻 Position and relations of the heart --- 109

245. 心脏的外形和血管（前面观）Outline form of the heart and its blood vessels（anterior aspect）----------------- 110

246. 心脏的外形和血管（后面观）Outline form of the heart and its blood vessels（posterior aspect）--------------- 110

247. 右心房（内面观）The right atrium（internal aspect）--- 111

248. 右心室（内面观）The right ventricle（internal aspect）-- 111

249. 左心房和左心室（内面观）The left atrium and left ventricle（internal aspect）------------------------------------ 112

250. 左心室（内面观）The left ventricle（internal aspect）--- 112

251. 心脏的瓣膜（上面观）Cardiac valves（superior aspect）--- 113

252. 房间隔和室间隔（切面）Interatrial septum and interventricular septum（section）----------------------------- 113

253. 心脏传导系统（右内面观）Conducting system of the heart（right internal aspect）--------------------------------- 114

254. 心脏传导系统（左内面观）Conducting system of the heart（left internal aspect）--------------------------------- 114

255. 心包腔（1）The pericardial cavity（1）--- 115

256. 心包腔（2）The pericardial cavity（2）--- 115

257. 肺根（前面观）Root of the lung（anterior aspect）-- 116

258. 肺根（后面观）Roots of the lungs（posterior aspect）--- 116

259. 肺循环的血管（模式图）Vessels of pulmonary circulation（diagram）--- 116

260. 主动脉弓分支和后纵隔的结构（前面观）The branches of the aortic arch and structures of posterior mediastinum
(anterior aspect) -- 117

261. 头、颈部的动脉 Arteries of the head and neck --- 118

262. 腋窝的动脉 Arteries of the axillary fossa --- 119

263. 上肢的动脉（前面观）Arteries of the upper limb（anterior aspect）--- 120

264. 上肢的动脉（后面观）Arteries of the upper limb（posterior aspect）-- 120

265. 右手掌面的动脉（浅层）Arteries of the palm of right hand（superficial layer）---------------------------------- 121

266. 右手掌面的动脉（深层）Arteries of the palm of right hand（deep layer）--------------------------------------- 121

267. 胸主动脉、腹主动脉及其分支 Thoracic aorta and abdominal aorta and their branches------------------------- 122

268. 腹腔干及其分支（1）Celiac trunk and its branches（1）-- 123

269. 腹腔干及其分支（2）Celiac trunk and its branches（2）-- 123

270. 肠系膜上动脉及其分支 The superior mesenteric artery and its branches -- 124

271. 肠系膜下动脉及其分支 The inferior mesenteric artery and its branches -- 124

272. 男性盆腔的动脉（正中矢状切面）Arteries of the male pelvic cavity（median sagittal section）----------------- 125

273. 女性盆腔的动脉（正中矢状切面）Arteries of the female pelvic cavity（median sagittal section）--------------- 125

274. 直肠和肛管的血管 Blood vessels of rectum and anal canal-- 126

275. 男性会阴部的动脉 Arteries of the male perineum --- 127

276. 女性会阴部的动脉 Arteries of the female perineum --- 127

277. 下肢的动脉（前面观）Arteries of the lower limb（anterior aspect）--- 128

278. 下肢的动脉（后面观）Arteries of the lower limb（posterior aspect）-- 128

279. 足背的动脉 Arteries of the dorsum of foot -- 129

280. 足底的动脉 Plantar arteries --- 129

281. 头、颈部的静脉 Veins of head and neck --- 130

282. 颅内、外静脉的交通 Communications between intracranial and extracranial veins ------------------------------ 131

283. 手背的浅静脉 Superficial veins of the back of hand --- 132

284. 上肢的浅静脉 Superficial veins of the upper limb --- 132

285. 上、下腔静脉及其属支 Superior vena cava, inferior vena cava and their tributaries------------------------------ 133

286. 胸、腹壁的浅静脉 Superficial veins of the thoracic and abdominal wall -------------------------------------- 134

287. 肝门静脉及其属支 Hepatic portal vein and its tributaries --- 135
288. 肝门静脉和门腔静脉吻合 Hepatic portal vein and portacaval anastomosis ------------------------- 136
289. 大隐静脉 The great saphenous vein --- 137
290. 小隐静脉 The small saphenous vein --- 137
291. 体腔后壁淋巴结和淋巴导管 Lymph nodes and lymphatic ducts of the posterior wall of the coelom ------------------- 138
292. 颈部浅层淋巴 Superficial cervical lymph --- 139
293. 颈部深层淋巴 Deep cervical lymph --- 140
294. 腋窝、乳腺的淋巴管和淋巴结 The lymphatic vessels and the lymph nodes of the axilla and the mammary glands --- 141
295. 气管、支气管和肺部的淋巴结 Lymph nodes of the trachea, the bronchi and the lungs ------------------------ 141
296. 胸骨旁淋巴结 The parasternal lymph nodes --- 141
297. 胃的淋巴（前面观）Lymph of stomach（anterior aspect）-- 142
298. 胃的淋巴（后面观）Lymph of stomach（posterior aspect）-- 142
299. 结肠的淋巴 Lymph of colon -- 143
300. 腹膜后隙的淋巴 The lymph of the retroperitoneal space --- 144
301. 女性生殖器的淋巴管和淋巴结（1）The lymphatic vessels and lymph nodes of the female genital organs（1）------ 145
302. 女性生殖器的淋巴管和淋巴结（2）The lymphatic vessels and lymph nodes of the female genital organs（2）------ 145
303. 上肢浅部淋巴管和淋巴结 Superficial lymphatic vessels and lymph nodes of upper limb ------------------ 146
304. 上肢深部淋巴管和淋巴结 Deep lymphatic vessels and lymph nodes of upper limb ----------------------- 146
305. 下肢浅部淋巴管和淋巴结 Superficial lymphatic vessels and lymph nodes of lower limb ------------------ 147
306. 腹股沟深部淋巴结 Deep inguinal lymph nodes --- 147
307. 脾（膈面）Spleen（diaphragmatic surface）--- 148
308. 脾（脏面）Spleen（visceral surface）--- 148

感觉器官 SENSATIVE ORGANS

309. 眼球水平切面（模式图）Horizontal section of the eyeball（diagram）------------------------------------- 150
310. 眼球前部水平切面（虹膜、睫状体、晶状体切面）Horizontal section of the anterior part of the eyeball
 （section through iris, ciliary body and lens）--- 150
311. 眼球前部（内面观）Anterior part of the eyeball（internal aspect）--- 151
312. 眼球后部（内面观）Posterior part of the eyeball（internal aspect）-- 151
313. 右侧泪器（前面观）Right lacrimal apparatus（anterior aspect）-- 152
314. 眼球外肌（外侧面观）The ocular muscles（lateral aspect）-- 152
315. 右侧眼球及眶矢状切面 Sagittal section through the right eyeball and orbital cavity ------------------------ 153
316. 眼球外肌（上面观）Extraocular muscles（superior aspect）--- 153
317. 眼的动脉 Arteries of eye -- 153
318. 眼球的血管 Blood vessels of eyeball --- 154
319. 前庭蜗器（切面）Vestibulocochlear organ（section）--- 155
320. 右侧鼓膜（外侧面观）Right tympanic membrane（lateral aspect）-- 155
321. 右侧听小骨 Right auditory ossicles -- 155
322. 右侧鼓室（内侧壁）Right tympanic cavity（medial walls）-- 156
323. 右侧鼓室（外侧壁）Right tympanic cavity（lateral walls）--- 156
324. 矢状窦、横窦和乙状窦的体表投影 The surface projection of the sagittal sinus, transverse sinus and
 the sigmoid sinus -- 157
325. 乳突、乙状窦和面神经的关系 Relations among the mastoid process, sigmoid sinusand the facial nerve -------------- 157
326. 右侧骨迷路和膜迷路（前外侧面观）Right bony labyrinth and membranous labyrinth（anterior lateral aspect）----- 158
327. 右侧骨迷路内腔 Internal cavity of the right osseous labyrinth -- 158

神经和内分泌系统 NERVOUS AND ENDOCRINE SYSTEMS

328. 神经系统概观 General view of the nervous system -- 160
329. 神经元的类型 Types of the neuron -- 161
330. 神经元的结构（电镜模式图）Structure of the neuron（diagram of electron microscope）------------------- 161
331. 脊髓颈段横切面 Transverse section through cervical segment of spinal cord ----------------------------------- 162
332. 脊髓的细胞构筑分层 Cytoarchitectonic layers of the spinal cord --- 162

333. 脊髓的被膜（后面观）Capsules of spinal cord（posterior aspect）-- 163

334. 脊髓的动脉 Arteries of spinal cord --- 163

335. 脊髓的血管 Blood vessels of spinal cord -- 164

336. 脊髓的静脉 Veins of spinal cord -- 164

337. 脑底面 Basal surface of the brain -- 165

338. 脑（外侧面观）Brain（lateral aspect）-- 166

339. 脑（内侧面观）Brain（medial aspect）-- 166

340. 脑干（腹侧面观）Brain stem（ventral aspect）-- 167

341. 脑干（背面观）Brain stem（dorsal aspect）--- 168

342. 延髓尾侧部水平切面（经锥体交叉）Horizontal section of the caudal part of the medulla oblongata
（through the pyramidal decussation）-- 169

343. 延髓水平切面（经内侧丘系交叉）Horizontal section of the medulla oblongata
（through the decussation of the medial lemniscus）-- 169

344. 延髓水平切面（经橄榄中部）Horizontal section of the medulla oblongata
（through the middle part of the olive）--- 170

345. 延髓水平切面（经橄榄上部）Horizontal section of the medulla oblongata
（through the superior part of the olive）--- 170

346. 脑桥水平切面（经脑桥中、下部）Horizontal section of the pons
（through the middle、inferior part of the pons）--- 171

347. 脑桥水平切面（经脑桥中部）Horizontal section of the pons（through the middle part of the pons）----------------- 171

348. 脑桥水平切面（经脑桥上部）The horizontal section of the pons（through the superior part of pons）--------------- 172

349. 中脑水平切面（经下丘）The horizontal section of midbrain（through the inferior colliculus）------------------------ 172

350. 中脑水平切面（经上丘颅侧部）The horizontal section of midbrain
（through the cranial part of superior colliculus）--- 173

351. 中脑上端与间脑之间水平切面（经后连合）The horizontal section between mesencephalic superior extremity
and diencephalon（through posterior commissure）--- 173

352. 小脑（上面观）Cerebellum（superior aspect）-- 174

353. 小脑（下面观）Cerebellum（inferior aspect）--- 174

354. 小脑深核 Deep cerebellar nucleus --- 175

355. 间脑（内侧面观）Diencephalon（medial aspect）--- 175

356. 间脑（后上面观）Diencephalon（posterosuperior aspect）-- 176

357. 间脑冠状切面（乳头体平面）Coronal section of diencephalon（level of the mammilary body）--------------------- 176

358. 下丘脑（下面观）Hypothalamus（inferior aspect）--- 176

359. 大脑半球内面的沟回 Gyruses and sulcuses of medial surface of the cerebral hemisphere --------------------------------- 177

360. 大脑岛叶的沟回 Sulcuses and gyri of cerebral insula --- 177

361. 脑的水平切面 Horizontal section of the brain -- 178

362. 脑的冠状切面 Coronal section of the brain --- 178

363. 大脑的动脉（内侧面观）Cerebral arteries（medial aspect）-- 179

364. 大脑的动脉（外侧面观）Cerebral arteries（lateral aspect）--- 179

365. 脑底部的动脉 Arteries at the base of the brain --- 180

366. 大脑中动脉的皮质支和中央支 The cortical and median branches of the middle cerebral artery---------------------------- 181

367. 大脑的深静脉（上面观）The deep cerebral veins（superior aspect）--- 181

368. 大脑表面的静脉和上矢状窦 Veins of cerebral surface and superior sagittal sinus -- 182

369. 蛛网膜及蛛网膜粒（上面观）Arachnoid mater and granulations（superior aspect）-------------------------------- 182

370. 大脑表面的静脉（外侧面观）superficial veins of cerebrum（lateral aspect）-- 182

371. 脑室铸型（上面观）Cast form of the cerebral ventridcle（superior aspect）--- 183

372. 脑室铸型（侧面观）Cast form of the cerebral ventricle（lateral aspect）--- 183

373. 侧脑室（上面观）Lateral ventricle（superior aspect）--- 183

374. 硬脑膜、硬脑膜窦和脑神经 Cerebral dura mater, sinuses of dura mater and cranial nerves ------------------------------ 184

375. 硬脑膜及硬脑膜静脉窦 Cerebral dura mater and venous sinuses of cerebral dura mater ----------------------------------- 185

376. 脑脊液循环（模式图）Cerebrospinal fluid circulation（diagram）--- 186

377. 脊神经的后支 Posterior branches of spinal nerves --- 187

378. 颈神经丛的皮支 Cutaneous branches of cervical plexus -- 188

379. 颈部浅层神经 Nerves of the superficial layer of the neck --- 188

380. 颈部深层神经 Nerves of the deep layer of the neck -- 189

381. 臂丛及毗邻（1）Brachial plexus and its relations（1）-- 189

382. 臂丛及毗邻（2）Brachial plexus and its relations（2）-- 190

383. 上肢的皮神经（前面观）Cutaneous nerves of upper limb（anterior aspect）------------------------------ 191

384. 上肢的皮神经（后面观）Cutaneous nerves of upper limb（posterior aspect）---------------------------- 191

385. 腋窝的神经及其毗邻（1）Nerves of axillary fossa and their neighbours（1）------------------------------ 192

386. 腋窝的神经及其毗邻（2）Nerves of axillary fossa and its neighbours（2）------------------------------- 192

387. 臂部的神经（前面观）（1）Nerves of the arm（anterior aspect）（1）------------------------------------- 193

388. 臂部的神经（前面观）（2）Nerves of the arm（anterior aspect）（2）------------------------------------- 193

389. 臂部的神经（后面观）Nerves of the arm（posterior aspect）-- 194

390. 臂部的神经（外侧面观）Nerves of the arm（lateral aspect）-- 194

391. 肘窝的神经（1）Nerves of cubital fossa（1）--- 195

392. 肘窝的神经（2）Nerves of cubital fossa（2）--- 195

393. 肘窝的神经（3）Nervers of cubital fossa（3）--- 196

394. 肘窝的神经（内侧面观）Nervers of cubital fossa（medial aspect）-- 196

395. 前臂的神经（前面观）（1）Nerves of the forearm（anterior aspect）（1）------------------------------- 197

396. 前臂的神经（前面观）（2）Nerves of the forearm（anterior aspect）（2）------------------------------- 197

397. 前臂的神经（前面观）（3）Nerves of the forearm（anterior aspect）（3）------------------------------- 198

398. 前臂的神经（前面观）（4）Nerves of the forearm（anterior aspect）（4）------------------------------- 198

399. 手部神经及血管的体表投影 Surface projection of the nerves and blood vessels of the hand ------------- 199

400. 手掌侧的神经及血管 Nerves and blood vessels of the palm of the hand -- 200

401. 手背部的神经及其毗邻结构（1）The nerves and neighboring structures of the dorsum of the hand（1）----------- 201

402. 手背部的神经及其毗邻结构（2）The nerves and adjacent structures of the dorsum of the hand（2）----------- 201

403. 肋间神经及其分布 Intercostal nerves and their distribution -- 202

404. 胸神经前支的配布 Distribution of anterior branches of thoracic nerves --------------------------------------- 202

405. 下肢的皮神经和节段分布（前面观）Cutaneous nerves and segmental distributions of the lower limb
（anterior view）-- 203

406. 下肢的皮神经和节段分布（后面观）Cutaneous nerves and segmental distributions of the lower limb
（posterior view）-- 203

407. 腰丛和骶丛 Lumbar plexus and sacral plexus --- 204

408. 骶尾丛及其毗邻结构 Sacrococcygeal plexus and its neighbours --- 204

409. 下肢的神经（前面观）Nerves of the lower limb（anterior aspect）--------------------------------------- 205

410. 下肢的神经（后面观）Nerves of the lower limb（posterior aspect）------------------------------------- 205

411. 股前部神经及其毗邻结构（1）Nerves of the anterior aspect of the thigh and their adjacent structures（1）---------- 206

412. 股前部神经及其毗邻结构（2）Nerves of the anterior aspect of the thigh and their adjacent structures（2）---------- 207

413. 臀部和股后部神经及其毗邻结构 The gluteal region and nerves of the posterior aspect of
the thigh and its adjacent structures -- 208

414. 小腿前部神经及其毗邻结构（1）Nerves of the anterior aspect of the leg and their adjacent structures（1）--------- 209

415. 小腿前部神经及其毗邻结构（2）Nerves of the anterior aspect of the leg and their adjacent structures（2）--------- 209

416. 小腿后部神经及其毗邻结构（1）Nerves of the posterior aspect of the leg and their adjacent strucures（1）--------- 210

417. 小腿后部神经及其毗邻结构（2）Nerves of the posterior aspect of the leg and their adjacent structures（2）-------- 210

418. 足背部的神经及静脉 Nerves and veins of the dorsum of the foot -- 211

419. 足背部的神经及动脉 Nerves and arteries of the dorsum of the foot -- 211

420. 足底部的神经及血管（1）Nerves and blood vessels of the sole of the foot（1）---------------------------- 212

421. 足底部的神经及血管（2）Nerves and blood vessels of the sole of the foot（2）---------------------------- 212

422. 男性会阴部的神经及其毗邻结构 Nerves in the male perineum and their adjacent structures------------------ 213

423. 女性会阴部的神经及其毗邻结构 Nerves in the female perineum and their adjacent structures -------------- 213

424. 右臂近侧 1/3 横切面（A）The transverse section through the porximal 1/3 of the right arm（A）------------- 214

425. 右臂中 1/3 横切面（B）The transverse section through the middle 1/3 of the right arm（B）---------------- 214

426. 右臂远侧 1/3 横切面（C）The transverse section through the distal 1/3 of the right arm（C）------------------ 214

427. 右前臂近侧 1/3 横切面 （A） The transverse section through the proximal 1/3 of right forearm （A） ------------------ 215

428. 右前臂中 1/3 横切面 （B） The transverse section through the middle 1/3 of right forearm （B） ------------------------ 215

429. 右前臂远侧 1/3 横切面 （C） The transverse section through the distal 1/3 of right forearm （C） ------------------ 215

430. 右大腿近侧 1/3 横切面 （A） The transverse section through the proximal 1/3 of the right thigh （A） ------------------ 216

431. 右大腿中 1/3 横切面 （B） The transverse section through the proximal 1/3 of the right thigh （B） ------------------ 216

432. 右大腿远侧 1/3 横切面 （C） The transverse section through the proximal 1/3 of the right thigh （C） ------------------ 216

433. 右小腿近侧 1/3 横切面 （A） The transverse section through the proximal 1/3 of the right leg （A） -------------------- 217

434. 右小腿中 1/3 横切面 （B） The transverse section through the middle 1/3 of the right leg （B） ------------------------ 217

435. 右小腿远侧 1/3 横切面 （C） The transverse section through the distal 1/3 of the right leg （C） ------------------------- 217

436. 十二对脑神经出颅部位 The inlet and exit points of the 12 pairs of cranial nerves ------------------------------------- 218

437. 鼻腔内的神经 Nerves in the nasal cavity -- 219

438. 眶腔内的神经 （上面观） Nerves in the orbit （superior aspect） -- 220

439. 眶腔内的神经 （外侧面观） Nerves in the orbit （lateral aspect） --- 220

440. 三叉神经及其分支 （1） The trigeminal nerve and its branches （1） --- 221

441. 三叉神经及其分支 （2） The trigeminal nerve and its branches （2） --- 222

442. 三叉神经的纤维成分及其分布 （模式图） Fiber compositions and distribution of the trigeminal nerve
（diagram） --- 223

443. 下颌神经的分支和下颌下神经节 Branches of mandibular nerve and submandibular gonglion ------------------------ 224

444. 面神经的分支及其毗邻结构 Branches and adjacent structures of the facial nerve -------------------------------------- 225

445. 面神经的纤维成分及其分布 （模式图） Fiber compositions and distribution of the facial nerve （diagram） ---------- 226

446. 睫状神经节、翼腭神经节、耳神经节及下颌下神经节和脑神经 Ciliary ganglion，
pterygopalatine ganglion， otic ganglion， submandibular ganglion and cranial nerves ------------------------ 227

447. 前庭蜗神经和面神经 （模式图） Vestibulocochlear nerve and facial nerve （diagram） ------------------------------- 228

448. 舌咽神经的纤维成分及其分布 Fiber composition and distribution of the glossopharyngeal nerve -------------------- 228

449. 舌咽神经、迷走神经、副神经和舌下神经 Glossopharyngeal nerve, vagus nerve,
accessory nerve and hypoglossal nerve -- 229

450. 左、右迷走神经颈胸部的分支 （后面观） Cervicothoracic branches of left and right vagus nerves
（posterior aspect） -- 230

451. 迷走神经的纤维成分及其分布 （模式图） Fiber compositions and distribution of the vagus nerve （diagram） ------- 231

452. 胸部自主神经 Autonomic nerves of the thorax -- 232

453. 腹、盆部的自主神经丛和节 Plexuses and ganglia of autonomic nerves in abdomen and pelvis --------------------- 233

454. 躯干、四肢痛、温、触觉传导路 The pain, thalpotic and pselaphesic conductive pathways of the trunk and limbs --- 234

455. 头面部痛、温、触觉传导路 Pathways of pain, thalposis, tactile sensation of head and face ------------------------- 234

456. 躯干、四肢本体感觉和精细触觉传导路 The proprioception and refined tactile sensation pathway
of trunk and limbs --- 235

457. 传向小脑的本体感觉传导路 Pathway of the proprioceptive sensibility conducting to the cerebellum --------------- 235

458. 视觉传导路 The visual pathway -- 236

459. 听觉传导路 The auditory pathway --- 236

460. 嗅觉传导路 The olfactory pathway -- 237

461. 平衡觉传导路 The pathway of the equilibrium sense -- 237

462. 锥体系 （皮质脊髓束） The pyramidal system （corticospinal tract） -- 238

463. 锥体系 （皮质核束） The pyramidal system （corticobulbar tract） -- 238

464. 锥体外系 （纹状体—苍白球系） Extrapyramidal system （corpus striatum-globus pallidus） ---------------------- 239

465. 锥体外系 （皮质—脑桥—小脑系） The extrapyramidal system （cortex-pons-cerebellum system） ----------------- 239

466. 自主神经系概观 General view of autonomic nervous system -- 240

467. 松果体 Pineal body --- 241

468. 甲状腺和甲状旁腺 Thyroid gland and parathyroid gland -- 241

469. 睾丸 Testis -- 241

470. 内分泌腺概观 General view of endocrine glands --- 241

471. 肾上腺 Suprarenal gland --- 241

472. 垂体的分部 Divisions of the hypophysis -- 241

473. 卵巢 Ovary -- 241

LOCOMOTOR SYSTEM

运动系统

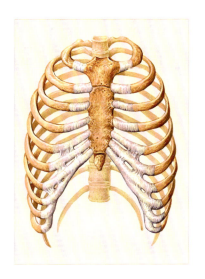

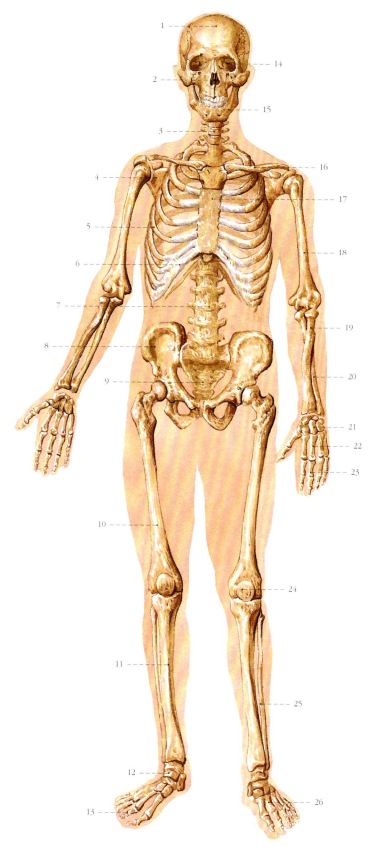

1. 人体骨骼（前面观）
The human skeleton (anterior aspect)

1.额骨 frontal bone
2.骨性鼻腔 bony nasal cavity
3.颈椎 cervical vertebrae
4.肩胛骨 scapula
5.肋骨 rib
6.肋弓 costal arch
7.腰椎 lumbar vertebrae
8.髋骨 hip bone
9.骶骨 sacrum
10.股骨 femur
11.胫骨 tibia
12.跗骨 tarsal bones
13.趾骨 phalanges of toes
14.眶腔 orbital cavity
15.下颌骨 mandible
16.锁骨 clavicle
17.胸骨 sternum
18.肱骨 humerus
19.桡骨 radius
20.尺骨 ulna
21.腕骨 carpal bones
22.掌骨 metacarpal bones
23.指骨 phalanges of fingers
24.髌骨 patella
25.腓骨 fibula
26.跖骨 metatarsal bones

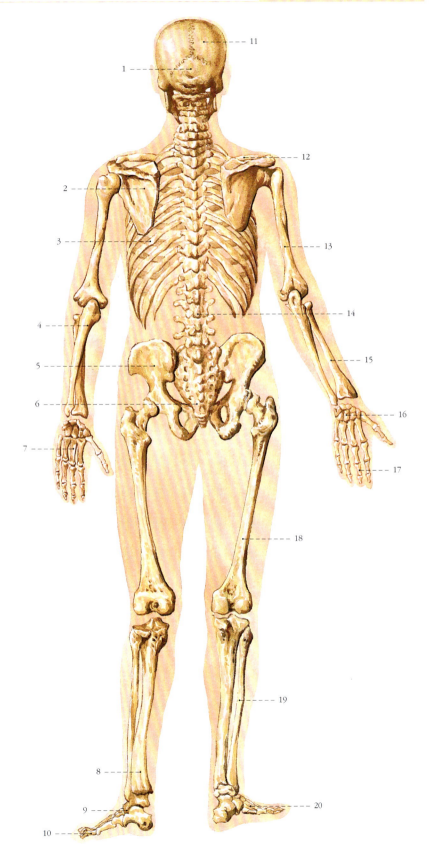

1.枕骨 occipital bone
2.肩胛骨 scapula
3.肋骨 costal bone
4.尺骨 ulna
5.髋骨 hip bone
6.骶骨 sacrum
7.掌骨 metacarpal bones
8.胫骨 tibia
9.跗骨 tarsal bones
10.趾骨 phalanges of toes
11.顶骨 parietal bone
12.锁骨 clavicle
13.肱骨 humerus
14.椎骨 vertebrae
15.桡骨 radius
16.腕骨 carpal bones
17.指骨 phalanges of fingers
18.股骨 femur
19.腓骨 fibula
20.跖骨 metatarsal bones

2. 人体骨骼（后面观）
The human skeleton (posterior aspect)

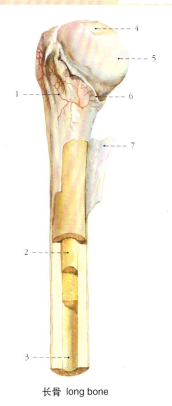

长骨 long bone

短骨 short bone

扁骨 flat bone

3. 骨的构造
Structure of the bones

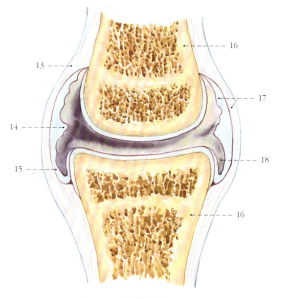

（关节连结）
The articular joint

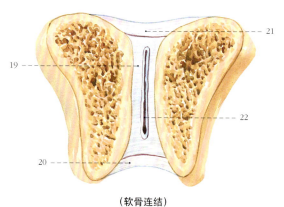

（软骨连结）
The cartilaginous joint

4. 骨的连结
The osseous joint

1.滋养动脉 nutrient arteries
2.骨髓 bone marrow
3.髓腔 medullary cavity
4.关节面 articular surface
5.关节软骨 articular cartilage
6.关节囊 articular capsule

7.骨膜 periosteum
8.压力曲线 pressure curve
9.小梁 trabeculae
10.外板 outer plate
11.板障 diplo
12.内板 inner plate

13.关节囊（纤维膜）articular
    capsule（fibrous membrane）
14.滑膜襞 synovial fold
15.关节囊（滑膜）articular
    capsule（synovial membrane）
16.骨 bone

17.关节囊 articular capsule
18.关节腔 articular cavity
19.耻骨间盘 interpubic disc
20.耻骨弓状韧带 arcuate pubic ligament
21.耻骨上韧带 superior pubic ligament
22.耻骨联合腔 cavity of pubic symphysis

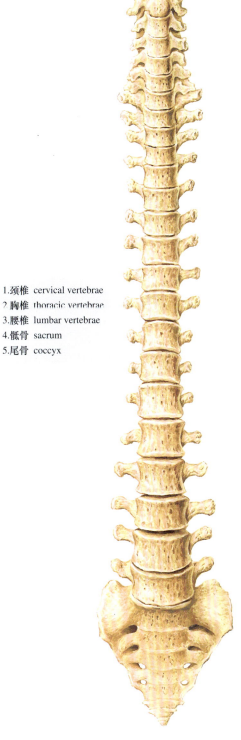

1.颈椎 cervical vertebrae
2.胸椎 thoracic vertebrae
3.腰椎 lumbar vertebrae
4.骶骨 sacrum
5.尾骨 coccyx

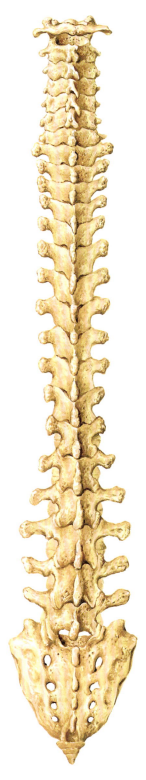

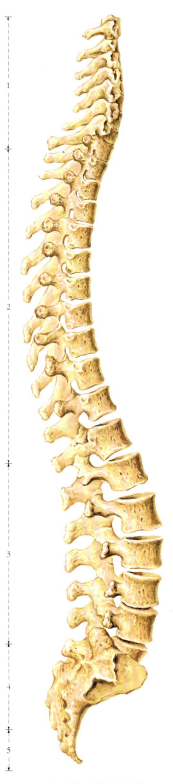

5. 脊柱（前面观）
The spinal column (anterior
aspect)

6. 脊柱（后面观）
The spinal column (posterior
aspect)

7. 脊柱（外侧面观）
The spinal column (lateral
aspect)

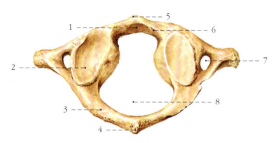

寰椎（上面观）
atlas（superior aspect）

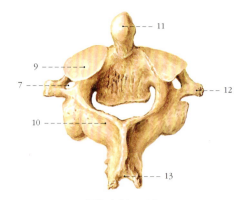

枢椎（后上面观）
axis（posterosuperior aspect）

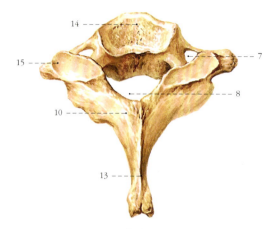

颈椎（上面观）
cervical vertebrae（superior aspect）

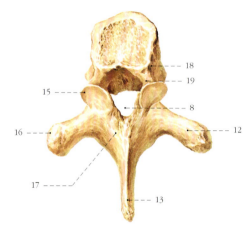

胸椎（上面观）
thoracic vertebrae（superior aspect）

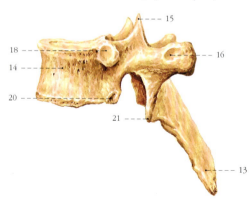

胸椎（左侧面观）
thoracic vertebrae（left lateral aspect）

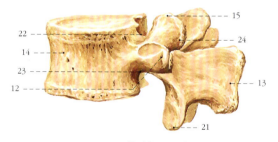

腰椎（左侧面观）
lumbar vertebrae（left lateral aspect）

8. 各部椎骨的形态
Features of the individual vertebrae

1.齿突凹 dental fovea	9.上关节面 superior articular surface	17.椎弓板 lamina of vertebral arch
2.上关节凹 superior articular fovea	10.椎弓 vertebral arch	18.上肋凹 superior costal fovea
3.后弓 posterior arch	11.齿突 dens	19.椎弓根 pedicle of vertebral arch
4.后结节 posterior tubercle	12.横突 transverse process	20.下肋凹 inferior costal fovea
5.前结节 anterior tubercle	13.棘突 spinous process	21.下关节突 inferior articular process
6.前弓 anterior arch	14.椎体 vertebral body	22.椎上切迹 superior vertebral notch
7.横突孔 transverse foramen	15.上关节突 superior articular process	23.椎下切迹 inferior vertebral notch
8.椎孔 vertebral foramen	16.横突肋凹 transverse costal fovea	24.乳突 mamillary process

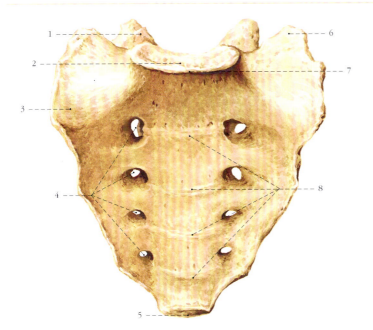

9. 骶骨（前面观）
The sacrum (anterior aspect)

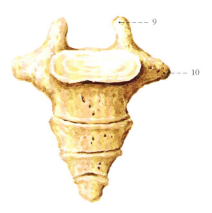

10. 尾骨（前面观）
The coccyx (anterior aspect)

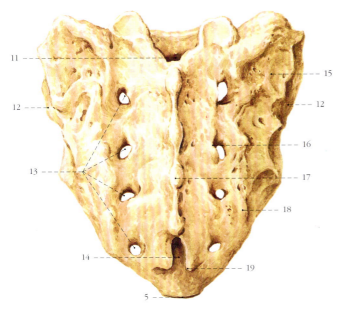

11. 骶骨（后面观）
The sacrum (posterior aspect)

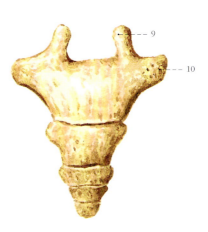

12. 尾骨（后面观）
The coccyx (posterior aspect)

1.上关节突 superior articular process
2.骶骨底 base of sacrum
3.侧部 lateral part
4.骶前孔 anterior sacral foramina
5.骶骨尖 apex of sacrum
6.骶翼 ala of sacrum
7.岬 promontory

8.横线 transverse lines
9.尾骨角 coccygeal cornu
10.横突 transverse process
11.骶管 sacral canal
12.耳状面 auricular surface
13.骶后孔 posterior sacral foramina
14.骶管裂孔 sacral hiatus

15.骶粗隆 sacral tuberosity
16.骶中间嵴 intermediate sacral crest
17.骶正中嵴 median sacral crest
18.骶外侧嵴 lateral sacral crest
19.骶角 sacral cornu

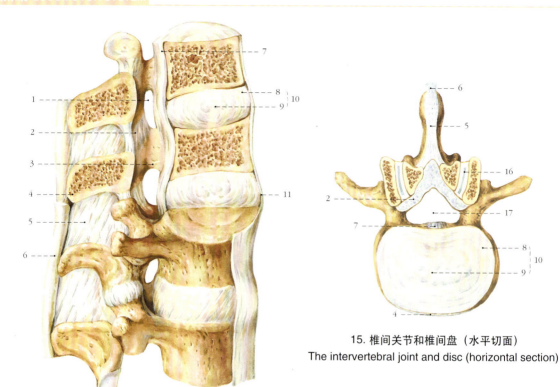

13. 椎骨的连结（正中矢状切面）
The intervertebral joints (median sagittal section)

15. 椎间关节和椎间盘（水平切面）
The intervertebral joint and disc (horizontal section)

1.椎间孔 intervertebral foramina
2.黄韧带 ligamenta flava
3.椎管 vertebral canal
4.棘突 spinous process
5.棘间韧带 interspinal ligament
6.棘上韧带 supraspinal ligament
7.后纵韧带 posterior longitudinal ligament
8.纤维环 anulus fibrosus
9.髓核 nucleus pulposus
10.椎间盘 intervertebral disc
11.前纵韧带 anterior longitudinal ligament
12.椎弓根 pedicle of vertebral arch
13.椎弓板 lamina of vertebral arch
14.横突 transverse process
15.上关节突 superior articular process
16.关节突关节 zygapophysial joint
17.椎孔 vertebral foramen

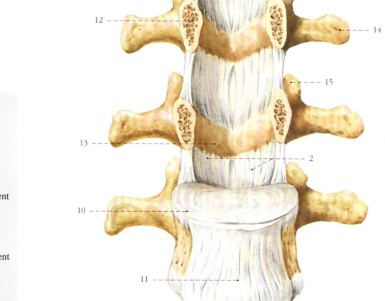

14. 椎骨的连结（前面观）
The intervertebral joints (anterior aspect)

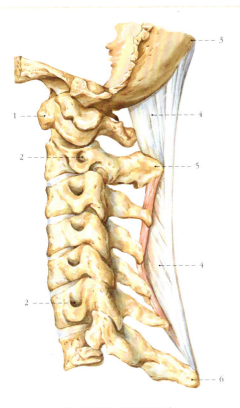

16. 项韧带（外侧面观）
Ligamentum nuchae (lateral aspect)

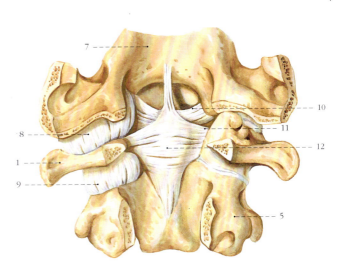

17. 寰枕和寰枢关节（后面观）
The atlantooccipital joint and atlantoaxial joint (posterior aspect)

1.寰椎 atlas
2.横突孔 transverse foramen
3.枕外隆凸 external occipital protuberance
4.项韧带 ligamentum nuchae
5.枢椎 axis
6.隆椎 vertebra prominens
7.枕骨（基底部）occipital bone（basilar part）
8.寰枕关节 atlantooccipital joint
9.寰枢外侧关节 lateral atlantoaxial joint
10.翼状韧带 alar ligament
11.寰椎横韧带 transverse ligament of atlas
12.寰椎十字韧带 cruciform ligament of atlas
13.第一胸椎 first thoracic vertebrae
14.胸廓上口 superior aperture of thorax
15.胸骨角 sternal angle
16.肋间隙 intercostal space
17.肋软骨 costal cartilage
18.肋骨 costal bone
19.肋弓 costal arch
20.第十一肋 eleventh rib
21.第一肋 first rib
22.胸骨柄 manubrium sterni
23.胸骨体 body of sternum
24.剑突 xiphoid process
25.胸骨下角 infrasternal angle
26.第十二胸椎 twelfth thoracic vertebrae
27.第十二肋 twelfth rib

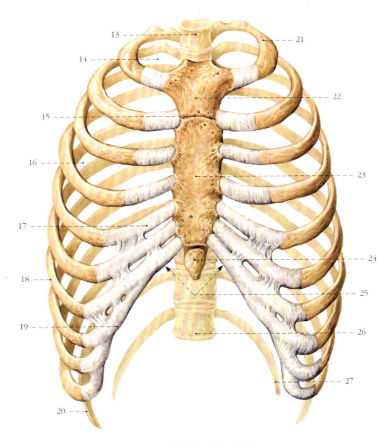

18. 骨性胸廓（前面观）
The osseous thorax (anterior aspect)

9

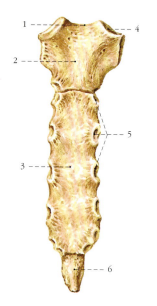

19. 胸骨（前面观）
The sternum (anterior aspect)

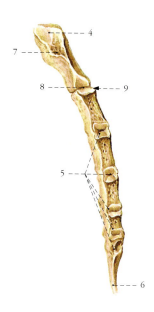

20. 胸骨（侧面观）
The sternum (lateral aspect)

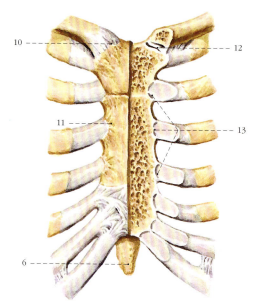

21. 胸肋关节（前面观）
Sternocostal joint (anterior aspect)

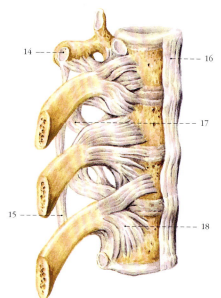

22. 肋椎关节（前面观）
Costovertebral joint (anterior aspect)

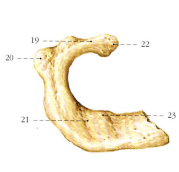

23. 第一肋骨
First rib

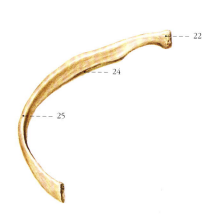

24. 第七肋骨
Seventh rib

1.颈静脉切迹 jugular notch	10.胸锁前韧带 anterior sternoclavicular ligament	19.肋颈 costal neck
2.胸骨柄 manubrium sterni	11.胸肋辐射韧带 radiate sternocostal ligament	20.肋结节 costal tubercle
3.胸骨体 body of sternum	12.关节盘 articular disc	21.锁骨下动脉沟 sulcus for subclavian artery
4.锁切迹 clavicular notch	13.胸肋关节 sternocostal joints	22.肋头 costal head
5.肋切迹 costal notches	14.横突肋凹 transverse costal fovea	23.前斜角肌结节 tubercle for scalenus anterior
6.剑突 xiphoid process	15.横突间韧带 intertransverse ligament	24.肋沟 costal groove
7.第一肋切迹 first costal notch	16.前纵韧带 anterior longitudinal ligament	25.肋体 shaft of rib
8.第二肋切迹 second costal notch	17.肋横突韧带 costotransverse ligament	
9.胸骨角 sternal angle	18.肋头辐状韧带 radiate ligament of costal head	

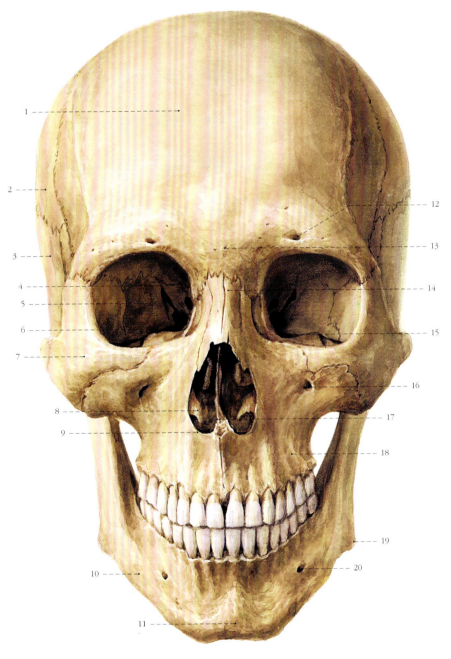

25. 颅（前面观）
The skull (anterior aspect)

1.额骨 frontal bone
2.顶骨 parietal bone
3.颞骨 temporal bone
4.眶上裂 superior orbital fissure
5.视神经管 optic canal
6.眶下裂 inferior orbital fissure
7.颧骨 zygomatic bone

8.下鼻甲 inferior nasal concha
9.梨状孔 piriform aperture
10.下颌骨 mandible
11.颏隆凸 mental protuberance
12.眶上孔（切迹）supraorbital foramen
  (notch)
13.眉间 glabella

14.鼻骨 nasal bone
15.泪囊窝 fossa for lacrimal sac
16.眶下孔 infraorbital foramen
17.骨鼻中隔 bony septum of nose
18.上颌骨 maxilla
19.下颌角 angle of mandible
20.颏孔 mental foramen

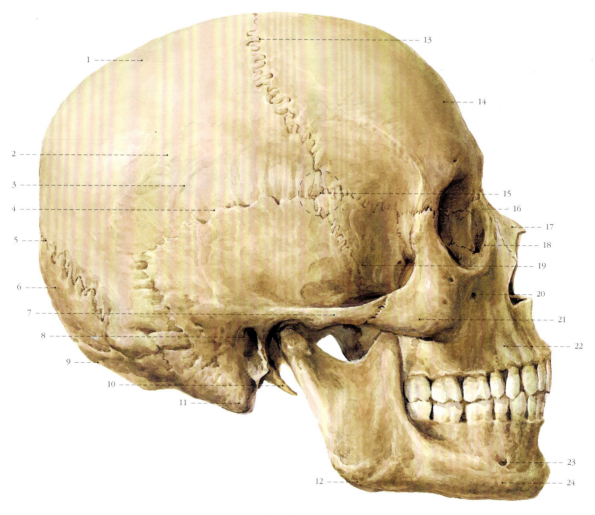

26. 颅（外侧面观）
The skull (lateral aspect)

1.顶骨 parietal bone
2.上颞线 superior temporal line
3.下颞线 inferior temporal line
4.顶颞缝 temporoparietal suture
5.人字缝 lambdoid suture
6.枕骨 occipital bone
7.颧弓 zygomatic arch
8.外耳门 external acoustic pore

9.枕外隆凸 external occipital protuberance
10.茎突 styloid process
11.乳突 mastoid process
12.下颌角 angle of mandible
13.冠状缝 coronal suture
14.额骨 frontal bone
15.翼点 pterion
16.泪骨 lacrimal bone

17.鼻骨 nasal bone
18.泪囊窝 fossa for lacrimal sac
19.蝶骨 sphenoid bone
20.眶下孔 infraorbital foramen
21.颧骨 zygomatic bone
22.上颌骨 maxilla
23.颏孔 mental foramen
24.下颌体 body of mandible

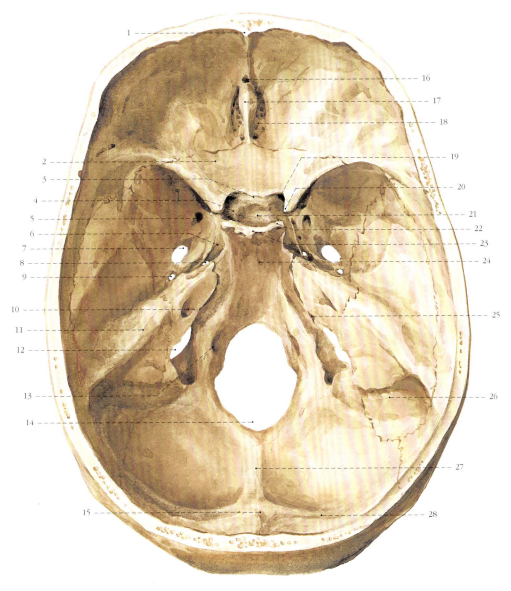

27. 颅底（内面观）
The base of the skull (internal aspect)

1.额嵴 frontal crest
2.蝶骨小翼 lesser wing of sphenoid bone
3.交叉前沟 sulcus prechiasmaticus
4.鞍结节 tuberculum sellae
5.圆孔 foramen rotundum
6.颈动脉沟 carotid sulcus
7.卵圆孔 foramen ovale
8.破裂孔 foramen lacerum
9.棘孔 foramen spinosum

10.内耳门 internal acoustic pore
11.岩上窦沟 sulcus for superior petrosal sinus
12.颈静脉孔 jugular foramen
13.舌下神经管 hypoglossal canal
14.枕骨大孔 foramen magnum of occipital bone
15.枕内隆凸 internal occipital protuberance
16.盲孔 foramen cecum
17.鸡冠 crista galli
18.筛板 cribriform plate
19.视神经管 optic canal

20.前床突 anterior clinoid process
21.垂体窝 hypophysial fossa
22.后床突 posterior clinoid process
23.鞍背 dorsum sellae
24.斜坡 clivus
25.岩下窦沟 sulcus for inferior petrosal sinus
26.乙状窦沟 sulcus for sigmoid sinus
27.枕内嵴 internal occipital crest
28.横窦沟 sulcus for transverse sinus

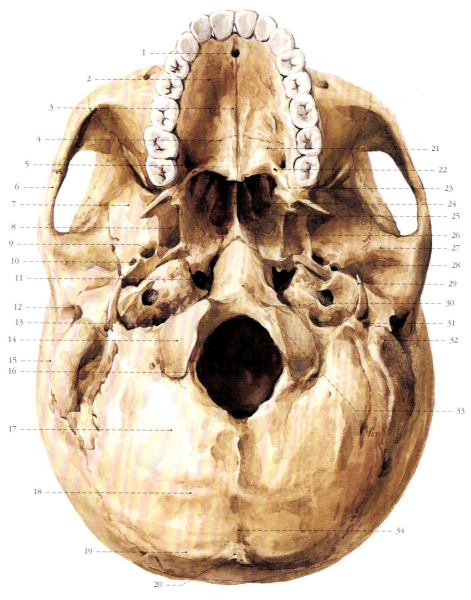

28. 颅底（外面观）
The base of the skull (external aspect)

1.切牙孔 incisive foramen
2.上颌骨腭突 palatine process of maxilla
3.腭中缝 median palatine suture
4.腭横缝 transverse palatine suture
5.腭大孔 greater palatine foramen
6.颧弓 zygomatic arch
7.蝶骨 sphenoid bone
8.翼窝 pterygoid fossa
9.卵圆孔 foramen ovale
10.棘孔 foramen spinosum
11.破裂孔 foramen lacerum
12.外耳门 external acoustic pore

13.颈静脉窝 jugular fossa
14.枕髁 occipital condyle
15.颞骨 temporal bone
16.枕骨大孔 foramen magnum of occipital bone
17.枕骨 occipital bone
18.下项线 inferior nuchal line
19.上项线 superior nuchal line
20.枕外隆凸 external occipital protuberance
21.腭骨水平板 horizontal plate of palatine bone
22.腭小孔 lesser palatine foramina

23.鼻后孔 posterior nasal apertures
24.犁骨 vomer
25.翼突内侧板 medial pterygoid plate
26.翼突外侧板 lateral pterygoid plate
27.关节结节 articular tubercle
28.下颌窝 mandibular fossa
29.茎突 styloid process
30.颈动脉管 carotid canal
31.茎乳孔 stylomastoid foramen
32.乳突 mastoid process
33.咽结节 pharyngeal tubercle
34.枕外嵴 external occipital crest

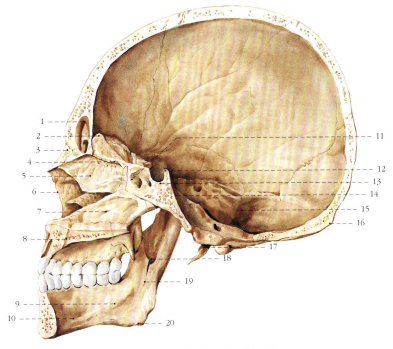

29. 颅骨（正中矢状切面）
The skull (median sagittal section)

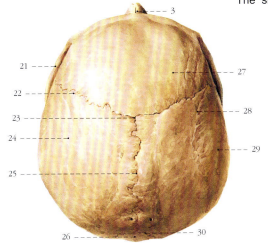

30. 颅（上面观）
The skull (superior aspect)

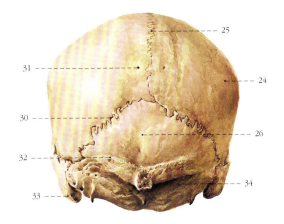

31. 颅（后面观）
The skull (posterior aspect)

1.额窦 frontal sinus
2.鸡冠 crista galli
3.鼻骨 nasal bone
4.筛板 cribriform plate
5.垂直板 perpendicular plate
6.梨状孔 piriform aperture
7.犁骨 vomer
8.切牙管 incisive canal
9.下颌舌骨肌线 mylohyoid line
10.舌下腺凹 sublingual fovea
11.蝶窦 sphenoidal sinus
12.鞍背 dorsum sellae

13.垂体窝 hypophysial fossa
14.斜坡 clivus
15.乙状窦沟 sulcus for sigmoid sinus
16.枕外隆凸 external occipital
　　protuberance
17.茎突 styloid process
18.下颌孔 mandibular foramen
19.下颌舌骨沟 mylohyoid groove
20.下颌角 angle of mandible
21.颧弓 zygomatic arch
22.冠状缝 coronal suture
23.前囟点 bregma

24.顶骨 parietal bone
25.矢状缝 sagittal suture
26.枕骨 occipital bone
27.额骨 frontal bone
28.上颞线 superior temporal line
29.下颞线 inferior temporal line
30.人字缝 lambdoid suture
31.顶孔 parietal foramen
32.上项线 superior nuchal line
33.乳突 mastoid process
34.枕外隆凸 external occipital protuberance

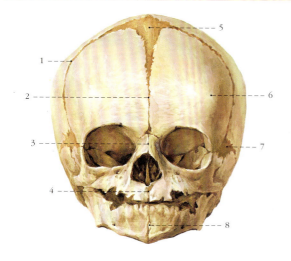

32. 新生儿颅（前面观）
The skull of a newborn infant (anterior aspect)

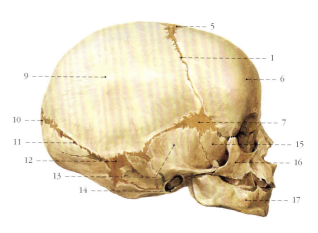

33. 新生儿颅（外侧面观）
The skull of a newborn infant (lateral aspect)

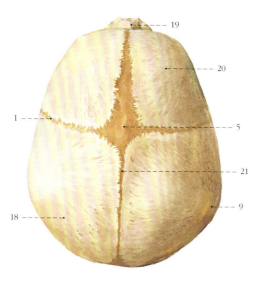

34. 新生儿颅（上面观）
The skull of a newborn infant (superior aspect)

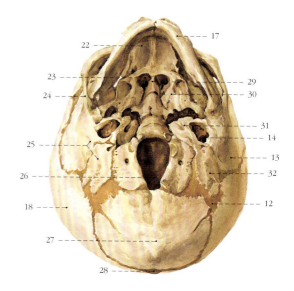

35. 新生儿颅底（下面观）
The base of skull of a newborn infant (inferior aspect)

1.冠状缝 coronal suture
2.额缝 frontal suture
3.鼻间缝 internasal suture
4.上颌间缝 intermaxillary suture
5.前囟 anterior fontanelle
6.额结节 frontal tuber
7.蝶囟 sphenoid fontanelle
8.下颌缝 mandibular suture
9.顶结节 parietal tuber
10.后囟 posterior fontanelle
11.人字缝 lambdoid suture

12.乳突囟 mastoid fontanelle
13.颞骨鳞部 squamous part of temporal bone
14.鼓环 tympanic anulus
15.蝶骨大翼 greater wing of sphenoid bone
16.颧骨 zygomatic bone
17.下颌体 body of mandible
18.顶骨 parietal bone
19.鼻骨 nasal bone
20.额骨 frontal bone
21.矢状缝 sagittal suture

22.上颌骨腭突 palatine process of maxilla
23.鼻后孔 posterior nasal apertures
24.颧弓 zygomatic arch
25.颧骨 zygomatic bone
26.枕骨大孔 foramen magnum of occipital bone
27.枕骨 occipital bone
28.后囟 posterior fontanelle
29.犁骨 vomer
30.蝶骨翼突 pterygoid process of sphenoid bone
31.颞骨岩部 petrous part of temporal bone
32.颞骨乳突 mastoid process of temporal bone

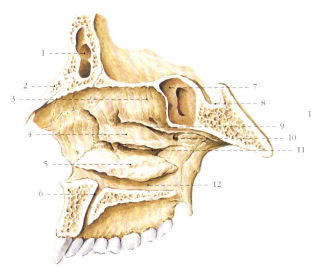

36. 骨性鼻腔外侧壁
The lateral wall of the bony nasal cavity

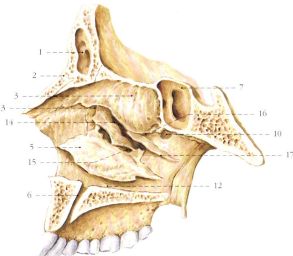

37. 骨性鼻腔外侧壁（示鼻旁窦的开口）
The lateral wall of the bony nasal cavity
(showing the apertures of the paranasal sinuses)

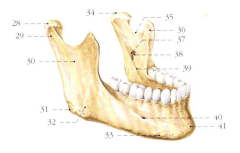

39. 下颌骨（外侧面观）
The mandible (lateral aspect)

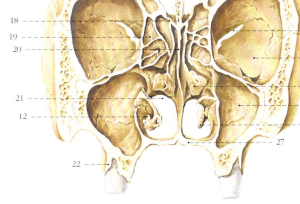

38. 颅冠状切面（前面观）
Coronary section of the skull (anterior aspect)

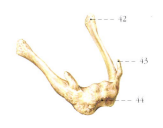

40. 舌骨
The hyoid bone

1.额窦 frontal sinus
2.鼻骨 nasal bone
3.上鼻甲 superior nasal concha
4.中鼻甲 middle nasal concha
5.下鼻甲 inferior nasal concha
6.切牙管 incisive canal
7.蝶窦 sphenoidal sinus
8.垂体窝 hypophysial fossa
9.上鼻道 superior nasal meatus
10.蝶腭孔 sphenopalatine foramen
11.中鼻道 middle nasal meatus
12.下鼻道 inferior nasal meatus

13.额窦开口 aperture of frontal sinus
14.筛窦开口 aperture of ethmoidal sinus
15.上颌窦开口 aperture of maxillary sinus
16.蝶窦口 aperture of sphenoidal sinus
17.中鼻甲（切缘）middle nasal concha（cutting edge）
18.筛板 cribriform plate
19.筛小房 ethmoidal cellules
20.垂直板 perpendicular plate
21.鼻腔 nasal cavity

22.牙槽突 alveolar process
23.鸡冠 crista galli
24.眶上裂 superior orbital fissure
25.眶腔 orbital cavity
26.上颌窦 maxillary sinus
27.硬腭 hard palate
28.下颌头 head of mandible
29.下颌颈 neck of mandible
30.下颌支 ramus of mandible
31.下颌角 angle of mandible
32.咬肌粗隆 masseteric tuberosity
33.下颌体 body of mandible

34.髁突 condylar process
35.下颌切迹 mandibular notch
36.冠突 coronoid process
37.下颌孔 mandibular foramen
38.下颌小舌 mandibular lingula
39.下颌舌骨沟 mylohyoid groove
40.颏孔 mental foramen
41.颏隆凸 mental protuberance
42.大角 greater horn
43.小角 lesser horn
44.舌骨体 body of hyoid bone

17

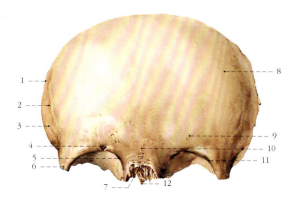

41. 额骨（前面观）
The frontal bone (anterior aspect)

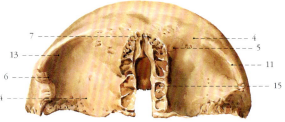

42. 额骨（下面观）
The frontal bone (inferior aspect)

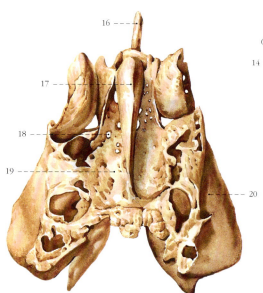

43. 筛骨（上面观）
The ethmoid bone (superior aspect)

1.额鳞 frontal squama
2.颞线 temporal line
3.颞面 temporal surface
4.眶上孔（切迹）supraorbital foramen（notch）
5.额切迹 frontal notch
6.颧突 zygomatic process
7.鼻缘 nasal margin
8.额结节 frontal tuber
9.眉弓 superciliary arch
10.眉间 glabella
11.眶上缘 supraorbital margin
12.鼻棘 nasal spine
13.泪腺窝 fossa for lacrimal gland
14.眶面 orbital surface
15.筛小房 ethmoidal cellules
16.垂直板 perpendicular plate
17.鸡冠 crista galli
18.筛孔 cribriform foramina
19.筛板 cribriform plate
20.眶板 orbital plate
21.鸡冠翼 ala of crista galli
22.中鼻甲 middle nasal concha
23.筛小房 ethmoidal cellules
24.上鼻甲 superior nasal concha
25.钩突 uncinate process

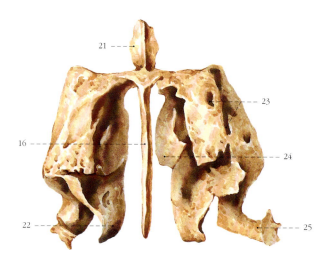

44. 筛骨（后面观）
The ethmoid bone (posterior aspect)

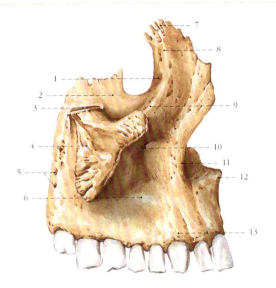

45. 上颌骨（外面观）
The maxilla (external aspect)

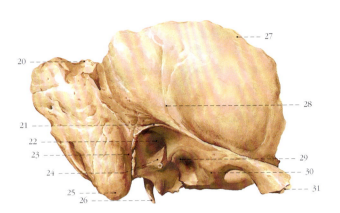

47. 颞骨（外面观）
The temporal bone (external aspect)

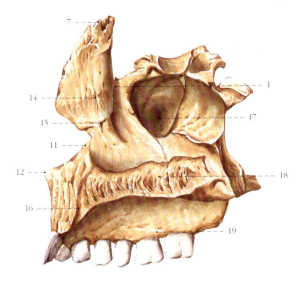

46. 上颌骨（内面观）
The maxilla (internal aspect)

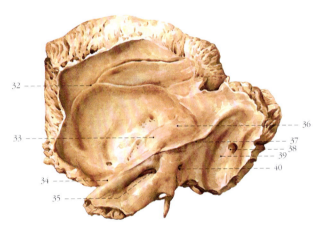

48. 颞骨（内面观）
The temporal bone (internal aspect)

1.泪沟 lacrimal sulcus
2.眶面 orbital surface
3.眶下沟 infraorbital groove
4.颧突 zygomatic process
5.牙槽孔 alveolar foramina
6.尖牙窝 canine fossa
7.额突 frontal process
8.泪前嵴 anterior lacrimal crest
9.眶下缘 infraorbital margin
10.眶下孔 infraorbital foramen
11.鼻切迹 nasal notch
12.鼻前棘 anterior nasal spine

13.牙槽轭 juga alveolaria
14.筛嵴 ethmoidal crest
15.鼻甲嵴 conchal crest
16.切牙孔 incisive foramen
17.上颌窦裂孔 maxillary hiatus
18.腭突 palatine process
19.牙槽突 alveolar process
20.顶切迹 parietal notch
21.道上棘 suprameatal spine
22.外耳门 external acoustic pore
23.鼓乳裂 tympanomastoid fissure
24.鼓部 tympanic part

25.乳突 mastoid process
26.茎突 styloid process
27.鳞部 squamous part
28.颞中动脉沟 sulcus for
  middle temporal artery
29.下颌窝 mandibular fossa
30.关节结节 articular tubercle
31.颧突 zygomatic process
32.脑膜中动脉沟 sulcus for
  middle meningeal artery
33.弓状隆起 arcuate
  eminence
34.三叉神经压迹 trigeminal

impression
35.内耳门 internal acoustic pore
36.鼓室盖 tegmen tympani
37.岩上窦沟 sulcus for superior
  petrosal sinus
38.乳突孔 mastoid foramen
39.乙状窦沟 sulcus for sigmoid
  sinus
40.前庭水管外口 external
  aperture of aqueduct of
  vestibule

1.颧突 zygomatic process
2.关节结节 articular tubercle
3.下颌窝 mandibular fossa
4.茎突 styloid process
5.外耳门 external acoustic pore
6.乳突 mastoid process
7.枕动脉沟 sulcus for occipital artery
8.颈动脉管 carotid canal
9.岩部尖 apex of petrous part
10.岩部 petrous part
11.岩鼓裂 petrotympanic fissure
12.颈静脉窝 jugular fossa
13.茎乳孔 stylomastoid foramen
14.乳突切迹 mastoid notch
15.枕缘 occipital margin
16.眶突 orbital process
17.蝶腭切迹 sphenopalatine notch
18.蝶突 sphenoidal process
19.垂直板 perpendicular plate
20.鼻甲嵴 conchal crest
21.鼻嵴 nasal crest
22.水平板 horizontal plate
23.腭大沟 greater palatine sulcus
24.锥突 pyramidal process
25.筛嵴 ethmoidal crest
26.鼻面 nasal surface

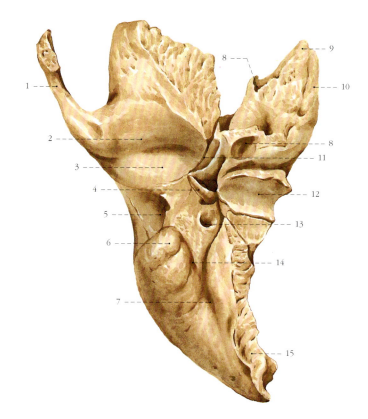

49. 颞骨（下面观）
The temporal bone (inferior aspect)

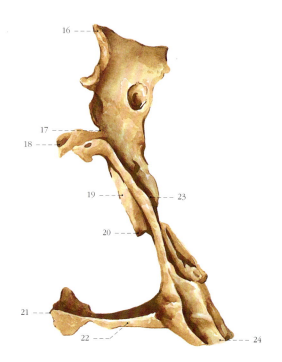

50. 腭骨（后面观）
The palatine bone (posterior aspect)

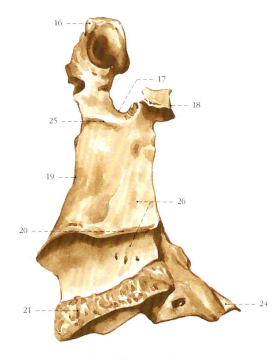

51. 腭骨（内面观）
The palatine bone (internal aspect)

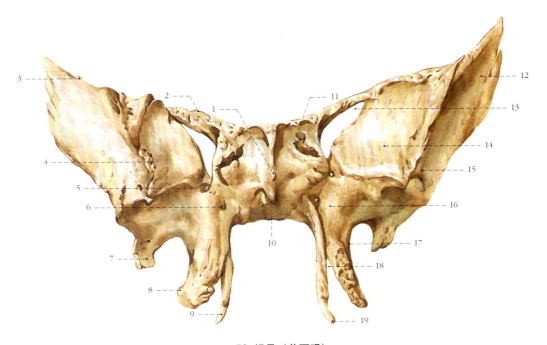

52. 蝶骨（前面观）
The sphenoid bone (anterior aspect)

53. 蝶骨（后面观）
The sphenoid bone (posterior aspect)

1.蝶嵴 sphenoidal crest
2.小翼 lesser wing
3.额缘 frontal margin
4.颧缘 zygomatic margin
5.圆孔 foramen rotundum
6.翼管 pterygoid canal
7.蝶棘 spine of sphenoid bone
8.翼突外侧板 lateral pterygoid plate
9.翼突内侧板 medial pterygoid plate

10.体 body
11.蝶窦口 aperture of sphenoidal sinus
12.颞面 temporal surface
13.眶上裂 superior orbital fissure
14.眶面 orbital surface
15.大翼 greater wing
16.上颌面 maxillary surface
17.翼突 pterygoid process
18.翼切迹 pterygoid fissure

19.翼钩 pterygoid hamulus
20.后床突 posterior clinoid process
21.斜坡 clivus
22.大脑面 cerebral surface
23.前床突 anterior clinoid process
24.颈动脉沟 carotid sulcus
25.翼窝 pterygoid fossa
26.蝶嘴 sphenoidal rostrum

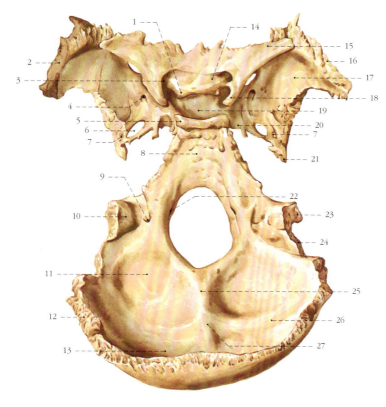

54. 枕骨和蝶骨（上面观）
The occipital bone and sphenoid bone (superior aspect)

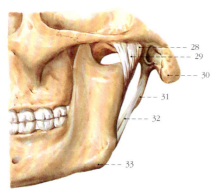

55. 颞下颌关节（外面观）
The temporomandibular joint
(external aspect)

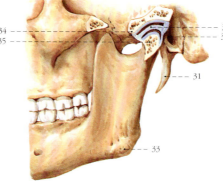

56. 颞下颌关节（矢状切面）
The temporomandibular joint
(sagittal section)

1.鞍结节 tuberculum sellae
2.蝶骨大翼 greater wing of sphenoid bone
3.视神经管 optic canal
4.圆孔 foramen rotundum
5.后床突 posterior clinoid process
6.卵圆孔 foramen ovale
7.棘孔 foramen spinosum
8.斜坡 clivus
9.髁管 condylar canal
10.乙状窦沟 sulcus for sigmoid sinus
11.小脑窝 cerebellar fossa
12.人字缘 lambdoid border
13.大脑窝 cerebral fossa
14.交叉前沟 sulcus prechiasmaticus
15.小翼 lesser wing
16.额缘 frontal margin
17.大脑面 cerebral surface
18.前床突 anterior clinoid process
19.垂体窝 hypophysial fossa
20.颈动脉沟 carotid sulcus
21.蝶棘 sphenoidal crest
22.舌下神经管 hypoglossal canal
23.颈静脉突 jugular process
24.乳突缘 mastoid border
25.枕内嵴 internal occipital crest
26.横窦沟 sulcus for transverse sinus
27.枕内隆凸 internal occipital protuberance
28.关节囊 articular capsule
29.外侧韧带 lateral ligament
30.乳突 mastoid process
31.茎突 styloid process
32.茎突下颌韧带 stylomandibular ligament
33.下颌角 angle of mandible
34.关节结节 articular tubercle
35.髁突 condylar process
36.关节盘 articular disc
37.外耳门 external acoustic pore

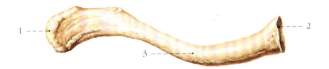

57. 锁骨（上面观）
The clavicle (superior aspect)

59. 锁骨（下面观）
The clavicle (inferior aspect)

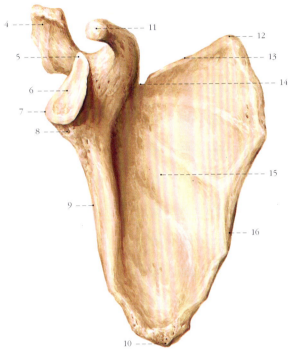

58. 肩胛骨（前面观）
The scapula (anterior aspect)

1.肩峰端 acromial end
2.胸骨端 sternal end
3.锁骨体 shaft of clavicle
4.肩峰 acromion
5.盂上结节 supraglenoid tubercle
6.关节盂 glenoid cavity
7.外侧角 lateral angle
8.盂下结节 infraglenoid tubercle
9.外侧缘 lateral border
10.下角 inferior angle
11.喙突 coracoid process
12.上角 superior angle
13.上缘 superior border
14.肩胛切迹 scapular notch
15.肩胛下窝 subscapular fossa
16.内侧缘 medial border
17.肋锁韧带压迹 impression for
    costoclavicular ligament
18.锥状结节 conoid tubercle
19.冈上窝 supraspinous fossa
20.肩胛冈 spine of scapula
21.冈下窝 infraspinous fossa
22.肩胛颈 neck of scapula

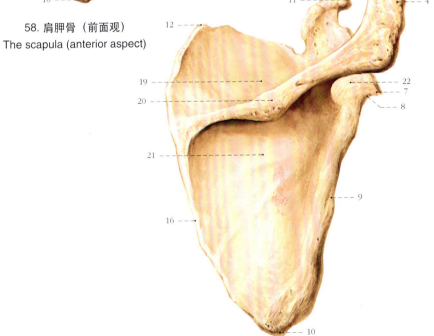

60. 肩胛骨（后面观）
The scapula (posterior aspect)

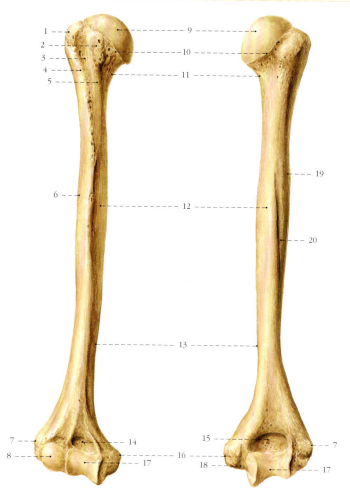

61. 肱骨（前面观）
The humerus (anterior aspect)

62. 肱骨（后面观）
The humerus (posterior aspect)

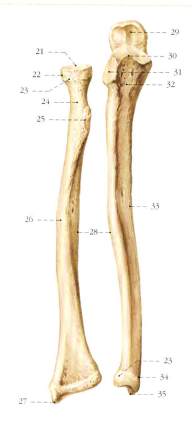

63. 桡骨和尺骨（前面观）
The radius and ulna (anterior aspect)

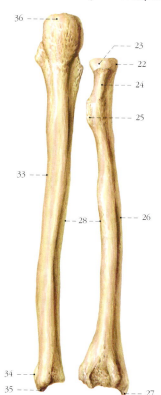

64. 桡骨和尺骨（后面观）
The radius and ulna (posterior aspect)

1.大结节 greater tubercle
2.小结节 lesser tubercle
3.结节间沟 intertubercular sulcus
4.大结节嵴 crest of greater tubercle
5.小结节嵴 crest of lesser tubercle
6.三角肌粗隆 deltoid tuberosity
7.外上髁 lateral epicondyle
8.肱骨小头 capitulum of humerus
9.肱骨头 head of humerus
10.解剖颈 anatomical neck
11.外科颈 surgical neck
12.肱骨体 shaft of humerus
13.内侧缘 medial border
14.冠突窝 coronoid fossa
15.鹰嘴窝 olecranon fossa
16.内上髁 medial epicondyle
17.肱骨滑车 trochlea of humerus
18.尺神经沟 sulcus for ulnar nerve
19.外侧缘 lateral border
20.桡神经沟 sulcus for radial nerve
21.关节凹 articular fovea
22.桡骨头 head of radius
23.环状关节面 articular circumference
24.桡骨颈 neck of radius
25.桡骨粗隆 radial tuberosity
26.桡骨体 shaft of radius
27.桡骨茎突 styloid process of radius
28.骨间缘 interosseous border
29.滑车切迹 trochlear notch
30.冠突 coronoid process
31.桡切迹 radial notch
32.尺骨粗隆 ulnar tuberosity
33.尺骨体 shaft of ulna
34.尺骨头 head of ulna
35.尺骨茎突 styloid process of ulna
36.鹰嘴 olecranon

1.远节指骨粗隆 tuberosity of distal phalanx
2.指骨体 shaft of phalanx
3.指骨底 base of phalanx
4.指骨滑车 trochlea of phalanx
5.第五掌骨 fifth metacarpal bone
6.钩骨钩 hamulus of hamate bone
7.钩骨 hamate bone
8.豌豆骨 pisiform bone
9.三角骨 triquetral bone
10.月骨 lunate bone
11.远节指骨 distal phalanx
12.中节指骨 middle phalanx
13.近节指骨 proximal phalanx
14.籽骨 sesamoid bone
15.第一掌骨 first metacarpal bone
16.小多角骨 trapezoid bone
17.大多角骨 trapezium bone
18.手舟骨 scaphoid bone
19.头状骨 capitate bone
20.掌骨头 head of metacarpal bone
21.掌骨体 shaft of metacarpal bone
22.掌骨底 base of metacarpal bone

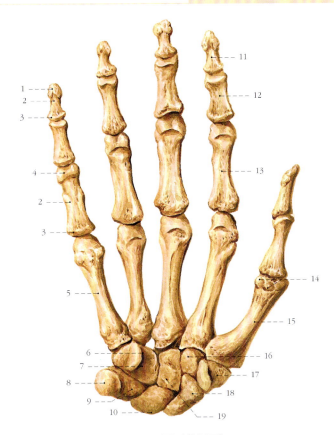

65. 手骨（掌侧面）
The bones of the hand (palmar aspect)

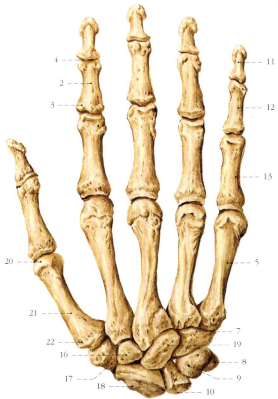

66. 手骨（背侧面）
The bones of the hand (dorsal aspect)

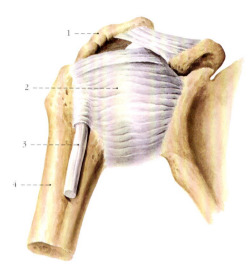

67. 肩关节（前面观）
The shoulder joint (anterior aspect)

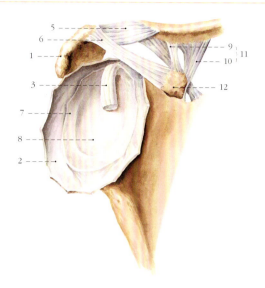

68. 肩关节（内面观，去掉肱骨）
The shoulder joint (internal aspect, without humerus)

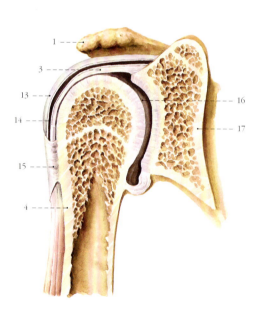

69. 肩关节（冠状切面）
The shoulder joint (coronal section)

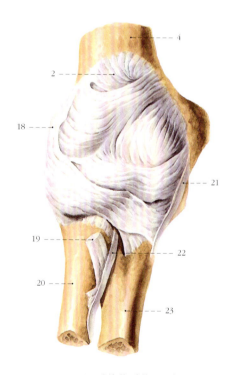

70. 肘关节（前面观）
The elbow joint (anterior aspect)

1.肩峰 acromion
2.关节囊 articular capsule
3.肱二头肌（长头腱）biceps brachii (long head tendon)
4.肱骨 humerus
5.肩锁韧带 acromioclavicular ligament
6.喙肩韧带 coracoacromial ligament
7.关节唇 articular labrum
8.关节盂 glenoid cavity

9.斜方韧带 trapezoid ligament
10.锥状韧带 conoid ligament
11.喙锁韧带 coracoclavicular ligament
12.喙突 coracoid process
13.关节囊（纤维膜）articular capsule (fibrous membrane)
14.关节囊（滑膜）articular capsule (synovial membrane)
15.结节间滑液鞘 intertubercular synovial sheath

16.关节腔 articular cavity
17.肩胛骨 scapula
18.桡侧副韧带 radial collateral ligament
19.肱二头肌腱 tendon of biceps brachii
20.桡骨 radius
21.尺侧副韧带 ulnar collateral ligament
22.斜索 oblique cord
23.尺骨 ulna

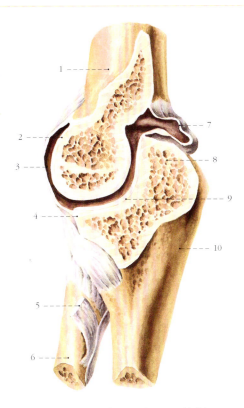

71. 肘关节矢状切面（示肱尺关节）
Sagittal section of the elbow joint
(showing the humeroulnar joint)

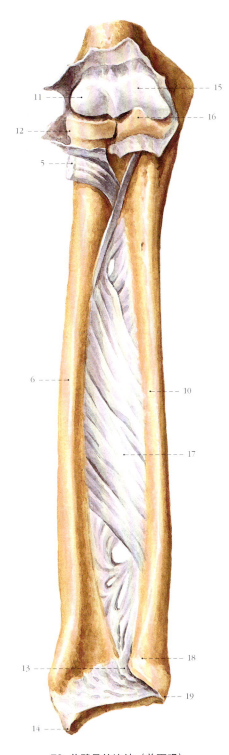

72. 前臂骨的连结（前面观）
The radioulnar syndesmosis
(anterior aspect)

1.肱骨 humerus
2.肱骨滑车（切面）trochlea of humerus（section）
3.关节腔 articular cavity
4.冠突（切面）coronoid process（section）
5.肱二头肌腱 tendon of biceps brachii
6.桡骨 radius
7.关节囊 articular capsule
8.鹰嘴（切面）olecranon（section）
9.滑车切迹（切面）trochlear notch（section）
10.尺骨 ulna
11.肱骨小头 capitulum of humerus
12.桡骨头 head of radius
13.桡尺远侧关节 distal radioulnar joint
14.桡骨茎突 styloid process of radius
15.肱骨滑车 trochlea of humerus
16.冠突 coronoid process
17.前臂骨间膜 interosseous membrane of forearm
18.尺骨头 head of ulna
19.尺骨茎突 styloid process of ulna

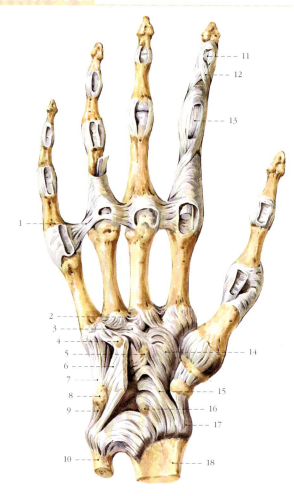

73. 手关节（掌面观）
The joints of the hand (palmar aspect)

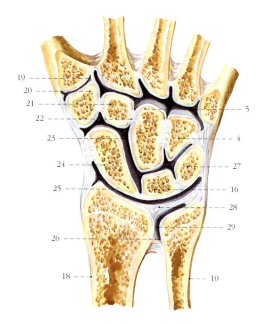

74. 腕关节（冠状切面）
The joints of the wrist (coronal section)

1.掌骨深横韧带 deep transverse metacarpal ligament
2.掌骨间掌侧韧带 palmar metacarpal ligament
3.腕掌掌侧韧带 palmar carpometacarpal ligament
4.钩骨 hamate bone
5.头状骨 capitate bone
6.豆钩韧带 pisohamate ligament
7.豆掌韧带 pisometacarpal ligament
8.豌豆骨 pisiform bone
9.腕尺侧副韧带 ulnar carpal collateral ligament
10.尺骨 ulna
11.指深屈肌腱 tendon of flexor digitorum profundus
12.指腱纤维鞘 fibrous sheaths of finger
13.指浅屈肌腱 tendon of flexor digitorum superficialis
14.腕辐状韧带 radiate carpal ligament
15.桡腕掌侧韧带 palmar radiocarpal ligament
16.月骨 lunate bone
17.腕桡侧副韧带 radial carpal collateral ligament
18.桡骨 radius
19.拇指腕掌关节 carpometacarpal joint of thumb
20.大多角骨 trapezium bone
21.小多角骨 trapezoid bone
22.腕骨间韧带 interosseous intercarpal ligaments
23.腕骨间关节 intercarpal joints
24.手舟骨 scaphoid bone
25.桡腕关节 radiocarpal joint
26.囊状隐窝 sacciform recess
27.三角骨 triquetral bone
28.关节盘 articular disc
29.桡尺远侧关节 distal radioulnar joint

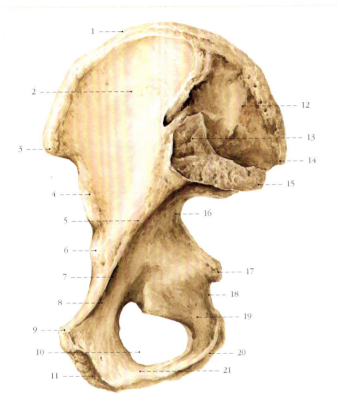

75. 髋骨（内面观）
The hip bone (internal aspect)

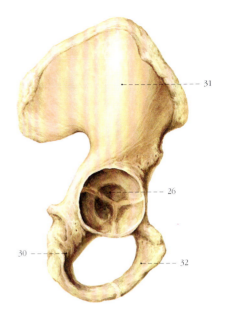

77. 小儿髋骨（外面观）
The hip bone of a child (external aspect)

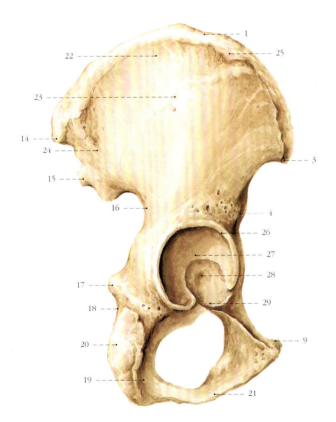

76. 髋骨（外面观）
The hip bone (external aspect)

1.髂嵴 iliac crest
2.髂窝 iliac fossa
3.髂前上棘 anterior superior iliac spine
4.髂前下棘 anterior inferior iliac spine
5.弓状线 arcuate line
6.髂耻隆起 iliopubic eminence
7.耻骨梳 pecten pubis
8.耻骨上支 superior ramus of pubis
9.耻骨结节 pubic tubercle
10.闭孔 obturator foramen
11.耻骨联合面 symphysial surface
12.髂粗隆 iliac tuberosity
13.耳状面 auricular surface
14.髂后上棘 posterior superior iliac spine
15.髂后下棘 posterior inferior iliac spine
16.坐骨大切迹 greater sciatic notch
17.坐骨棘 ischial spine
18.坐骨小切迹 lesser sciatic notch
19.坐骨支 ramus of ischium
20.坐骨结节 ischial tuberosity
21.耻骨下支 inferior ramus of pubis
22.髂骨翼 ala of ilium
23.臀前线 anterior gluteal line
24.臀后线 posterior gluteal line
25.髂结节 tubercle of iliac crest
26.髋臼 acetabulum
27.月状面 lunate surface
28.髋臼窝 acetabular fossa
29.髋臼切迹 acetabular notch
30.坐骨 ischium
31.髂骨 ilium
32.耻骨 pubis

29

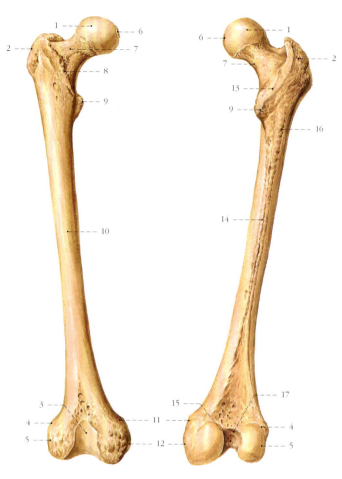

78. 股骨（前面观）
The femur (anterior aspect)

79. 股骨（后面观）
The femur (posterior aspect)

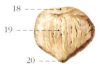

80. 髌骨（前面观）
The patella
(anterior aspect)

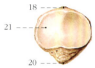

81. 髌骨（后面观）
The patella
(posterior aspect)

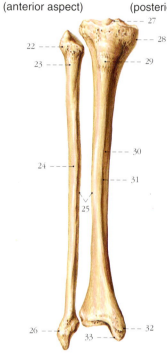

82. 胫骨和腓骨（前面观）
The tibia and fibula (anterior aspect)

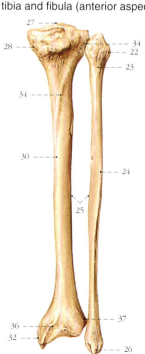

83. 胫骨和腓骨（后面观）
The tibia and fibula (posterior aspect)

1.股骨头 femoral head
2.大转子 greater trochanter
3.髌面 patellar surface
4.外上髁 lateral epicondyle
5.外侧髁 lateral condyle
6.股骨头凹 fovea of femoral head
7.股骨颈 neck of femur
8.转子间线 intertrochanteric line
9.小转子 lesser trochanter
10.股骨体 shaft of femur
11.内上髁 medial epicondyle
12.内侧髁 medial condyle
13.转子间嵴 intertrochanteric crest
14.粗线 linea aspera
15.髁间窝 intercondylar fossa
16.臀肌粗隆 gluteal tuberosity
17.髁间线 intercondylar line
18.髌底 base of patella
19.前面 anterior surface

20.髌尖 apex of patella
21.关节面 articular surface
22.腓骨头 fibular head
23.腓骨颈 neck of fibula
24.腓骨体 shaft of fibula
25.骨间缘 interosseous border
26.外踝 lateral malleolus
27.髁间隆起 intercondylar eminence
28.内侧髁 medial condyle
29.胫骨粗隆 tibial tuberosity
30.胫骨体 shaft of tibia
31.前缘 anterior border
32.内踝 medial malleolus
33.内踝关节面 articular facet of medial malleolus
34.腓骨头关节面 articular surface of fibular head
35.比目鱼肌线 soleal line
36.踝沟 malleolar sulcus
37.腓骨切迹 fibular notch

13.内侧楔骨　medial cuneiform bone
14.跖骨底　base of metatarsal bone
15.跖骨体　shaft of metatarsal bone
16.跖骨头　head of metatarsal bone
17.趾骨底　base of phalanx
18.趾骨体　body of phalanx
19.趾骨滑车　trochlea of phalanx
20.第一跖骨　first metatarsal bone
21.籽骨　sesamoid bone
22.跟骨结节　calcaneal tuberosity

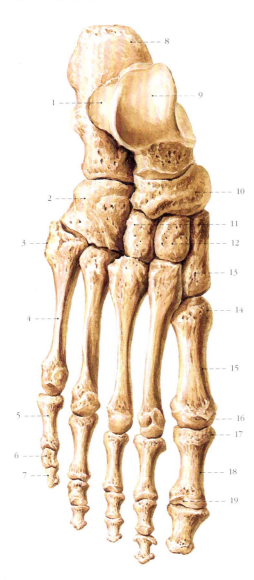

84. 足骨（背面观）
Bones of the foot (dorsal aspect)

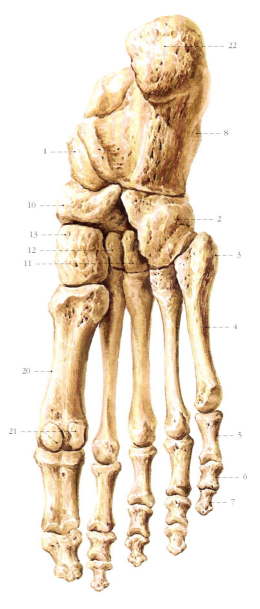

85. 足骨（跖面观）
Bones of the foot (plantar aspect)

1.距骨　talus
2.骰骨　cuboid bone
3.第五跖骨粗隆　tuberosity of fifth metatarsal bone
4.第五跖骨　fifth metatarsal bone
5.近节趾骨　proximal phalanx
6.中节趾骨　middle phalanx
7.远节趾骨　distal phalanx
8.跟骨　calcaneum bone
9.距骨滑车　trochlea of talus
10.足舟骨　navicular bone
11.外侧楔骨　lateral cuneiform bone
12.中间楔骨　intermediate cuneiform bone

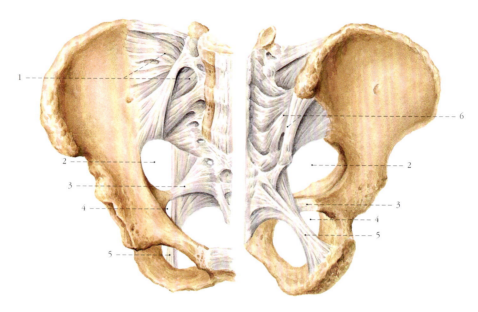

86. 骨盆的韧带（前面观和后面观）
The ligaments of the pelvis (anterior aspect and posterior aspect)

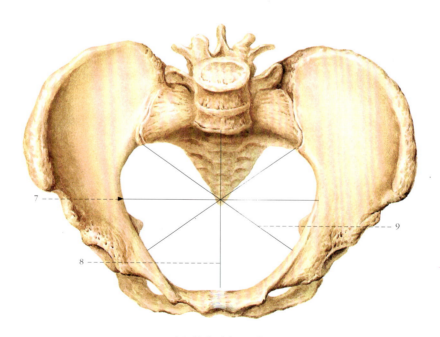

87. 骨盆（上面观）
The pelvis (superior aspect)

1.髂腰韧带 iliolumbar ligament
2.坐骨大孔 greater sciatic foramen
3.骶棘韧带 sacrospinous ligament
4.坐骨小孔 lesser sciatic foramen
5.骶结节韧带 sacrotuberous ligament
6.骶髂后韧带 posterior sacroiliac ligaments
7.横径 transverse diameter
8.前后径 anteroposterior diameter
9.斜径 oblique diameter

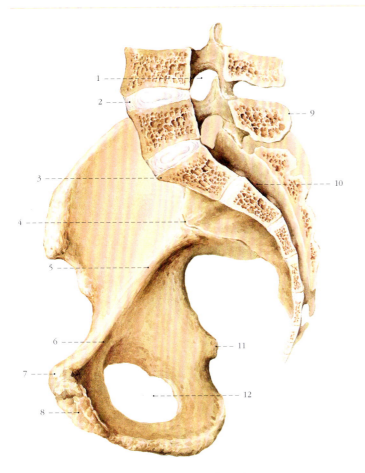

1.椎间孔 intervertebral foramen
2.椎间盘 intervertebral disc
3.岬 promontory
4.骶髂关节 sacroiliac joint
5.弓状线 arcuate line
6.耻骨梳 pecten pubis
7.耻骨结节 pubic tubercle
8.耻骨联合面 symphysial surface
9.棘突 spinous process
10.骶管 sacral canal
11.坐骨棘 ischial spine
12.闭孔 obturator foramen
13.髂股韧带 iliofemoral ligament
14.大转子 greater trochanter
15.关节囊 articular capsule
16.耻股韧带 pubofemoral ligament
17.闭孔膜 obturator membrane
18.小转子 lesser trochanter
19.坐股韧带 ischiofemoral ligament
20.坐骨结节 ischial tuberosity
21.股骨颈 neck of femur
22.转子间嵴 intertrochanteric crest

88. 骨盆（正中矢状切面）
The pelvis (median sagittal section)

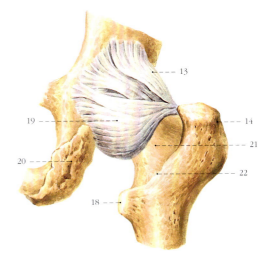

90. 髋关节（后面观）
The hip joint (posterior aspect)

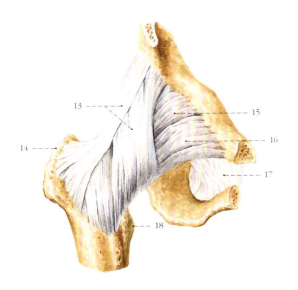

89. 髋关节（前面观）
The hip joint (anterior aspect)

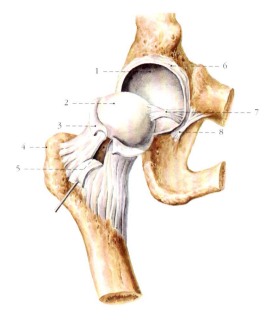

91. 切开关节囊（示髋关节腔内面）
The opened articular capsule (showing the internal
surface of the hip joint cavity)

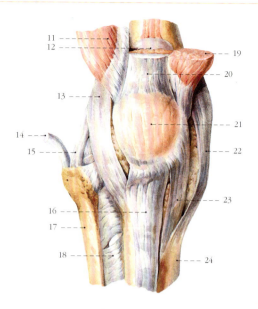

93. 膝关节（前面观）
The knee joint (anterior aspect)

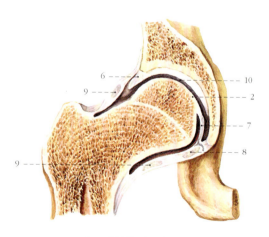

92. 髋关节（冠状切面）
The hip joint (coronal section)

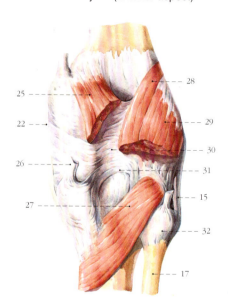

94. 膝关节（后面观）
The knee joint (posterior aspect)

1. 月状面 lunate surface
2. 股骨头 femoral head
3. 关节囊 articular capsule
4. 大转子 greater trochanter
5. 股骨颈 neck of femur
6. 髋臼唇 acetabular labrum
7. 股骨头韧带 ligament of head of femur
8. 髋臼横韧带 transverse acetabular ligament
9. 轮匝带 zona orbicularis
10. 关节腔 articular cavity

11. 股外侧肌 vastus lateralis
12. 髌上囊 suprapatellar bursa
13. 髌外侧支持带 lateral patellar retinaculum
14. 股二头肌腱 tendon of biceps femoris
15. 腓侧副韧带 fibular collateral ligament
16. 髌韧带 patellar ligament
17. 腓骨 fibula
18. 小腿骨间膜 crural interosseous membrane
19. 股内侧肌 vastus medialis
20. 股直肌 rectus femoris

21. 髌骨 patella
22. 胫侧副韧带 tibial collateral ligament
23. 髌内侧支持带 medial patellar retinaculum
24. 胫骨 tibia
25. 腓肠肌（内侧头）gastrocnemius（medial head）
26. 半膜肌腱 tendon of semimembranosus
27. 腘肌 popliteus
28. 跖肌 plantaris
29. 腓肠肌（外侧头）gastrocnemius（lateral head）
30. 腘斜韧带 oblique popliteal ligament
31. 腘弓状韧带 arcuate popliteal ligament
32. 腓骨头 fibular head

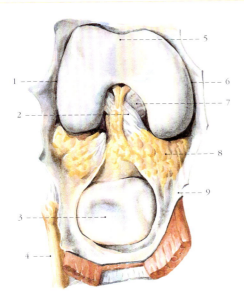

95. 切开关节囊前部（示膝关节腔内面）
The anterior aspect of the opened articular capsule (showing
the internal surface of the knee joint cavity)

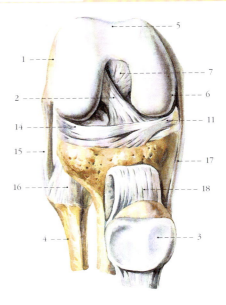

97. 膝关节前面观（切除关节囊）
The anterior aspect of the knee joint
(without the articular capsule)

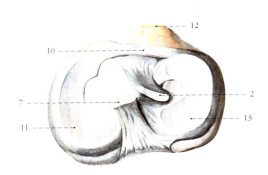

96. 膝关节半月板和交叉韧带（上面观）
The articular meniscus and cruciate ligament of the
knee joint (superior aspect)

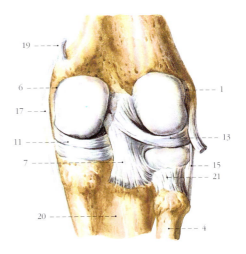

98. 膝关节后面观（切除关节囊）
The posterior aspect of the knee joint
(without the articular capsule)

1.外侧髁 lateral condyle

2.前交叉韧带 anterior cruciate ligament

3.关节面 articular surface

4.腓骨 fibula

5.髌面 patellar surface

6.内侧髁 medial condyle

7.后交叉韧带 posterior cruciate ligament

8.翼状襞 alar folds

9.关节囊 articular capsule

10.膝横韧带 transverse ligament of knee

11.内侧半月板 medial meniscus

12.胫骨粗隆 tibial tuberosity

13.外侧半月板 lateral meniscus

14.外侧半月板 lateral meniscus

15.腓侧副韧带 fibular collateral ligament

16.腓骨头前韧带 anterior ligament of

fibular head

17.胫侧副韧带 tibial collateral ligament

18.髌韧带 patellar ligament

19.大收肌腱 tendon of adductor
magnus

20.胫骨 tibia

21.腓骨头后韧带 posterior ligament of
fibular head

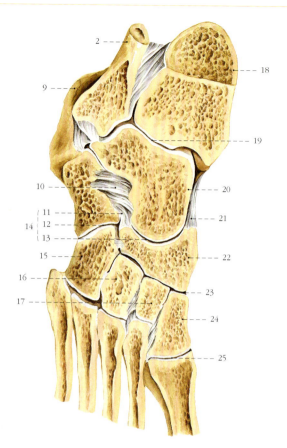

99. 足关节（切面）
The joints of foot (section)

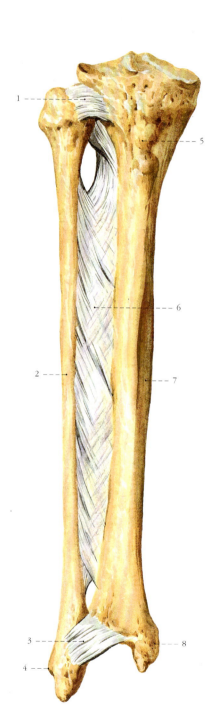

100. 小腿骨连结（前面观）
The tibiofibular syndesmosis (anterior aspect)

1.腓骨头前韧带 anterior ligament of fibular head
2.腓骨 fibula
3.胫腓前韧带 anterior tibiofibular ligament
4.外踝 lateral malleolus
5.胫骨粗隆 tibial tuberosity
6.小腿骨间膜 interosseous membrane of leg
7.胫骨 tibia
8.内踝 medial malleolus
9.跟骨 calcaneus
10.距跟骨间韧带 interosseous talocalcaneal ligament
11.跟舟韧带 calcaneonavicular ligament
12.跟骰关节 calcaneocuboid joint
13.距跟舟关节 talocalcaneonavicular joint
14.跗横关节 transverse tarsal joint
15.骰骨 cuboid bone
16.外侧楔骨 lateral cuneiform bone
17.中间楔骨 intermediate cuneiform bone
18.胫骨 tibia
19.距小腿关节 talocrural joint
20.距骨 talus
21.胫舟部 tibionavicular part
22.足舟骨 navicular bone
23.楔舟关节 cuneonavicular joint
24.内侧楔骨 medial cuneiform bone
25.跗跖关节 tarsometatarsal joint

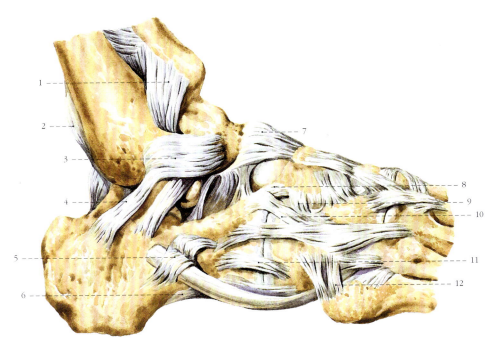

101. 距小腿关节和足关节（外侧面观）
The talocrural joint and the joints of foot (lateral aspect)

1.胫腓前韧带 anterior tibiofibular ligament
2.胫腓后韧带 posterior tibiofibular ligament
3.距腓前韧带 anterior talofibular ligament
4.跟腓韧带 calcaneofibular ligament
5.腓骨肌下支持带 inferior peroneal retinaculum
6.足底长韧带 long plantar ligament
7.距舟韧带 talonavicular ligament
8.跟舟韧带 calcaneonavicular ligament
9.骰舟背侧韧带 dorsal cuboideonavicular ligament
10.跟骰韧带 calcaneocuboid ligament
11.跟骰背侧韧带 dorsal calcaneocuboid ligament
12.跗跖背侧韧带 dorsal tarsometatarsal ligament
13.趾长屈肌腱 tendon of flexor digitorum longus
14.胫骨后肌腱 tendon of tibialis posterior
15.跟舟足底韧带 plantar calcaneonavicular ligament
16.骰舟足底韧带 plantar cuboideonavicular ligament
17.足舟骨 navicular bone
18.楔舟足底韧带 plantar cuneonavicular ligament
19.内侧楔骨 medial cuneiform bone
20.胫骨前肌腱 tendon of tibialis anterior
21.跟骨 calcaneus
22.姆长屈肌腱 tendon of flexor hallucis longus
23.腓骨短肌腱 tendon of peroneus brevis
24.腓骨长肌腱 tendon of peroneus longus
25.跖骨足底韧带 plantar metatarsal ligament

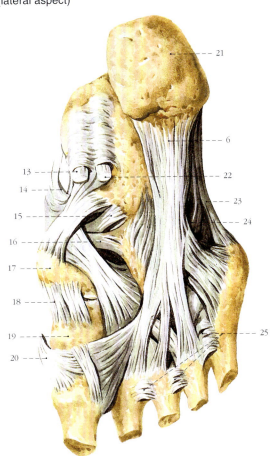

102.足关节（下面观）
The joints of foot (inferior aspect)

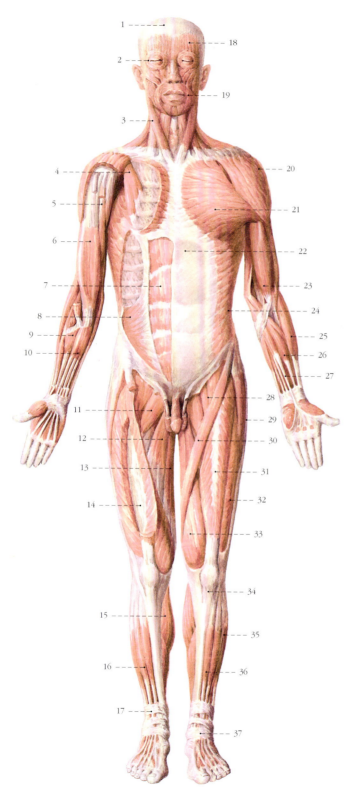

1.帽状腱膜 galea aponeurotica
2.眼轮匝肌 orbicularis oculi
3.胸锁乳突肌 sternocleidomastoid
4.胸小肌 pectoralis minor
5.喙肱肌 coracobrachialis
6.肱肌 brachialis
7.腹直肌 rectus abdominis
8.腹内斜肌 obliquus internus abdominis
9.拇长屈肌 flexor pollicis longus
10.指深屈肌 flexor digitorum profundus
11.耻骨肌 pectineus
12.长收肌 adductor longus
13.大收肌 adductor magnus
14.股中间肌 vastus intermedius
15.腓肠肌 gastrocnemius
16.趾长伸肌 extensor digitorum longus
17.伸肌上支持带 superior extensor retinaculum
18.枕额肌（额腹）occipitofrontalis (frontal belly)
19.口轮匝肌 orbicularis oris
20.三角肌 deltoid
21.胸大肌 pectoralis major
22.腹直肌鞘 sheath of rectus abdominis
23.肱二头肌 biceps brachii
24.腹外斜肌 obliquus externus abdominis
25.肱桡肌 brachioradialis
26.桡侧腕屈肌 flexor carpi radialis
27.掌长肌腱 tendon of palmaris longus
28.髂腰肌 iliopsoas
29.阔筋膜张肌 tensor fasciae latae
30.缝匠肌 sartorius
31.股直肌 rectus femoris
32.股外侧肌 vastus lateralis
33.股内侧肌 vastus medialis
34.髌韧带 patellar ligament
35.腓骨长肌 peroneus longus
36.胫骨前肌 tibialis anterior
37.伸肌下支持带 inferior extensor retinaculum

103. 全身肌肉（前面观）
Muscles of the whole body (anterior aspect)

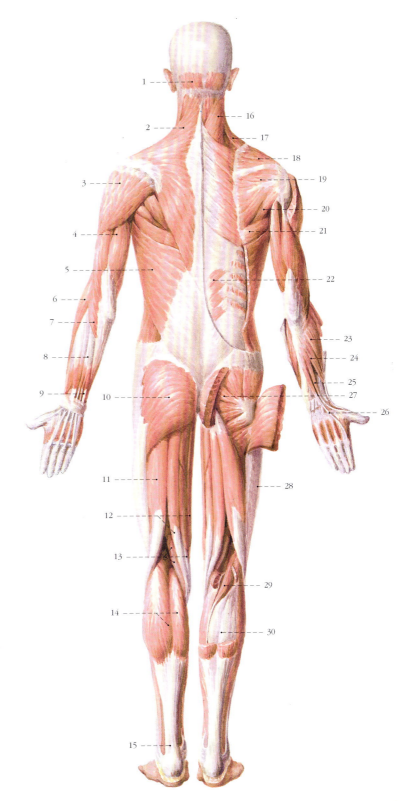

1.枕额肌（枕腹）occipitofrontalis
  （occipital belly）
2.斜方肌 trapezius
3.三角肌 deltoid
4.肱三头肌 triceps brachii
5.背阔肌 latissimus dorsi
6.肱桡肌 brachioradialis
7.肘肌 anconeus
8.指伸肌 extensor digitorum
9.尺侧腕伸肌 extensor carpi ulnaris
10.臀大肌 gluteus maximus
11.股二头肌 biceps femoris
12.半腱肌 semitendinosus
13.半膜肌 semimembranosus
14.腓肠肌 gastrocnemius
15.跟腱 tendo calcaneus
16.头夹肌 splenius capitis
17.肩胛提肌 levator scapulae
18.冈上肌 supraspinatus
19.冈下肌 infraspinatus
20.小圆肌 teres minor
21.大圆肌 teres major
22.下后锯肌 serratus posterior inferior
23.旋后肌 supinator
24.拇长展肌 abductor pollicis longus
25.拇长伸肌 extensor pollicis longus
26.示指伸肌腱 tendon of extensor indicis
27.梨状肌 piriformis
28.髂胫束 iliotibial tract
29.跖肌 plantaris
30.比目鱼肌 soleus

104. 全身肌肉（后面观）
Muscles of the whole body (posterior aspect)

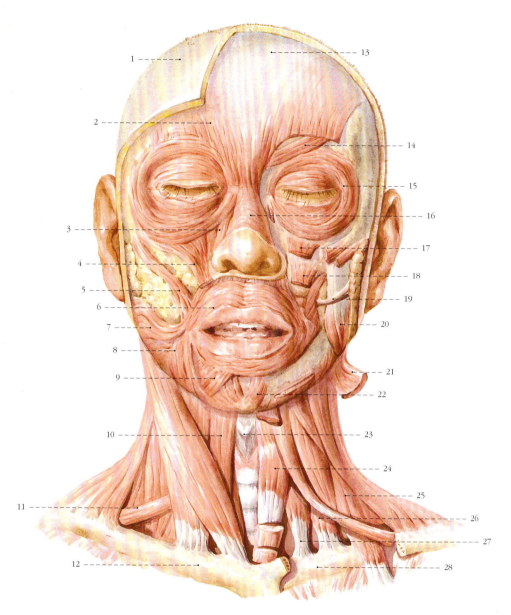

105. 头颈肌（前面观）
Muscles of the head and neck (anterior aspect)

1.皮肤 skin	11.肩胛舌骨肌 omohyoid	20.咬肌 masseter
2.枕额肌（额腹）occipitofrontalis（frontal belly）	12.锁骨 clavicle	21.胸锁乳突肌 sternocleidomastoid
3.提上唇鼻翼肌 levator labii superioris alaeque nasi	13.帽状腱膜 galea aponeurotica	22.颏肌 mentalis
4.颧小肌 zygomaticus minor	14.皱眉肌 corrugator supercilii	23.喉结 laryngeal prominence
5.颧大肌 zygomaticus major	15.眼轮匝肌 orbicularis oculi	24.胸骨甲状肌 sternothyroid
6.口轮匝肌 orbicularis oris	16.鼻肌 nasalis	25.后斜角肌 scalenus posterior
7.笑肌 risorius	17.提上唇肌 levator labii superioris	26.中斜角肌 scalenus medius
8.降口角肌 depressor anguli oris	18.提口角肌 levator anguli oris	27.前斜角肌 scalenus anterior
9.降下唇肌 depressor labii inferioris	19.腮腺管 parotid duct	28.第一肋 first rib
10.胸骨舌骨肌 sternohyoid		

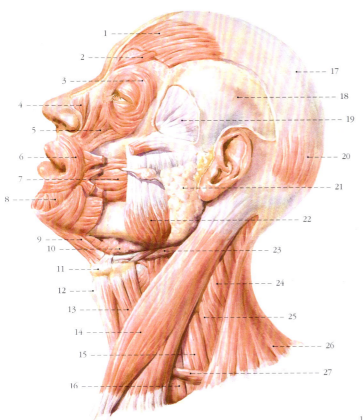

1.枕额肌（额腹）occipitofrontalis（frontal belly）
2.皱眉肌 corrugator supercilii
3.眼轮匝肌 orbicularis oculi
4.鼻肌 nasalis
5.提上唇肌 levator labii superioris
6.口轮匝肌 orbicularis oris
7.颊肌 buccinator
8.降下唇肌 depressor labii inferioris
9.二腹肌（前腹）digastric（anterior belly）
10.下颌下腺 submandibular gland
11.舌骨 hyoid bone
12.喉结 laryngeal prominence
13.肩胛舌骨肌（上腹）omohyoid（superior belly）
14.胸锁乳突肌 sternocleidomastoid
15.中斜角肌 scalenus medius
16.前斜角肌 scalenus anterior
17.帽状腱膜 galea aponeurotica
18.颞筋膜（深层）temporal fascia（deep layer）

106. 头颈肌的浅层（外侧面观）
Superficial layer of the muscles of the head and neck
(lateral aspect)

19.颞肌 temporalis
20.枕额肌（枕腹）occipitofrontalis（occipital belly）
21.腮腺 parotid gland
22.咬肌 masseter
23.二腹肌（后腹）digastric（posterior belly）
24.肩胛提肌 levator scapulae
25.后斜角肌 scalenus posterior
26.斜方肌 trapezius
27.肩胛舌骨肌（下腹）omohyoid（inferior belly）
28.甲状腺 thyroid gland
29.胸骨舌骨肌 sternohyoid
30.胸骨甲状肌 sternothyroid
31.气管 trachea
32.食管 esophagus
33.头夹肌 splenius capitis
34.咽中缩肌 middle constrictor of pharynx
35.咽下缩肌 inferior constrictor of pharynx
36.肩胛提肌 levator scapulae
37.第一肋 first rib

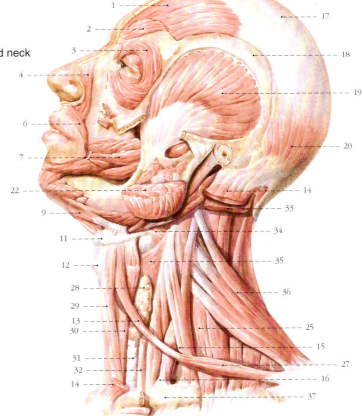

107. 头颈肌的深层（外侧面观）
Deep layer of muscles of the head and neck (lateral aspect)

1.头长肌 longus capitis
2.前斜角肌 scalenus anterior
3.中斜角肌 scalenus medius
4.后斜角肌 scalenus posterior
5.寰椎横突 transverse process of atlas
6.颈长肌 longus colli
7.第一肋 first rib
8.第二肋 second rib
9.气管 trachea
10.胸锁乳突肌 sternocleidomastoid
11.锁骨 clavicle
12.胸小肌 pectoralis minor
13.胸大肌 pectoralis major
14.前锯肌 serratus anterior
15.肱二头肌 biceps brachii
16.肋间外肌 intercostales externi
17.肋间外膜 external intercostal membrane

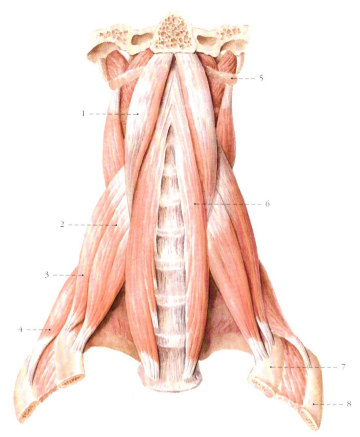

108. 颈深肌群（前面观）
Deep cervical muscle group (anterior aspect)

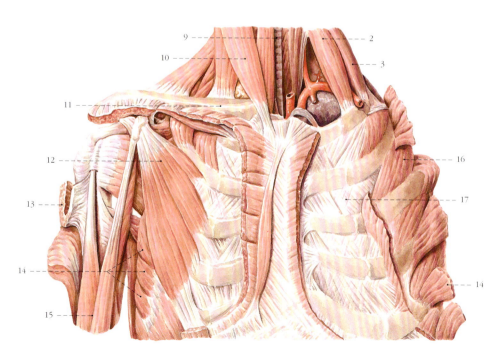

109. 胸部肌深层（前面观）
Muscles of the deep layer of the thorax (anterior aspect)

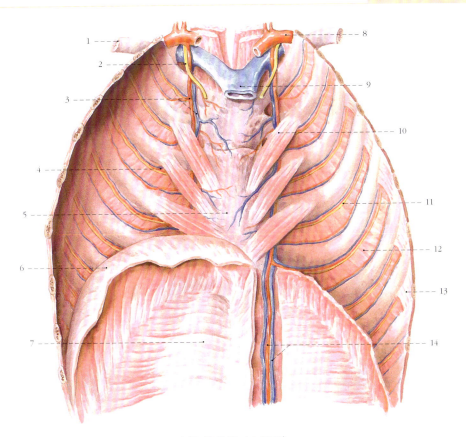

110. 胸前壁（内面观）
The anterior thoracic wall (internal aspect)

1.锁骨 clavicle
2.膈神经 phrenic nerve
3.胸廓内动、静脉 internal thoracic artery and vein
4.肋间前动、静脉 anterior intercostal artery and vein
5.胸骨 sternum
6.膈 diaphragm
7.腹直肌鞘后层 posterior layer of sheath of rectus abdominis
8.锁骨下动脉 subclavian artery
9.上腔静脉 superior vena cava
10.胸横肌 transversus thoracis
11.肋间神经 intercostal nerve
12.肋间内肌 intercostales interni
13.肋间最内肌 intercostales intimi
14.腹壁上动、静脉 superior epigastric artery and vein
15.第一肋 first rib
16.肋间外肌 intercostales externi
17.前斜角肌 scalenus anterior
18.中斜角肌 scalenus medius
19.斜角肌间隙 scalenus space
20.颈长肌 longus colli
21.脊柱 vertebral column

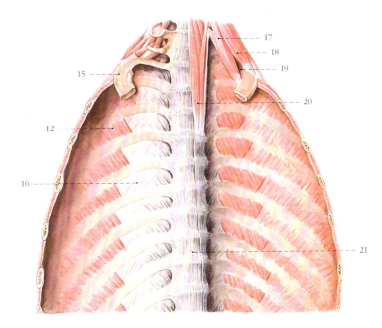

111. 胸后壁（内面观）
The posterior thoracic wall (internal aspect)

43

1.前锯肌 serratus anterior
2.腹外斜肌 obliquus externus abdominis
3.腹直肌鞘（前层）sheath of rectus abdominis（anterior layer）
4.腹内斜肌 obliquus internus abdominis
5.腱划 tendinous intersection
6.腹直肌鞘（后层）sheath of rectus abdominis（posterior layer）
7.白线 linea alba
8.弓状线 arcuate line
9.腹直肌 rectus abdominis
10.锥状肌 pyramidalis
11.腔静脉孔 vena caval foramen
12.内侧弓状韧带 medial arcuate ligament
13.外侧弓状韧带 lateral arcuate ligament
14.右脚 right crus
15.腹横肌 transversus abdominis

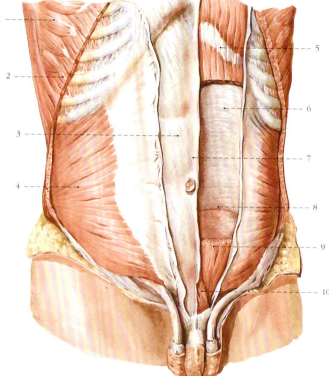

112. 腹前外侧壁肌（前面观）
Muscles of the anterolateral abdominal wall (anterior aspect)

113. 腹后壁肌及膈（前面观）
Muscles of the posterior abdominal wall and the diaphragm (anterior aspect)

16.髂肌 iliacus
17.腰大肌 psoas major
18.阔筋膜张肌 tensor fasciae latae
19.髂腰肌 iliopsoas
20.耻骨肌 pectineus
21.长收肌 adductor longus
22.中心腱 central tendon
23.食管裂孔 esophageal hiatus
24.正中弓状韧带 median arcuate ligament
25.主动脉裂孔 aortic hiatus
26.左脚 left crus
27.腰方肌 quadratus lumborum
28.腰小肌 psoas minor
29.髂筋膜 iliac fascia
30.腹股沟韧带 inguinal ligament
31.缝匠肌 sartorius
32.股薄肌 gracilis

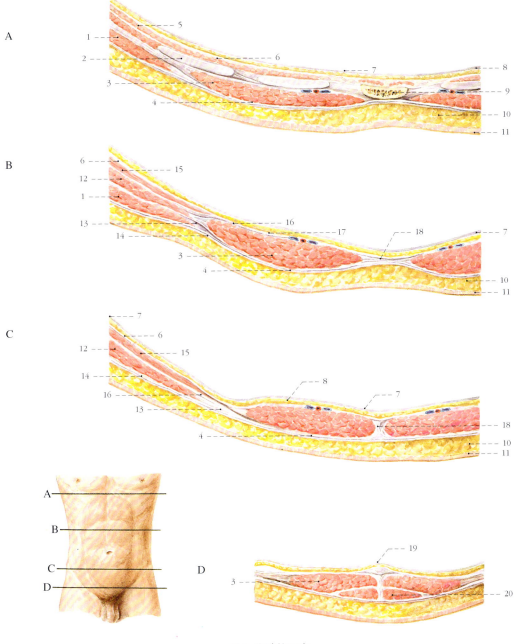

114. 腹壁的层次
The layers of the abdominal wall

1.腹外斜肌 obliquus externus abdominis
2.肋软骨 costal cartilage
3.腹直肌 rectus abdominis
4.腹直肌鞘前层 anterior layer of sheath of rectus abdominis
5.膈 diaphragm
6.腹横筋膜 transversalis fascia
7.壁腹膜 parietal peritoneum
8.腹膜下筋膜 subperitoneal fascia

9.胸骨 sternum
10.浅筋膜 superficial fascia
11.皮肤 skin
12.腹内斜肌 obliquus internus abdominis
13.腹内斜肌腱膜 aponeurosis of obliquus internus abdominis
14.腹外斜肌腱膜 aponeurosis of obliquus externus abdominis
15.腹横肌 transversus abdominis

16.腹横肌腱膜 aponeurosis of transversus abdominis
17.腹直肌鞘后层 posterior layer of sheath of rectus abdominis
18.白线 linea alba
19.脐正中襞 median umbilical fold
20.锥状肌 pyramidalis

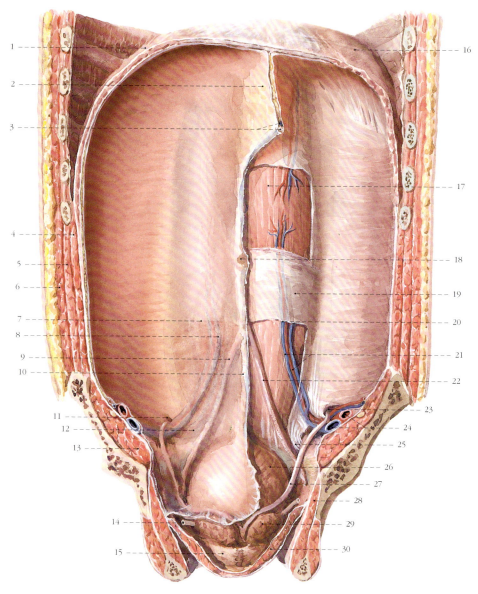

115. 腹前壁的内面
The internal aspect of the anterior abdominal wall

1.胸膜 pleura
2.镰状韧带 falciform ligament of liver
3.肝圆韧带、附脐静脉 ligamentum teres hepatis, paraumbilical veins
4.腹横肌 transversus abdominis
5.腹内斜肌 obliquus internus abdominis
6.腹外斜肌 obliquus externus abdominis
7.弓状线 arcuate line
8.脐外侧襞 lateral umbilical fold
9.脐内侧襞 medial umbilical fold
10.脐正中襞、脐尿管 median umbilical fold, urachus

11.腹股沟外侧窝 lateral inguinal fossa
12.腹股沟内侧窝 medial inguinal fossa
13.髂腰肌 iliopsoas
14.输尿管 ureter
15.前列腺 prostate
16.膈 diaphragm
17.腹直肌 rectus abdominis
18.脐 umbilicus
19.腹直肌鞘后层 posterior layer of sheath of rectus abdominis
20.弓状线 arcuate line
21.腹壁下动、静脉 inferior epigastric

artery and vein
22.脐内侧韧带 medial umbilical ligament
23.腹股沟深环 deep inguinal ring
24.髂外动、静脉 external iliac artery and vein
25.联合腱 conjoined tendon
26.膀胱 urinary bladder
27.输精管 ductus deferens
28.闭孔内肌 obturator internus
29.精囊 seminal vesicle
30.肛提肌 levator ani

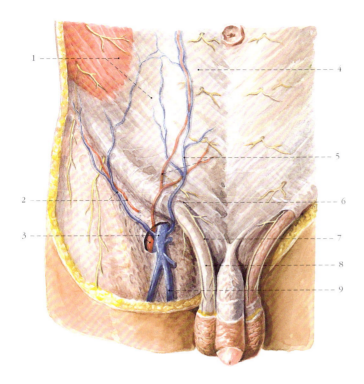

1.腹外斜肌、腱膜 aponeurosis of obliquus externus abdominis
2.旋髂浅动、静脉 superficial iliac circumflex artery and vein
3.股动、静脉 femoral artery and vein
4.腹直肌鞘前层 anterior layer of sheath of rectus abdominis
5.腹壁浅动、静脉 superficial epigastric artery and vein
6.浅环 superficial inguinal ring
7.髂腹股沟神经 ilioinguinal nerve
8.精索 spermatic cord
9.大隐静脉 great saphenous vein
10.腹内斜肌 obliquus internus abdominis
11.腹股沟韧带 inguinal ligament
12.髂腹下神经 iliohypogastric nerve
13.联合腱 conjoined tendon

116. 腹股沟区 （1）
Inguinal region (1)

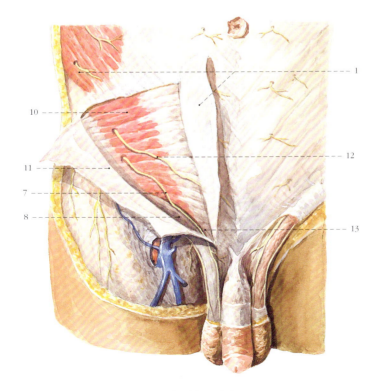

117. 腹股沟区 （2）
Inguinal region (2)

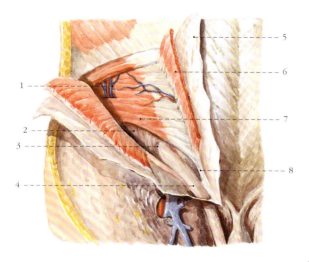

118. 腹股沟区（3）
Inguinal region (3)

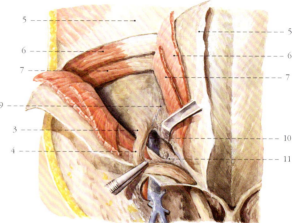

119. 腹股沟区（4）
Inguinal region (4)

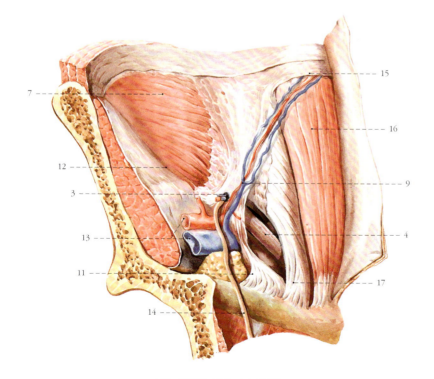

120. 腹股沟三角（内面观）
Inguinal triangle (internal aspect)

1.旋髂深动、静脉 deep iliac circumflex artery and vein
2.腹横筋膜 transversalis fascia
3.深环 deep inguinal ring
4.精索 spermatic cord
5.腹外斜肌腱膜 aponeurosis of obliquus externus abdominis
6.腹内斜肌 obliquus internus abdominis
7.腹横肌 transversus abdominis
8.联合腱 conjoined tendon
9.腹壁下动、静脉 inferior epigastric artery and vein
10.髂外静脉 external iliac vein
11.腔隙韧带 lacunar ligament
12.腹股沟韧带 inguinal ligament
13.髂外动、静脉 external iliac artery and vein
14.输精管 ductus deferens
15.弓状线 arcuate line
16.腹直肌 rectus abdominis
17.腹股沟镰 inguinal falx

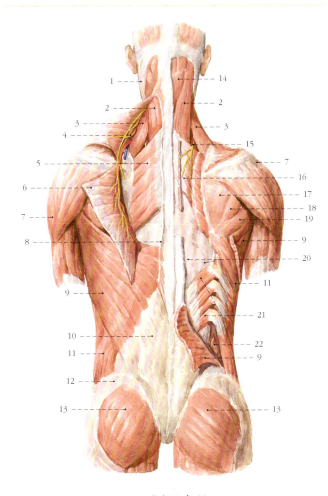

1.胸锁乳突肌 sternocleidomastoid
2.头夹肌 splenius capitis
3.肩胛提肌 levator scapulae
4.副神经 accessory nerve
5.菱形肌 rhomboideus
6.斜方肌 trapezius
7.三角肌 deltoid
8.竖脊肌鞘 sheath of erector spinae
9.背阔肌 latissimus dorsi
10.胸腰筋膜 thoracolumbar fascia
11.腹外斜肌 obliquus externus abdominis
12.臀筋膜 gluteal fascia
13.臀大肌 gluteus maximus
14.头半棘肌 semispinalis capitis
15.肩胛背神经 dorsal scapular nerve
16.上后锯肌 serratus posterior superior
17 冈下肌 infraspinatus
18.小圆肌 teres minor
19.大圆肌 teres major
20.竖脊肌 erector spinae
21.下后锯肌 serratus posterior inferior
22.腹内斜肌 obliquus internus abdominis

121. 背部肌肉 (1)
Muscles of the back (1)

23.头后小直肌 rectus capitis posterior minor
24.头后大直肌 rectus capitis posterior major
25.寰椎后结节 posterior tubercle of atlas
26.枢椎棘突 spinous process of axis
27.第七颈椎棘突 spinous process of the seventh cervical vertebra
28.第一肋 first rib
29.肋间外肌 intercostales externi
30.胸半棘肌 semispinalis thoracis
31.第十二胸椎棘突 spinous process of the twelfth thoracic vertebra
32.第十二肋 twelfth rib
33.腹横肌 transversus abdominis
34.多裂肌 multifidi
35.头上斜肌 superior obliquus capitis
36.枕下三角 suboccipital triangle
37.头下斜肌 inferior obliquus capitis
38.头最长肌 longissimus capitis
39.颈棘肌 spinalis cervicis
40.颈最长肌 longissimus cervicis
41.颈髂肋肌 iliocostalis cervicis
42.胸棘肌 spinalis thoracis
43.胸髂肋肌 iliocostalis thoracis
44.胸最长肌 longissimus thoracis
45.腹横肌腱膜 aponeurosis of transversus abdominis

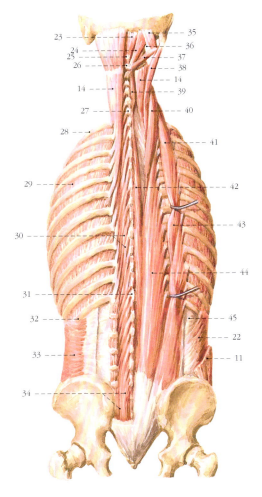

122. 背部肌肉 (2)
Muscles of the back (2)

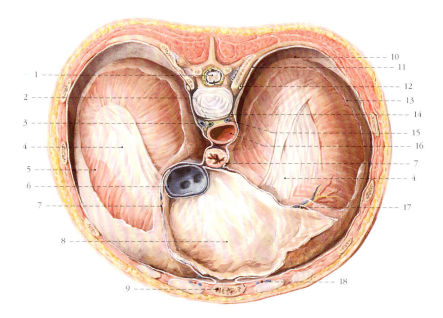

123. 膈（上面观）
The diaphragm (superior aspect)

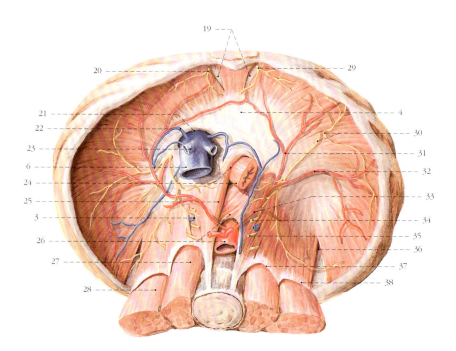

124. 膈（下面观）
The diaphragm (inferior aspect)

1.脊髓 spinal cord
2.胸导管 thoracic duct
3.奇静脉 azygos vein
4.中心腱 central tendon
5.膈 diaphragm
6.下腔静脉 inferior vena cava
7.纵隔胸膜 mediastinal pleura
8.心包膈部 diaphragmatic part of the pericardium
9.胸骨 sternum
10.肋膈隐窝 costodiaphragmatic recess
11.肋胸膜 costal pleura
12.交感神经干 sympathetic trunk
13.膈胸膜 diaphragmatic pleura
14.内脏大神经 greater splanchnic nerve
15.半奇静脉 hemiazygos vein
16.胸主动脉 thoracic aorta
17.心包膈血管、膈神经 pericardiacophrenic vessels, phrenic nerves
18.胸廓内动、静脉 internal thoracic artery and vein
19.胸肋三角 sternocostal triangle
20.右膈神经前支 anterior branch of right phrenic nerve
21.腔静脉孔 vena caval foramen
22.右膈下静脉 right inferior phrenic vein
23.肝静脉 hepatic vein
24.食管裂孔、食管 esophageal hiatus, esophagus
25.右脚 right crus
26.主动脉、主动脉裂孔 aorta, aortic hiatus
27.腰大肌 psoas major
28.腰方肌 quadratus lumborum
29.左膈神经前支 anterior branch of left phrenic nerve
30.左膈神经 left phrenic nerve
31.前支 anterior branch
32.后支 posterior branch
33.左膈下动脉 left inferior phrenic artery
34.内脏大神经 greater splanchnic nerve
35.内脏小神经 lesser splanchnic nerve
36.腰肋三角 lumbocostal trigone
37.内侧弓状韧带 medial arcuate ligament
38.外侧弓状韧带 lateral arcuate ligament

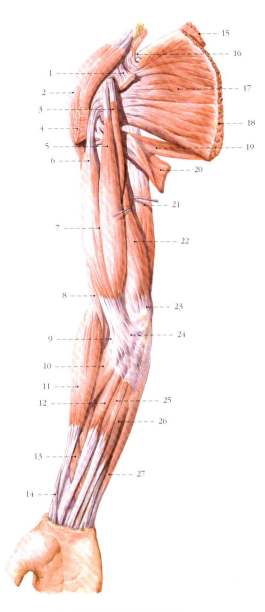

125. 上肢肌（前面观）（1）
Muscles of the upper limb (anterior aspect) (1)

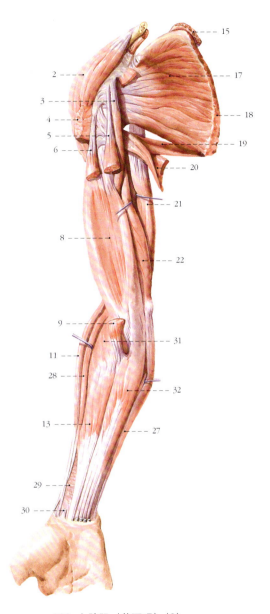

126. 上肢肌（前面观）（2）
Muscles of the upper limb (anterior aspect) (2)

1.胸小肌 pectoralis minor
2.三角肌 deltoid
3.喙肱肌 coracobrachialis
4.胸大肌 pectoralis major
5.肱二头肌（短头）biceps brachii (short head)
6.肱二头肌（长头）biceps brachii (long head)
7.肱二头肌 biceps brachii
8.肱肌 brachialis
9.肱二头肌腱 tendon of biceps brachii
10.旋前圆肌 pronator teres

11.肱桡肌 brachioradialis
12.桡侧腕屈肌 flexor carpi radialis
13.拇长屈肌 flexor pollicis longus
14.拇长展肌腱 tendon of abductor pollicis longus
15.肩胛提肌 levator scapulae
16.肩胛上横韧带 superior transverse scapular ligament
17.肩胛下肌 subscapularis
18.前锯肌 serratus anterior
19.大圆肌 teres major
20.背阔肌 latissimus dorsi

21.肱三头肌（长头）triceps brachii (long head)
22.肱三头肌（内侧头）triceps brachii (medial head)
23.内上髁 medial epicondyle
24.肱二头肌腱膜 bicipital aponeurosis
25.掌长肌 palmaris longus
26.指浅屈肌 flexor digitorum superficialis
27.尺侧腕屈肌 flexor carpi ulnaris
28.桡侧腕长伸肌 extensor carpi radialis longus
29.旋前方肌 pronator quadratus
30.桡侧腕屈肌腱 tendon of flexor carpi radialis
31.旋后肌 supinator
32.指深屈肌 flexor digitorum profundus

1.肱三头肌（长头）triceps brachii
  （long head）
2.肱三头肌（外侧头）triceps
  brachii（lateral head）
3.肱三头肌（内侧头）triceps
  brachii（medial head）
4.肱三头肌腱 tendon of triceps
  brachii
5.鹰嘴 olecranon
6.肘肌 anconeus
7.尺侧腕伸肌 extensor carpi
  ulnaris
8.指伸肌 extensor digitorum
9.拇短伸肌 extensor pollicis brevis
10.伸肌支持带 extensor
   retinaculum
11.桡侧腕短伸肌腱 tendon of
   extensor carpi radialis brevis
12.桡侧腕长伸肌腱 tendon of
   extensor carpi radialis longus

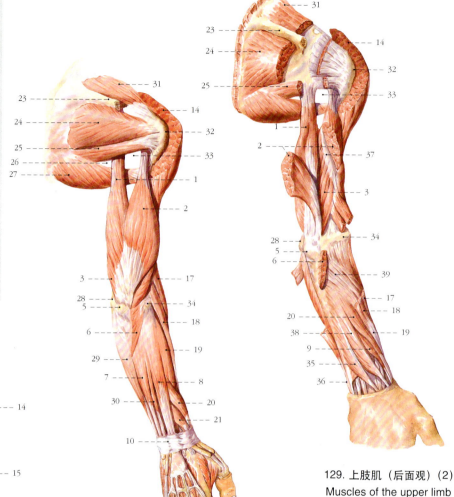

129. 上肢肌（后面观）（2）
Muscles of the upper limb
(posterior aspect) (2)

128. 上肢肌（后面观）（1）
Muscles of the upper limb
(posterior aspect) (1)

127. 上肢肌（外侧面观）
Muscles of the upper limb (lateral aspect)

13.指伸肌腱 tendon of extensor
   digitorum
14.三角肌 deltoid
15.肱二头肌 biceps brachii
16.肱肌 brachialis
17.肱桡肌 brachioradialis
18.桡侧腕长伸肌 extensor carpi
   radialis longus
19.桡侧腕短伸肌 extensor carpi
   radialis brevis
20.拇长展肌 abductor pollicis longus
21.拇短伸肌腱 tendon of extensor
   pollicis brevis
22.拇长伸肌腱 tendon of extensor
   pollicis longus
23.肩胛冈 spine of scapula

24.冈下肌 infraspinatus
25.小圆肌 teres minor
26.三边孔 triangular space
27.大圆肌 teres major
28.内上髁 medial epicondyle
29.尺侧腕屈肌 flexor carpi ulnaris
30.小指伸肌 extensor digiti minimi
31.冈上肌 supraspinatus
32.大结节 greater tubercle
33.四边孔 quadrangular space
34.外上髁 lateral epicondyle
35.示指伸肌 extensor indicis
36.尺侧腕屈肌 flexor carpi ulnaris
37.桡神经沟 sulcus for radial nerve
38.拇长伸肌 extensor pollicis longus
39.旋后肌 supinator

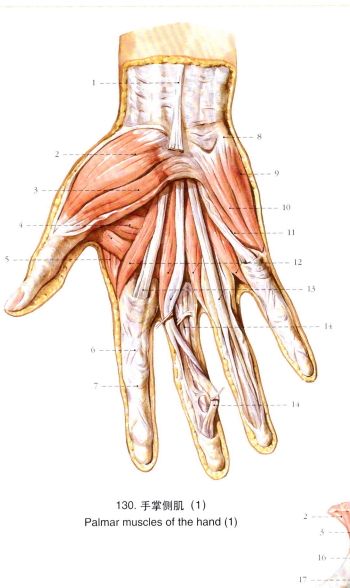

1.掌长肌 palmaris longus
2.拇短展肌 abductor pollicis brevis
3.拇短屈肌 flexor pollicis brevis
4.拇收肌 adductor pollicis
5.第一骨间背侧肌 first dorsal interossei
6.纤维鞘交叉部 cruciform part of fibrous sheath
7.纤维鞘环状部 annular part of fibrous sheath
8.豌豆骨 pisiform bone
9.小指展肌 abductor digiti minimi
10.小指短屈肌 flexor digiti minimi brevis
11.小指对掌肌 opponens digiti minimi
12.蚓状肌 lumbricales

130. 手掌侧肌（1）
Palmar muscles of the hand (1)

13.指浅屈肌腱 tendon of flexor digitorum superficialis
14.指深屈肌腱 tendon of flexor digitorum profundus
15.屈肌支持带 flexor retinaculum
16.骨间背侧肌 dorsal interossei
17.拇长屈肌腱 tendon of flexor pollicis longus
18.指深屈肌 flexor digitorum profundus
19.拇收肌（斜头）adductor pollicis (oblique head)
20.骨间掌侧肌 palmar interossei
21.拇收肌（横头）adductor pollicis (transverse head)

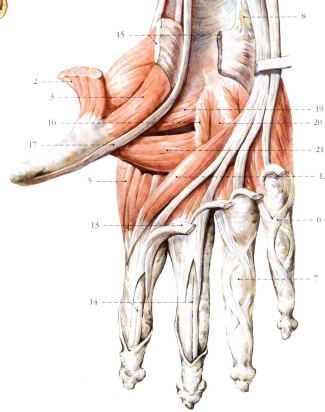

131. 手掌侧肌（2）
Palmar muscles of the hand (2)

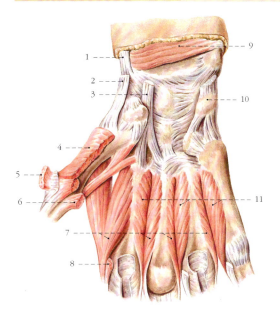

132. 手掌侧肌（3）
Palmar muscles of the hand (3)

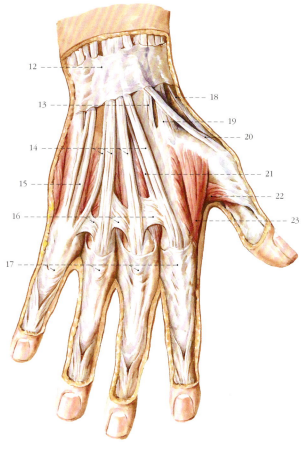

133. 手背侧肌（1）
Dorsal muscles of the hand (1)

1.肱桡肌腱 tendon of brachioradialis
2.拇长展肌腱 tendon of abductor pollicis longus
3.桡侧腕屈肌腱 tendon of flexor carpi radialis
4.拇对掌肌 opponens pollicis
5.拇短展肌 abductor pollicis brevis
6.拇长屈肌腱 tendon of flexor pollicis longus
7.骨间背侧肌 dorsal interossei
8.蚓状肌腱 tendon of lumbricales
9.旋前方肌 pronator quadratus
10.豌豆骨 pisiform bone
11.骨间掌侧肌 palmar interossei
12.伸肌支持带 extensor retinaculum
13.桡侧腕短伸肌 extensor carpi radialis brevis
14.指伸肌腱 tendon of extensor digitorum
15.小指伸肌腱 tendon of extensor digiti minimi
16.腱间结合 intertendinous connections
17.指背腱膜 dorsal digital aponeurosis
18.拇短伸肌腱 tendon of extensor pollicis brevis
19.桡侧腕长伸肌腱 tendon of extensor carpi radialis longus
20.拇长伸肌腱 tendon of extensor pollicis longus
21.示指伸肌腱 tendon of extensor indicis
22.拇收肌 adductor pollicis
23.第一骨间背侧肌 first dorsal interossei
24.小指展肌 abductor digiti minimi

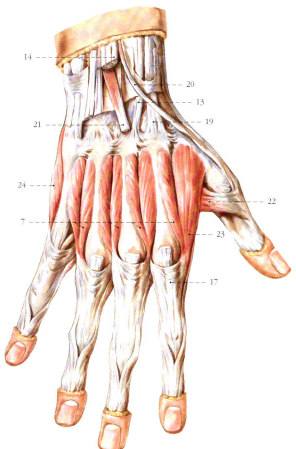

134. 手背侧肌（2）
Dorsal muscles of the hand (2)

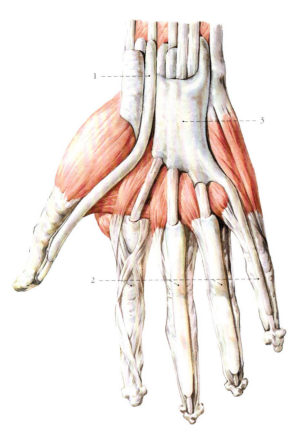

1.拇长屈肌腱鞘 tendinous sheath of flexor pollicis longus
2.指腱鞘 tendinous sheaths of fingers
3.屈肌总腱鞘 common flexor sheath
4.尺侧腕伸肌腱鞘 tendinous sheath of extensor carpi ulnaris
5.指伸肌和示指伸肌腱鞘 tendinous sheath of extensor digitorum and extensor indicis

135. 手掌侧腱鞘
The tendinous sheaths of the palmar side of the hand

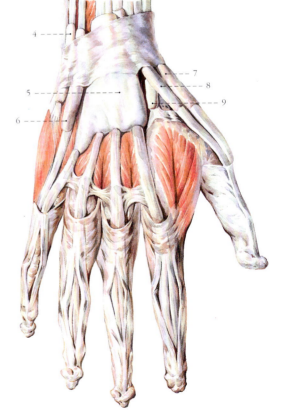

6.小指伸肌腱鞘 tendinous sheath of extensor digiti minimi
7.拇长展肌和拇短伸肌腱鞘 tendinous sheath of abductor pollicis longus and extensor pollicis brevis
8.拇长伸肌腱鞘 tendinous sheath of extensor pollicis longus
9.桡侧腕伸肌腱鞘 tendinous sheath of extensores carpi radiales

136. 手背侧腱鞘
The tendinous sheaths of the dorsal side of the hand

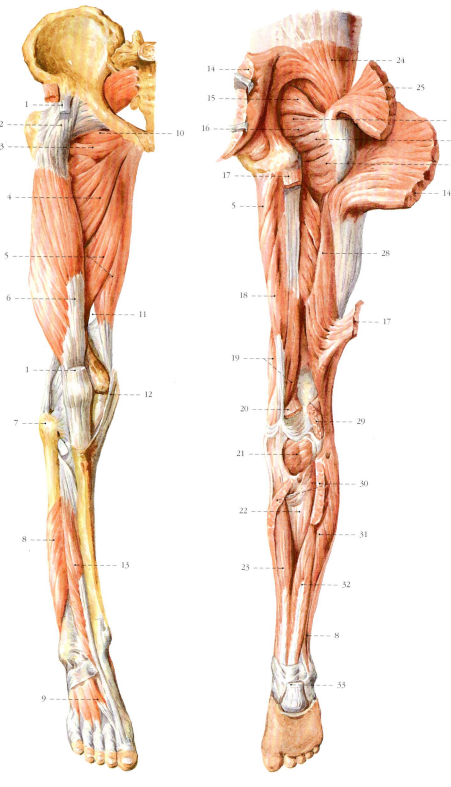

137. 下肢肌深层（前面观）
Deep layer of the muscles of the lower limb
(anterior aspect)

138. 下肢肌深层（后面观）
Deep layer of the muscles of the lower limb
(posterior aspect)

1.股直肌 rectus femoris
2.髂股韧带 iliofemoral ligament
3.股方肌 quadratus femoris
4.小收肌 adductor minimus
5.大收肌 adductor magnus
6.股中间肌 vastus intermedius
7.腓骨头 fibular head
8.腓骨短肌 peroneus brevis
9.踇短伸肌 extensor hallucis brevis
10.闭孔外肌 obturator externus
11.收肌腱裂孔 adductor tendinous opening
12.缝匠肌 sartorius
13.踇长伸肌 extensor hallucis longus
14.臀大肌 gluteus maximus
15.梨状肌 piriformis
16.闭孔内肌 obturator internus
17.股二头肌（长头）biceps femoris (long head)
18.半腱肌 semitendinosus
19.半膜肌 semimembranosus
20.腓肠肌（内侧头）gastrocnemius (lateral head)
21.腘肌 popliteus
22.胫骨后肌 tibialis posterior
23.趾长屈肌 flexor digitorum longus
24.臀小肌 gluteus minimus
25.臀中肌 gluteus medius
26.上孖肌 gemellus superior
27.下孖肌 gemellus inferior
28.股二头肌（短头）biceps femoris (short head)
29.腓肠肌（外侧头）gastrocnemius (lateral head)
30.比目鱼肌 soleus
31.腓骨长肌 peroneus longus
32.踇长屈肌 flexor hallucis longus
33.跟腱 tendo calcaneus

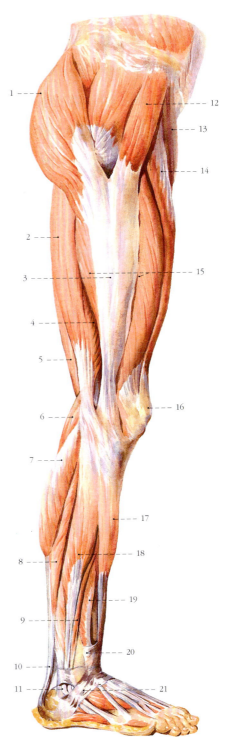

1.臀大肌 gluteus maximus
2.股二头肌（长头）biceps femoris（long head）
3.髂胫束 iliotibial tract
4.股二头肌（短头）biceps femoris（short head）
5.半膜肌 semimembranosus
6.跖肌 plantaris
7.腓肠肌（外侧头）gastrocnemius（lateral head）
8.比目鱼肌 soleus
9.腓骨短肌 peroneus brevis
10.跟腱 tendo calcaneus
11.腓骨长肌腱 tendon of peroneus longus
12.阔筋膜张肌 tensor fasciae latae
13.缝匠肌 sartorius
14.股直肌 rectus femoris
15.股外侧肌 vastus lateralis
16.髌骨 patella
17.胫骨前肌 tibialis anterior
18.腓骨长肌 peroneus longus
19.趾长伸肌 extensor digitorum longus
20.伸肌上支持带 superior extensor retinaculum
21.伸肌下支持带 inferior extensor retinaculum

139. 下肢肌（外侧面观）
Muscles of the lower limb (lateral aspect)

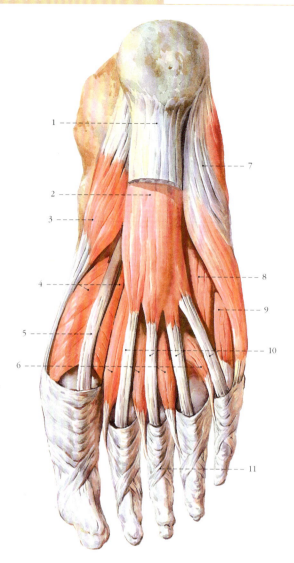

140. 足底肌（1）
Plantar muscles (1)

1.足底腱膜 plantar aponeurosis
2.趾短屈肌 flexor digitorum brevis
3.踇展肌 abductor hallucis
4.踇短屈肌 flexor hallucis brevis
5.踇长屈肌腱 tendon of flexor hallucis longus
6.蚓状肌 lumbricales
7.小趾展肌 abductor digiti minimi
8.骨间足底肌 plantar interossei
9.小趾短屈肌 flexor digiti minimi brevis
10.趾短屈肌腱 tendon of flexor digitorum brevis
11.纤维鞘交叉部 cruciform part of fibrous sheath
12.胫骨后肌腱 tendon of tibialis posterior
13.趾长屈肌腱 tendon of flexor digitorum longus
14.足底方肌 quadratus plantae

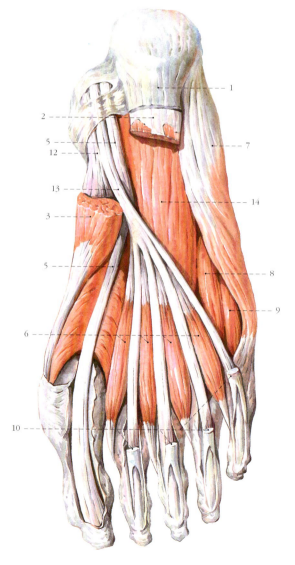

141. 足底肌（2）
Plantar muscles (2)

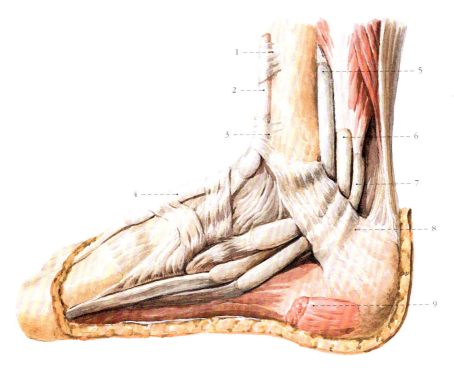

142. 足腱鞘（内侧面观）
The tendinous sheaths of the foot (medial aspect)

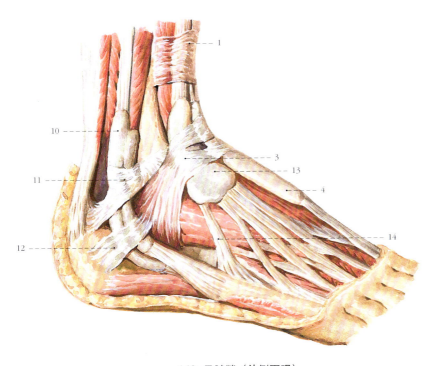

143. 足腱鞘（外侧面观）
The tendinous sheaths of the foot (lateral aspect)

1.伸肌上支持带　superior extensor retinaculum
2.胫骨前肌腱鞘　tendinous sheath of tibialis anterior
3.伸肌下支持带　inferior extensor retinaculum
4.踇长伸肌腱鞘　tendinous sheath of extensor hallucis longus
5.胫骨后肌腱鞘　tendinous sheath of tibialis posterior
6.趾长屈肌腱鞘　tendinous sheath of flexor digitorum longus
7.踇长屈肌腱鞘　tendinous sheath of flexor hallucis longus
8.屈肌支持带　flexor retinaculum
9.踇展肌　abductor hallucis
10.腓骨肌总腱鞘　common sheath of peronei
11.腓骨肌上支持带　superior peroneal retinaculum
12.腓骨肌下支持带　inferior peroneal retinaculum
13.趾长伸肌腱鞘　tendinous sheath of extensor digitorum longus
14.第3腓骨肌腱　peroneus tertius tendon

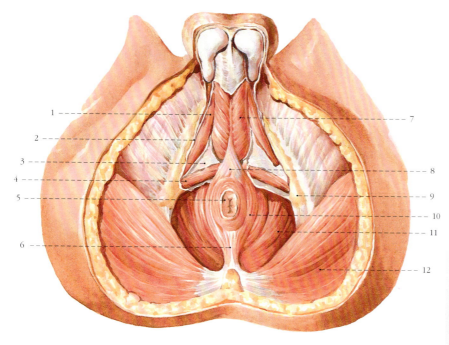

144. 男性会阴肌
Male perineal muscles

1.坐骨海绵体肌 ischiocavernosus
2.会阴浅筋膜 superficial fascia of perineum
3.尿生殖膈下筋膜 inferior fascia of urogenital diaphragm
4.会阴浅横肌 superficial transverse muscle of perineum
5.肛门 anus
6.肛尾韧带 anococcygeal ligament
7.球海绵体肌 bulbocavernosus
8.会阴中心腱 perineal central tendon
9.坐骨结节 ischial tuberosity
10.肛门外括约肌 sphincter ani externus
11.肛提肌 levator ani
12.臀大肌 gluteus maximus
13.阴蒂头 glans of clitoris
14.尿道外口 external orifice of urethra
15.阴道口 vaginal orifice
16.阴蒂包皮 prepuce of clitoris
17.小阴唇 lesser lip of pudendum
18.尾骨 coccyx

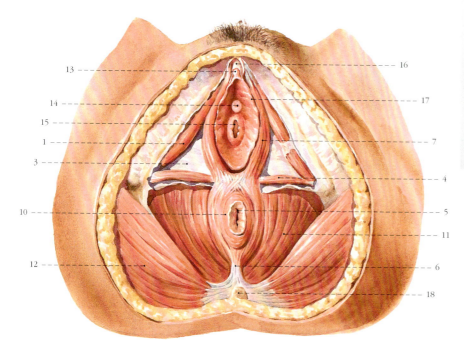

145. 女性会阴肌
Female perineal muscles

SPLANCHNOLOGY
内脏学

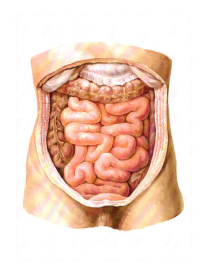

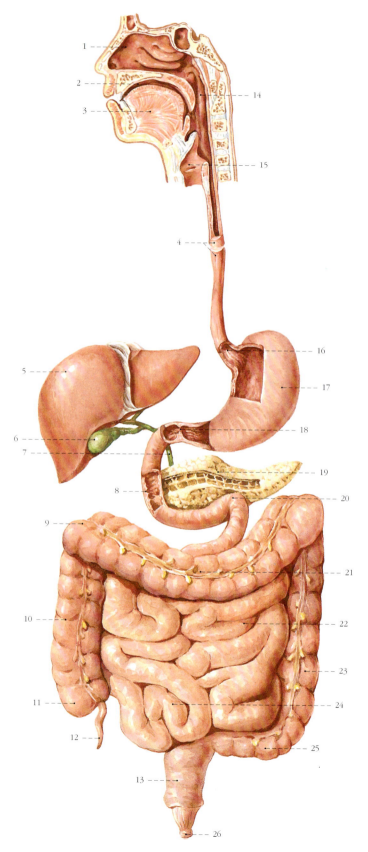

146. 消化系统全貌
General arrangement of the alimentary system

1.鼻腔 nasal cavity
2.口腔 oral cavity
3.舌 tongue
4.食管 esophagus
5.肝 liver
6.胆囊 gallbladder
7.胆总管 common bile duct
8.十二指肠 duodenum
9.结肠右曲 right colic flexure
10.升结肠 ascending colon
11.盲肠 cecum
12.阑尾 vermiform appendix
13.直肠 rectum
14.咽 pharynx
15.喉 larynx
16.贲门 cardiac orifice
17.胃 stomach
18.幽门口 pyloric orifice
19.胰 pancreas
20.十二指肠空肠曲 duodenojejunal flexure
21.横结肠 transverse colon
22.空肠 jejunum
23.降结肠 descending colon
24.回肠 ileum
25.乙状结肠 sigmoid colon
26.肛门 anus

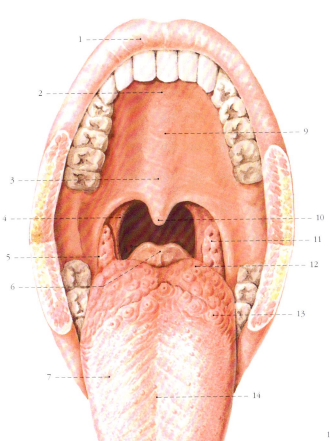

1. 上唇 upper lip
2. 硬腭 hard palate
3. 软腭 soft palate
4. 腭咽弓 palatopharyngeal arch
5. 腭舌弓 palatoglossal arch
6. 会厌 epiglottis
7. 舌体 body of tongue
8. 舌尖 apex of tongue
9. 腭缝 palatine raphe
10. 腭垂 uvula
11. 腭扁桃体 palatine tonsil

147. 口腔的结构（1）
Structure of the oral cavity (1)

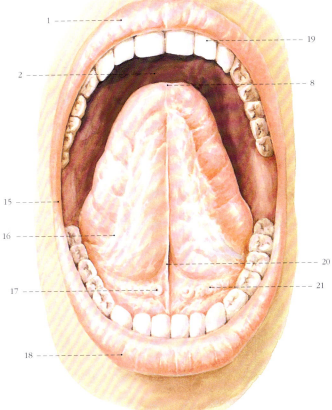

12. 舌根 root of tongue
13. 轮廓乳头 vallate papillae
14. 舌正中沟 median sulcus of tongue
15. 唇联合 labial commissure
16. 伞襞 fimbriated fold
17. 舌下阜 sublingual caruncle
18. 下唇 lower lip
19. 上牙弓 upper dental arch
20. 舌系带 frenulum of tongue
21. 舌下襞 sublingual fold

148. 口腔的结构（2）
Structure of the oral cavity (2)

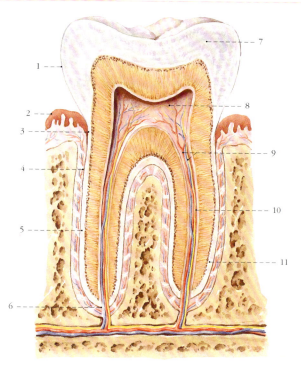

149. 牙的构造（模式图）
The structure of tooth (schema chart)

1.牙冠 crown of tooth
2.牙龈 gum
3.牙颈 neck of tooth
4.牙周膜 periodontal membrane
5.牙根 root of tooth
6.牙根尖孔 apical foramen
7.釉质 enamel
8.牙腔 dental cavity
9.牙髓 dental pulp
10.牙根管 root canal
11.牙骨质 cementum
12.切牙孔 incisive foramina
13.腭正中缝 median palatine suture
14.腭突 palatine process

150. 上颌恒牙的排列（下面观）
Arrangement of the permanent teeth of maxilla
(inferior aspect)

15.腭横缝 transverse palatine suture
16.水平板 horizontal plate
17.腭大孔 greater palatine foramen
18.中切牙 central incisor
19.侧切牙 lateral incisor
20.尖牙 canine tooth
21.第一前磨牙 first premolar
22.第二前磨牙 second premolar
23.第一磨牙 first molar
24.第二磨牙 second molar
25.第三磨牙 third molar
26.鼻后棘 posterior nasal spine

151. 下颌恒牙的排列（上面观）
Arrangement of the permanent teeth of mandible
(superior aspect)

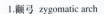

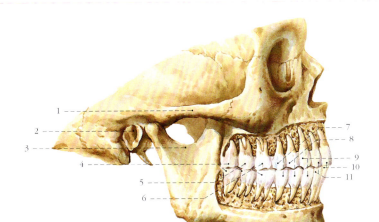

152. 恒牙（外面观）
The permanent teeth (external aspect)

1. 颧弓 zygomatic arch
2. 外耳门 external acoustic pore
3. 下颌支 ramus of mandible
4. 第三磨牙 third molar
5. 第二磨牙 second molar
6. 第一磨牙 first molar
7. 第二前磨牙 second premolar
8. 第一前磨牙 first premolar
9. 尖牙 canine tooth
10. 中切牙 central incisor
11. 侧切牙 lateral incisor
12. 舌粘膜 lingual mucous membrane
13. 上纵肌 superior longitudinal muscle
14. 舌中隔 septum of tongue
15. 颏舌肌 genioglossus
16. 舌横肌 transverse muscle of tongue
17. 下纵肌 inferior longitudinal muscle
18. 舌下腺 sublingual gland
19. 舌前腺 anterior lingual gland
20. 颏舌骨肌 geniohyoid
21. 舌腺 lingual glands
22. 会厌 epiglottis
23. 舌骨 hyoid bone

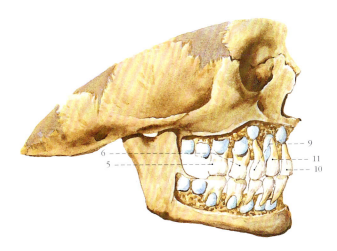

153. 乳牙（外面观）
The deciduous teeth (external aspect)

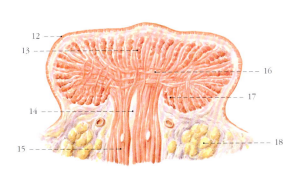

154. 舌（冠状切面）
The tongue (coronal section)

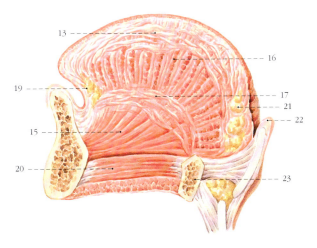

155. 舌（正中矢状切面）
The tongue (median sagittal section)

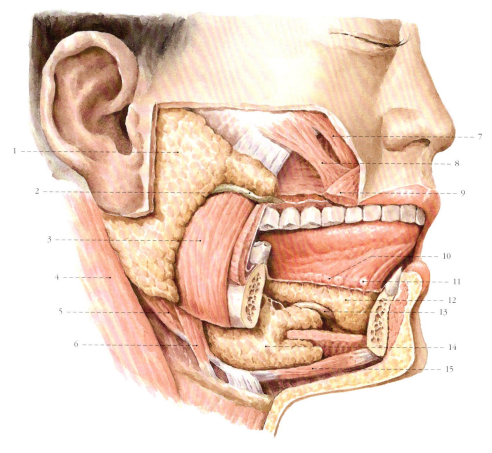

156. 腮腺、下颌下腺和舌下腺
The parotid gland, submandibular gland and sublingual gland

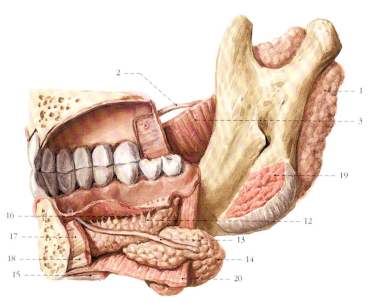

157. 腮腺、下颌下腺和舌下腺（内面观）
The parotid gland, submandibular gland and sublingual gland (internal aspect)

1.腮腺 parotid gland
2.腮腺管 parotid duct
3.咬肌 masseter
4.胸锁乳突肌 sternocleidomastoid
5.二腹肌后腹 posterior belly of digastric
6.茎突舌骨肌 stylohyoid
7.提上唇肌 levator labii superioris
8.颧肌 zygomaticus
9.口轮匝肌 orbicularis oris
10.舌下襞 sublingual fold
11.舌下阜 sublingual caruncle
12.舌下腺 sublingual gland
13.下颌下腺管 submandibular duct
14.下颌下腺 submandibular gland
15.二腹肌前腹 anterior belly of digastric
16.舌下腺小管 minor sublingual ducts
17.颏舌肌 genioglossus
18.颏舌骨肌 geniohyoid
19.翼内肌 medial pterygoid
20.下颌舌骨肌 mylohyoid

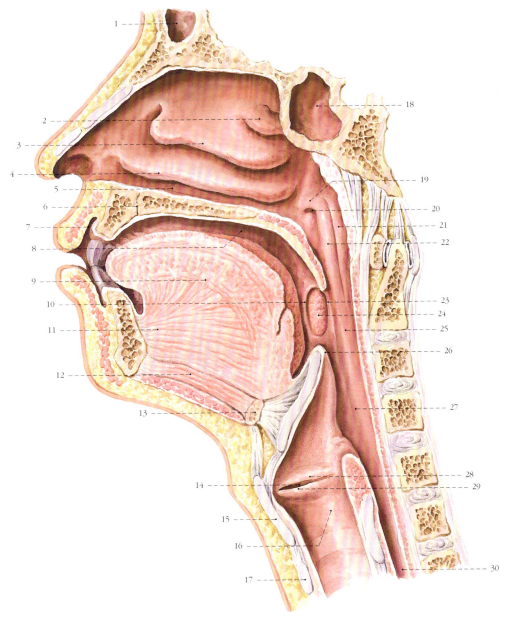

158. 咽与鼻、口、喉的交通

Connection of the pharynx and nose, mouth, larynx

1.额窦　frontal sinus	11.颏舌肌　genioglossus	21.咽隐窝　pharyngeal recess
2.上鼻甲　superior nasal concha	12.颏舌骨肌　geniohyoid	22.鼻咽　nasopharynx
3.中鼻甲　middle nasal concha	13.舌骨　hyoid bone	23.腭咽弓　palatopharyngeal arch
4.下鼻甲　inferior nasal concha	14.喉室　ventricle of larynx	24.腭扁桃体　palatine tonsil
5.下鼻道　inferior nasal meatus	15.甲状软骨　thyroid cartilage	25.口咽　oropharynx
6.切牙管　incisive canal	16.喉　larynx	26.会厌　epiglottis
7.口腔前庭　oral vestibule	17.环状软骨　cricoid cartilage	27.喉咽　laryngopharynx
8.固有口腔　proper oral cavity	18.蝶窦　sphenoidal sinus	28.前庭襞　vestibular fold
9.舌　tongue	19.咽鼓管圆枕　tubal torus	29.声襞　vocal fold
10.腭舌弓　arcus palatoglossus	20.咽鼓管咽口　pharyngeal opening of auditory tube	30.食管　esophagus

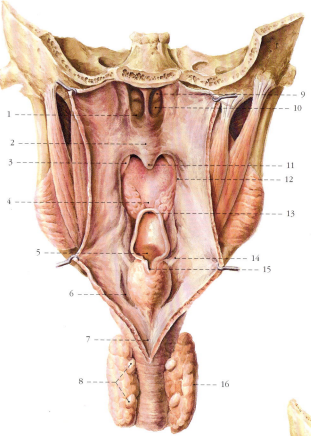

1.鼻后孔 choanae
2.软腭 soft palate
3.腭扁桃体 palatine tonsil
4.舌根 root of tongue
5.喉口 aperture of larynx
6.梨状隐窝 piriform recess
7.食管 esophagus
8.甲状旁腺 parathyroid gland
9.中鼻甲 middle nasal concha
10.下鼻甲 inferior nasal concha
11.腭垂 uvula
12.腭咽弓 palatopharyngeal arch
13.会厌 epiglottis
14.喉神经襞 fold of laryngeal nerve
15.杓间切迹 interarytenoid notch
16.甲状腺 thyroid gland

159. 咽腔（后面观）
The pharyngeal cavity (posterior aspect)

17.腭帆张肌 tensor veli palatini
18.茎突咽肌 stylopharyngeus
19.茎突舌骨肌 stylohyoid
20.二腹肌（后腹）digastric（posterior belly）
21.腭垂肌 musculus uvulae
22.咽上缩肌 superior constrictor of pharynx
23.腭咽肌 palatopharyngeus
24.翼内肌 medial pterygoid
25.咽中缩肌 middle constrictor of pharynx
26.小角结节 corniculate tubercle
27.咽下缩肌 inferior constrictor of pharynx
28.咽鼓管咽肌 salpingopharyngeus
29.腭帆提肌 levator veli palatini
30.杓状会厌襞 aryepiglottic fold
31.楔状结节 cuneiform tubercle

160. 咽肌（内面观）
The pharyngeal muscles (internal aspect)

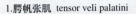

1.腭帆张肌 tensor veli palatini
2.颊肌 buccinator
3.咽上缩肌 superior constrictor of pharynx
4.茎突舌肌 styloglossus
5.舌骨 hyoid bone
6.喉结 laryngeal prominence
7.甲状软骨 thyroid cartilage
8.环状软骨 cricoid cartilage
9.气管 trachea
10.茎突咽肌 stylopharyngeus
11.咽中缩肌 middle constrictor of pharynx
12.舌骨舌肌 hyoglossus
13.舌骨（大角） hyoid bone（greater cornu）

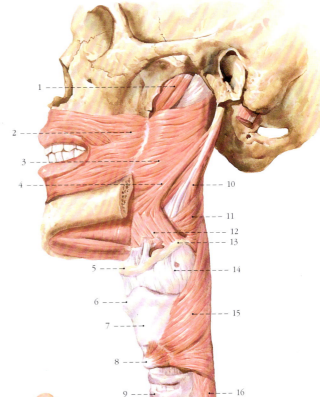

161. 咽肌（外侧面观）
The pharyngeal muscles (lateral aspect)

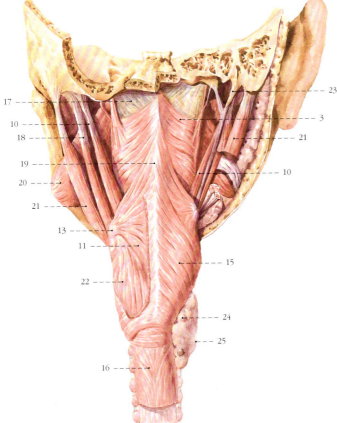

162. 咽肌（后面观）
The pharyngeal muscles (posterior aspect)

14.甲状舌骨膜 thyrohyoid membrane
15.咽下缩肌 inferior constrictor of pharynx
16.食管 esophagus
17.咽颅底筋膜 pharyngobasilar fascia
18.茎突舌骨肌 stylohyoid
19.咽缝 raphe of pharynx
20.翼内肌 medial pterygoid
21.二腹肌（后腹）digastric（posterior belly）
22.腭咽肌 palatopharyngeus
23.茎突 styloid process
24.甲状旁腺 parathyroid gland
25.甲状腺 thyroid gland

69

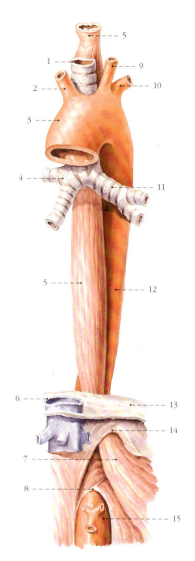

163. 食管的位置及毗邻
Position and relations of the esophagus

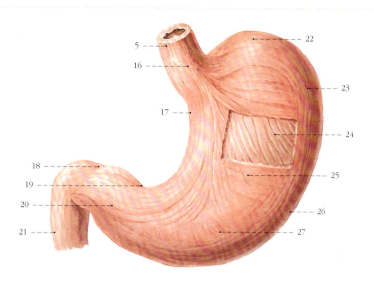

164. 胃的肌肉
The gastric muscles

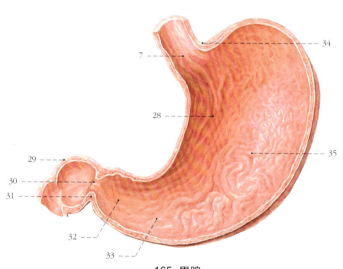

165. 胃腔
The gastric lumen

1.气管 trachea
2.头臂干 brachiocephalic trunk
3.主动脉 aorta
4.右主支气管 right principal bronchus
5.食管 esophagus
6.下腔静脉 inferior vena cava
7.贲门 cardia
8.主动脉裂孔 aortic hiatus
9.左颈总动脉 left common carotid artery
10.左锁骨下动脉 left subclavian artery
11.左主支气管 left principal bronchus
12.胸主动脉 thoracic aorta

13.膈 diaphragm
14.食管裂孔 esophageal hiatus
15.腹主动脉 abdominal aorta
16.贲门部 cardiac part
17.胃小弯 lesser curvature of stomach
18.幽门 pylorus
19.角切迹 angular incisure
20.幽门部 pyloric part
21.十二指肠 duodenum
22.胃底 fundus of stomach
23.纵层 longitudinal layer
24.斜纤维 oblique fibers

25.胃体 body of stomach
26.胃大弯 greater curvature of stomach
27.环层 circular layer
28.胃道 gastric canal
29.十二指肠上部 superior part of duodenum
30.幽门口 pyloric orifice
31.幽门括约肌 pyloric sphincter
32.幽门管 pyloric canal
33.幽门窦 pyloric antrum
34.贲门切迹 cardiac incisure
35.粘膜皱襞 mucosal plica

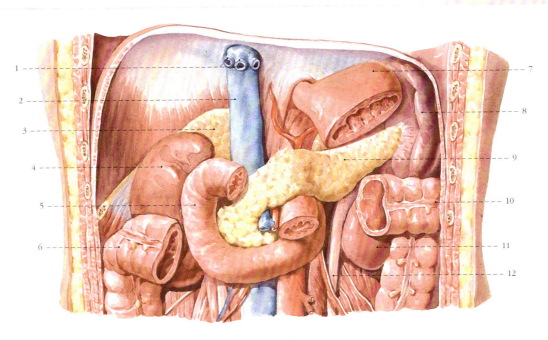

166. 十二指肠及毗邻（前面观）
The duodenum and its relations (anterior aspect)

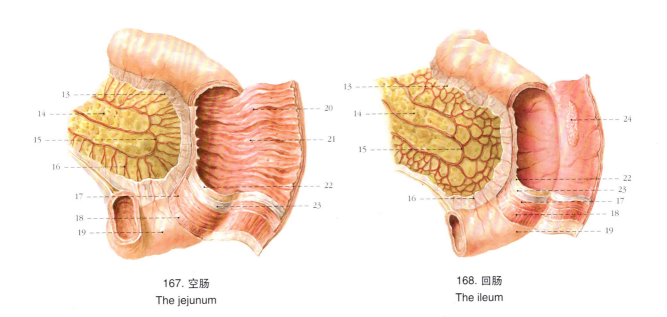

167. 空肠
The jejunum

168. 回肠
The ileum

1.肝静脉 hepatic veins	9.胰 pancreas	17.环层 circular layer
2.下腔静脉 inferior vena cava	10.结肠左曲 left colic flexure	18.纵层 longitudinal layer
3.肾上腺 adrenal gland	11.左肾 left kidney	19.浆膜层 serosa
4.右肾 right kidney	12.输尿管 ureter	20.环状襞 circular folds
5.十二指肠 duodenum	13.肠系膜 mesentery	21.孤立淋巴滤泡 solitary lymphatic follicles
6.结肠右曲 right colic flexure	14.脂肪 fat	22.粘膜层 mucosa
7.胃 stomach	15.动脉弓 arterial arch	23.粘膜下层 submucosa
8.脾 spleen	16.直动脉 straight artery	24.集合淋巴滤泡 aggregated lymphatic follicles

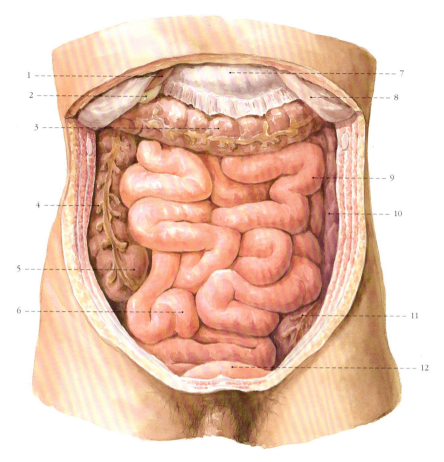

1.肝 liver
2.胆囊 gallbladder
3.横结肠 transverse colon
4.升结肠 ascending colon
5.盲肠 cecum
6.回肠 ileum
7.胃 stomach
8.肋弓 costal arch
9.空肠 jejunum
10.降结肠 descending colon
11.乙状结肠 sigmoid colon
12.膀胱 urinary bladder
13.独立带 free band
14.盲肠襞 cecal folds
15.网膜带 omental band
16.盲肠后支 posterior cecal branches
17.盲肠皱襞 cecal plica
18.回结肠动脉 ileocolic artery
19.阑尾 vermiform appendix
20.阑尾动脉 appendicular artery
21.结肠系膜带 mesocolic band
22.脂肪垂 epiploic appendices
23.结肠袋 haustra of colon
24.半月襞 semilunar fold
25.回盲瓣口 orifice of ileocecal valve
26.阑尾口 orifice of vermiform appendix
27.回盲瓣 ileocecal valve

169. 小肠和大肠（前面观）
The small intestine and the large intestine (anterior aspect)

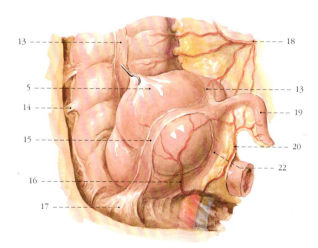

170. 盲肠和阑尾
The cecum and vermiform appendix

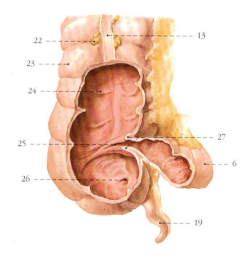

171. 回盲部（内面观）
The ileocecal part (internal aspect)

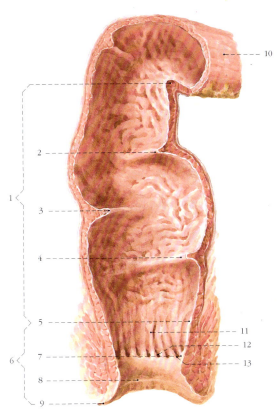

172. 直肠（冠状切面）
The rectum (coronal section)

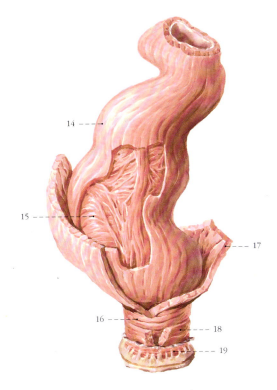

173. 直肠和肛管的肌肉
Muscles of the rectum and the anal canal

1.直肠 rectum
2.上直肠横襞 superior transverse fold of rectum
3.中直肠横襞 middle transverse fold of rectum
4.下直肠横襞 inferior transverse fold of rectum
5.肛直肠线 anorectal line
6.肛管 anal canal
7.齿状线 dentate line
8.白线 white line
9.肛门 anus
10.乙状结肠 sigmoid colon
11.肛柱 anal columns
12.肛窦 anal sinuses
13.肛瓣 anal valves
14.直肠纵层肌 rectal longitudinal muscle
15.直肠环层肌 rectal circular muscle
16.肛门外括约肌深部 deep part of sphincter ani externus
17.肛提肌 levator ani muscle
18.肛门外括约肌浅部 superficial part of sphincter ani externus
19.肛门外括约肌皮下部 subcutaneous part of sphincter ani externus
20.盆膈上筋膜 superior fascia of pelvic diaphragm
21.直肠内静脉丛 internal rectal venous plexus
22.肛门内括约肌 sphincter ani internus
23.直肠筋膜 rectal fascia
24.盆膈下筋膜 inferior fascia of pelvic diaphragm
25.直肠外静脉丛 external rectal venous plexus

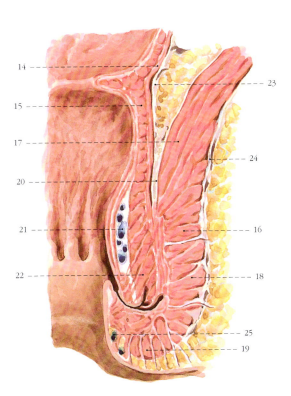

174. 肛门括约肌（冠状切面）
The anal sphincter (coronal section)

73

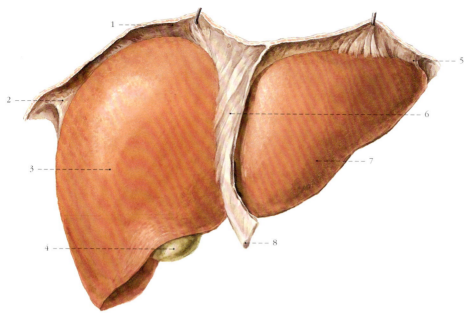

175. 肝（前面观）
The liver (anterior aspect)

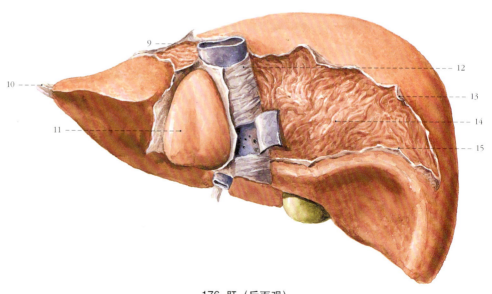

176. 肝（后面观）
The liver (posterior aspect)

1.冠状韧带 coronary ligament
2.右三角韧带 right triangular ligament
3.肝右叶 right lobe of liver
4.胆囊 gallbladder
5.左三角韧带 left triangular ligament
6.镰状韧带 falciform ligament of liver
7.肝左叶 left lobe of liver
8.肝圆韧带 ligamentum teres hepatis

9.下腔静脉 inferior vena cava
10.肝纤维附件 fibrous appendix of liver
11.尾状叶 caudate lobe
12.腔静脉韧带 vena caval ligament
13.冠状韧带上层 superior layer of coronary ligament
14.裸区 bare area of liver
15.冠状韧带下层 inferior layer of coronary ligament

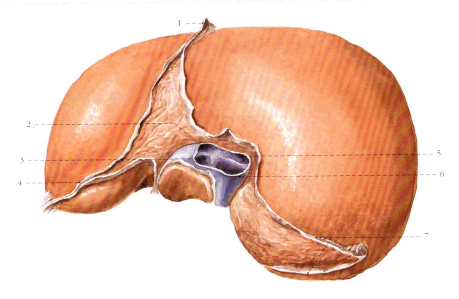

177. 肝（上面观）
The liver (superior aspect)

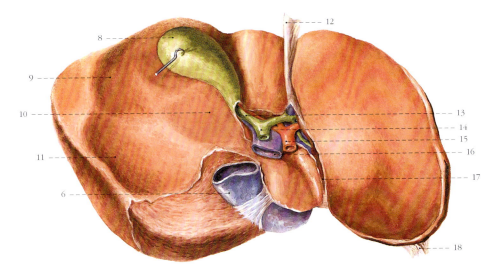

178. 肝（下面观）
The liver (inferior aspect)

1.镰状韧带 falciform ligament of liver
2.肝中静脉 middle hepatic vein
3.肝左静脉 left hepatic vein
4.左三角韧带 left triangular ligament
5.肝右静脉 right hepatic vein
6.下腔静脉 inferior vena cava
7.冠状韧带 coronary ligament
8.胆囊 gallbladder
9.结肠压迹 colic impression

10.十二指肠压迹 duodenal impression
11.肾压迹 renal impression
12.肝圆韧带 ligamentum teres hepatis
13.胆囊管 cystic duct
14.胆总管 common bile duct
15.肝固有动脉 proper hepatic artery
16.肝门静脉 hepatic portal vein
17.静脉韧带 venous ligament
18.肝纤维附件 fibrous appendix of liver

75

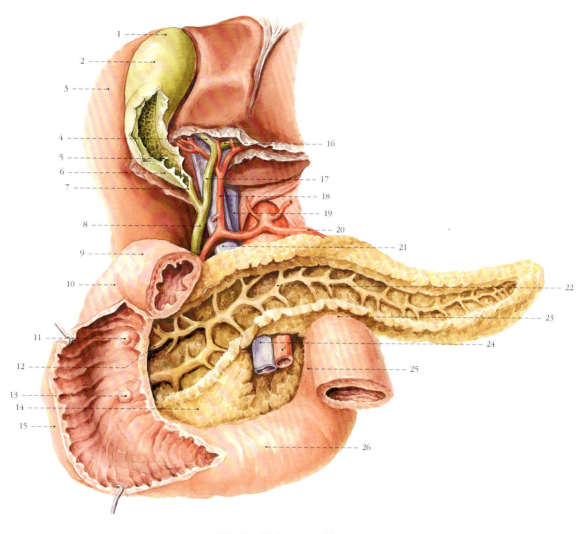

179. 输胆管道及开口（前面观）
The bile passage and its openings (anterior aspect)

1.胆囊底 fundus of gallbladder
2.胆囊体 body of gallbladder
3.肝 liver
4.肝右管 right hepatic duct
5.螺旋襞 spiral fold
6.胆囊颈 neck of gallbladder
7.胆囊管 cystic duct
8.胆总管 common bile duct
9.十二指肠上部 superior part of duodenum

10.十二指肠上曲 superior duodenal flexure
11.十二指肠小乳头 minor duodenal papilla
12.副胰管 accessory pancreatic duct
13.十二指肠大乳头 major duodenal papilla
14.胰头 head of pancreas
15.十二指肠降部 descending part of duodenum
16.肝左管 left hepatic duct
17.肝总管 common hepatic duct
18.肝固有动脉 proper hepatic artery
19.下腔静脉 inferior vena cava

20.脾动脉 splenic artery
21.肝门静脉 hepatic portal vein
22.胰管 pancreatic duct
23.十二指肠空肠曲 duodenojejunal flexure
24.肠系膜上动、静脉 superior mesenteric artery and vein
25.十二指肠升部 ascending part of duodenum
26.十二指肠水平部 horizontal part of duodenum

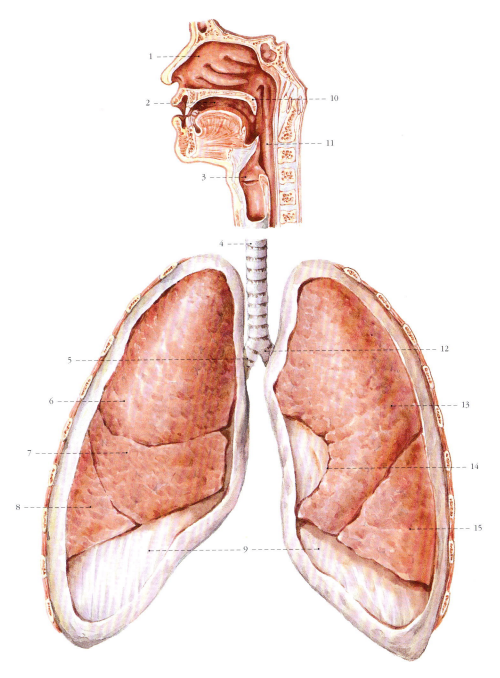

180. 呼吸系全貌

General arrangement of respiratory system

1.鼻腔 nasal cavity
2.口腔 oral cavity
3.喉 larynx
4.气管 trachea
5.右主支气管 right principal bronchus
6.右肺上叶 superior lobe of right lung
7.右肺中叶 middle lobe of right lung
8.右肺下叶 inferior lobe of right lung

9.膈 diaphragm
10.软腭 soft palate
11.咽 pharynx
12.左主支气管 left principal bronchus
13.左肺上叶 superior lobe of left lung
14.心切迹 cardiac impression
15.左肺下叶 inferior lobe of left lung

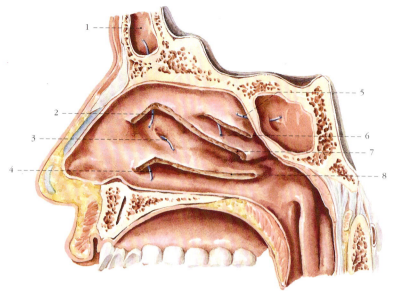

181. 鼻旁窦的开口
The openings of paranasal sinuses

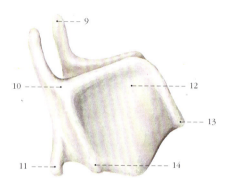

182. 甲状软骨（侧面观）
The thyroid cartilage (lateral aspect)

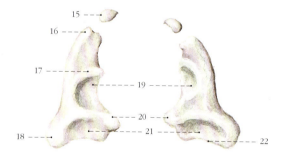

183. 杓状软骨和小角软骨（前面观）
The arytenoid and corniculate (anterior aspect)

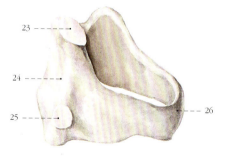

184. 环状软骨（侧面观）
The cricoid cartilage (lateral aspect)

1.额窦 frontal sinus
2.探针通额窦 probe into the frontal sinus
3.探针通上颌窦 probe into the maxillary sinus
4.探针通鼻泪管 probe into the nasolacrimal duct
5.探针通蝶窦 probe into the sphenoid sinus
6.探针通筛窦 probe into the ethmoid sinus
7.中鼻甲（切缘）middle nasal concha (cuting edge)

8.下鼻甲（切缘）inferior nasal concha (cuting edge)
9.上角 superior cornu
10.上结节 superior thyroid tubercle
11.下角 inferior cornu
12.右板 right lamina
13.喉结 laryngeal prominence
14.下结节 inferior thyroid tubercle
15.小角软骨 corniculate cartilage
16.杓状软骨尖 apex of arytenoid cartilage

17.弓状嵴 arcuate crest
18.肌突 muscular process
19.三角凹 triangular fovea
20.声带突 vocal process
21.椭圆凹 oblong fovea
22.杓状软骨底 base of arytenoid cartilage
23.杓关节面 arytenoid articular surface
24.环状软骨板 lamina of cricoid cartilage
25.甲关节面 thyroid articular surface
26.环状软骨弓 arch of cricoid cartilage

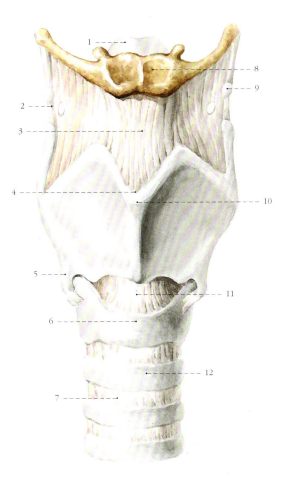

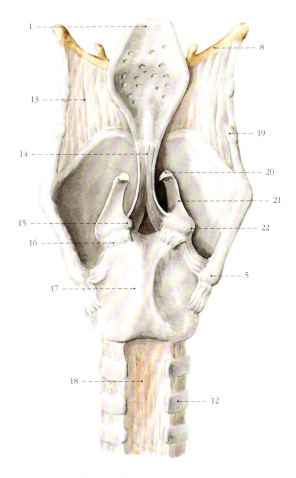

1.会厌软骨 epiglottic cartilage
2.甲状舌骨外侧韧带 lateral thyrohyoid ligament
3.甲状舌骨正中韧带 median thyrohyoid ligament
4.上切迹 superior thyroid notch
5.下角 inferior cornu
6.环状软骨 cricoid cartilage
7.环状韧带 annular ligament
8.舌骨 hyoid bone
9.麦粒软骨 triticeal cartilage
10.喉结 laryngeal prominence
11.环甲正中韧带 median cricothyroid ligament

185. 喉软骨和韧带（前面观）
The cartilages and ligaments of larynx
(anterior aspect)

12.气管软骨 tracheal cartilage
13.甲状舌骨膜 thyrohyoid membrane
14.甲状会厌韧带 thyroepiglottic ligament
15.声带突 vocal process
16.环杓后韧带 posterior cricoarytenoid ligament
17.环状软骨板 lamina of cricoid cartilage
18.膜壁 membranous wall
19.上角 superior cornu
20.小角软骨 corniculate cartilage
21.杓状软骨 arytenoid cartilage
22.肌突 muscular process

186. 喉软骨和韧带（后面观）
The cartilages and ligaments of larynx
(posterior aspect)

79

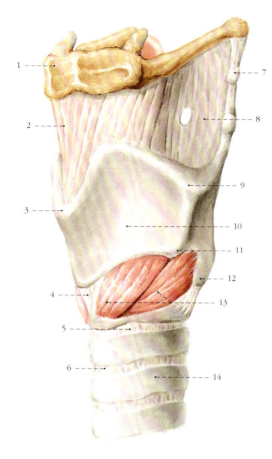

1.舌骨　hyoid bone
2.甲状舌骨正中韧带　median thyrohyoid ligament
3.喉结　laryngeal prominence
4.环甲正中韧带　median cricothyroid ligament
5.环状软骨气管韧带　cricotracheal ligament
6.环状韧带　annular ligaments
7.麦粒软骨　triticeal cartilage
8.甲状舌骨膜　thyrohyoid membrane
9.上结节　superior thyroid tubercle
10.左板　left lamina
11.下结节　inferior thyroid tubercle
12.下角　inferior cornu
13.环甲肌　cricothyroid
14.气管软骨　tracheal cartilage

187. 喉软骨和韧带（外侧面观）
The cartilages and ligaments of larynx
(lateral aspect)

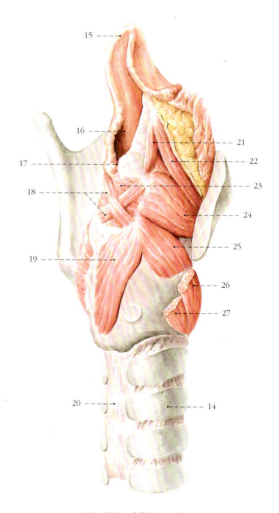

188. 喉肌（外侧面观）
Muscles of the larynx (lateral aspect)

15.会厌　epiglottis
16.喉口　aperture of larynx
17.杓间切迹　interarytenoid notch
18.杓斜肌　oblique arytenoid
19.环杓后肌　posterior cricoarytenoid
20.膜壁　membranous wall
21.杓会厌肌　aryepiglottic muscle
22.甲状会厌肌　thyroepiglottis
23.杓横肌　transverse arytenoid
24.甲杓肌　thyroarytenoid
25.环杓侧肌　lateral cricoarytenoid
26.环甲肌直部　straight part of cricothyroid
27.环甲肌斜部　oblique part of cricothyroid

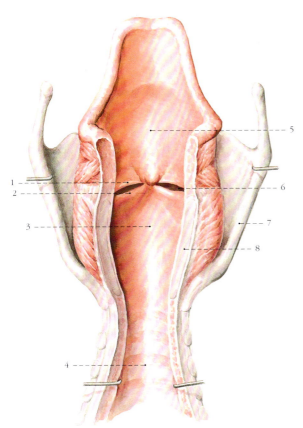

189. 喉腔（后面观）
The laryngeal cavity (posterior aspect)

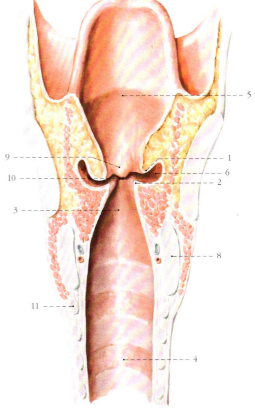

190. 喉腔冠状切面（后面观）
Coronal section through the laryngeal cavity (posterior aspect)

1.前庭襞 vestibular fold
2.声襞 vocal fold
3.声门下腔 infraglottic cavity
4.气管 trachea
5.喉前庭 laryngeal vestibule
6.喉室 ventricle of larynx
7.甲状软骨 thyroid cartilage
8.环状软骨 cricoid cartilage
9.会厌结节 tubercle of epiglottis
10.喉中间腔 intermedial cavity of larynx
11.气管软骨 tracheal cartilage

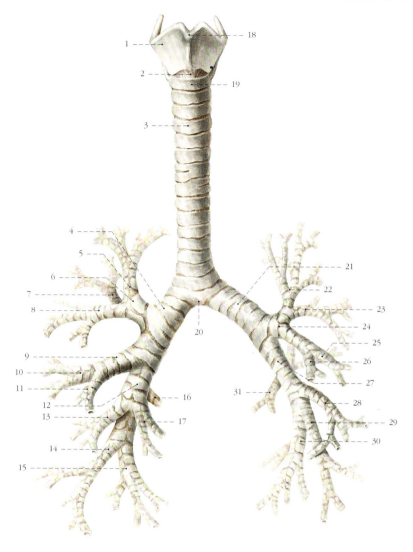

191. 气管和肺段支气管

The trachea and segmental bronchi

1.甲状软骨 thyroid cartilage
2.环甲正中韧带 median cricothyroid ligament
3.气管 trachea
4.右主支气管 right principal bronchus
5.尖段支气管（BⅠ）apical segmental bronchus（BⅠ）
6.右肺上叶支气管 right superior lobar bronchus
7.后段支气管（BⅡ）posterior segmental bronchus（BⅡ）
8.前段支气管（BⅢ）anterior segmental bronchus（BⅢ）
9.右肺中叶支气管 right middle lobar bronchus
10.外段支气管（BⅣ）lateral segmental bronchus（BⅣ）
11.内段支气管（BⅤ）medial segmental bronchus（BⅤ）
12.右肺下叶支气管 right inferior lobar bronchus
13.前底段支气管（BⅧ）anterior basal segmental bronchus（BⅧ）
14.外侧底段支气管（BⅨ）lateral basal segmental bronchus（BⅨ）
15.后底段支气管（BⅩ）posterior basal segmental bronchus（BⅩ）
16.尖（上）段支气管（BⅥ）apical（superior）segmental bronchus（BⅥ）
17.内侧（心）底段支气管（BⅦ）medial（cardiac）basal segmental bronchus（BⅦ）
18.喉结 laryngeal prominence
19.环状软骨 cricoid cartilage
20.气管杈 bifurcation of trachea
21.左主支气管 left principal bronchus
22.尖后段支气管（BⅠ+Ⅱ）apicoposterior segmental bronchus（BⅠ+Ⅱ）
23.前段支气管（BⅢ）anterior segmental bronchus（BⅢ）
24.左肺上叶支气管 left superior lobar bronchus
25.上舌段支气管（BⅣ）superior lingular bronchus（BⅣ）
26.下舌段支气管（BⅤ）inferior lingular bronchus（BⅤ）
27.左肺下叶支气管 left inferior lobar bronchus
28.前内侧底段支气管（BⅦ+Ⅷ）anteromedial basal segmental bronchus（BⅦ+Ⅷ）
29.外侧底段支气管（BⅨ）lateral basal segmental bronchus（BⅨ）
30.后底段支气管（BⅩ）posterior basal segmental bronchus（BⅩ）
31.上段支气管 （BⅥ）superior segmental bronchus（BⅥ）

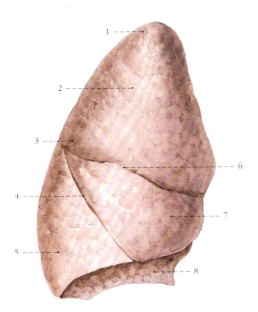

192. 右肺（前面观）
Right lung (anterior aspect)

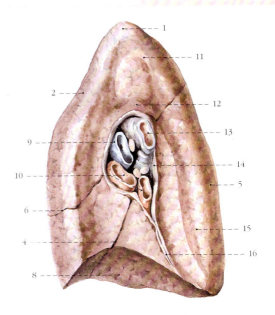

193. 右肺（内侧面观）
Right lung (medial aspect)

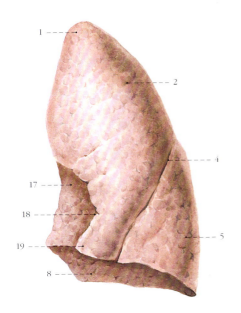

194. 左肺（前面观）
Left lung (anterior aspect)

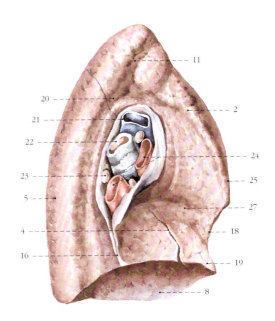

195. 左肺（内侧面观）
Left lung (medial aspect)

1.肺尖 apex of lung
2.上叶 superior lobe
3.肋面 costal surface
4.斜裂 oblique fissure
5.下叶 inferior lobe
6.水平裂 horizontal fissure
7.中叶 middle lobe
8.膈面 diaphragmatic surface
9.右肺动脉 right pulmonary artery

10.右肺静脉 right pulmonary vein
11.锁骨下动脉沟 sulcus for subclavian artery
12.奇静脉沟 sulcus for azygos vein
13.右主支气管 right principal bronchus
14.肺门 hilum of lung
15.食管沟 esophageal sulcus
16.肺韧带 pulmonary ligament
17.内侧面 medial surface
18.心切迹 cardiac notch

19.左肺小舌 lingula of left lung
20.主动脉沟 aortic sulcus
21.左肺动脉 left pulmonary artery
22.左主支气管 left principal bronchus
23.支气管肺门淋巴结 bronchopulmonary
    hilar lymph nodes
24.左肺静脉 left pulmonary vein
25.前缘 anterior border
26.心压迹 cardiac impression

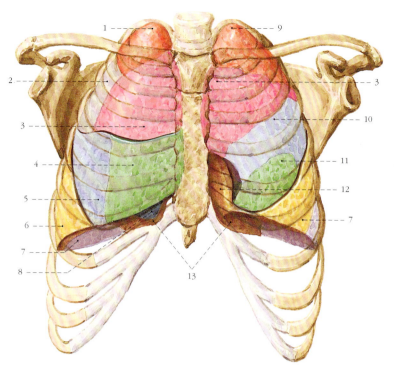

196. 支气管肺段（前面观）
The bronchopulmonary segments (anterior aspect)

1.尖段（S I）apical segment（S I）

2.后段（S II）posterior segment（S II）

3.前段（S III）anterior segment（S III）

4.内侧段（S V）medial segment（S V）

5.外侧段（S IV）lateral segment（S IV）

6.前底段（S VIII）anterior basal segment
（S VIII）

7.外侧底段（S IX）lateral basal segment
（S IX）

8.内侧底段（S VII）medial basal segment
（S VII）

9.尖后段（S I + S II）apicoposterior segment
（S I + S II）

10.上舌段（S IV）superior lingular segment
（S IV）

11.下舌段（S V）inferior lingular segment
（S V）

12.前内侧底段（S VII + S VIII）anteromedial
basal segment（S VII + S VIII）

13.后底段（S X）posterior basal segment
（S X）

14.上段（S VI）superior segment（S VI）

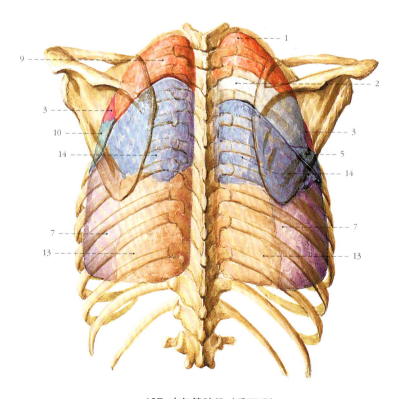

197. 支气管肺段（后面观）
The bronchopulmonary segments (posterior aspect)

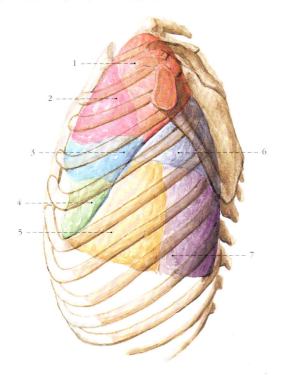

198. 支气管肺段（左外侧面观）
The bronchopulmonary segments (left lateral aspect)

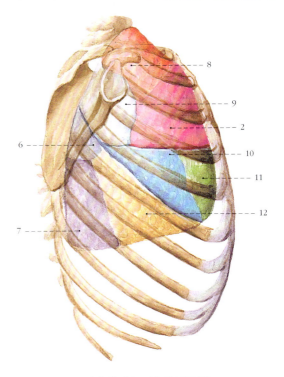

199. 支气管肺段（右外侧面观）
The bronchopulmonary segments (right lateral aspect)

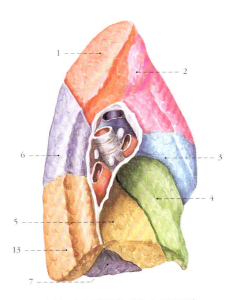

200. 支气管肺段（左内侧面观）
The bronchopulmonary segments (left medial aspect)

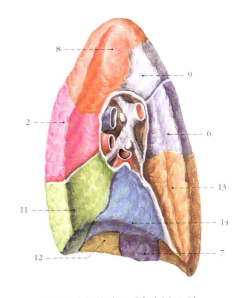

201. 支气管肺段（右内侧面观）
The bronchopulmonary segments (right medial aspect)

1.尖后段（SⅠ+SⅡ）apicoposterior segment（SⅠ+SⅡ）
2.前段（SⅢ）anterior segment（SⅢ）
3.上舌段（SⅣ）superior lingular segment（SⅣ）
4.下舌段（SⅤ）inferior lingular segment（SⅤ）
5.前内侧底段（SⅦ+SⅧ）anterior medial basal segment（SⅦ+SⅧ）
6.上段（SⅥ）superior segment（SⅥ）
7.外侧底段（SⅨ）lateral basal segment（SⅨ）

8.尖段（SⅠ）apical segment（SⅠ）
9.后段（SⅡ）posterior segment（SⅡ）
10.外侧段（SⅣ）lateral segment（SⅣ）
11.内侧段（SⅤ）medial segment（SⅤ）
12.前底段（SⅧ）anterior basal segment（SⅧ）
13.后底段（SⅩ）posterior basal segment（SⅩ）
14.内侧底段（SⅦ）medial basal segment（SⅦ）

85

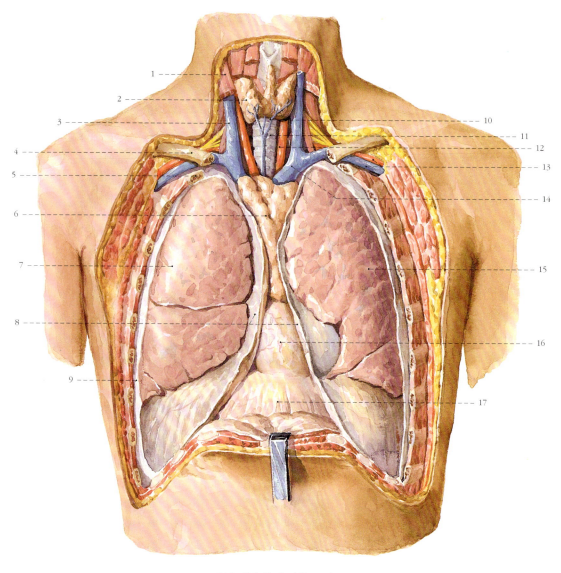

202. 肺和胸膜（前面观）
The lungs and the pleura (anterior aspect)

1.胸锁乳突肌 sternocleidomastoid

2.甲状腺 thyroid gland

3.颈内静脉 internal jugular vein

4.锁骨 clavicle

5.第一肋 first rib

6.胸腺 thymus

7.右肺 right lung

8.纵隔胸膜 mediastinal pleura

9.肋胸膜 costal pleura

10.甲状腺下静脉 inferior thyroid vein

11.气管 trachea

12.颈总动脉 common carotid artery

13.锁骨下动、静脉 subclavian artery and vein

14.头臂静脉 brachiocephalic vein

15.左肺 left lung

16.心包 pericardium

17.膈 diaphragm

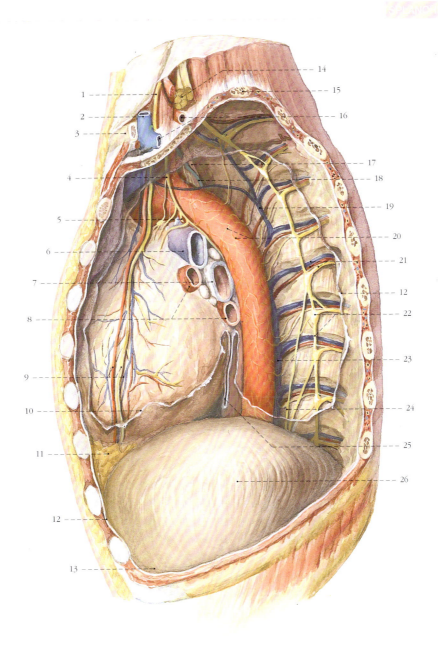

203. 纵隔（左外侧面观）

The mediastinum (left lateral aspect)

1.膈神经 phrenic nerve

2.颈内静脉 internal jugular vein

3.锁骨 clavicle

4.左迷走神经 left vagus nerve

5.喉返神经 recurrent laryngeal nerve

6.左肺动脉 left pulmonary artery

7.左主支气管 left principal bronchus

8.左肺静脉 left pulmonary vein

9.膈神经，心包膈动、静脉 phrenic nerve, pericardiacophrenic artery and veins

10.纵隔胸膜 mediastinal pleura

11.胸膜下脂肪体 subpleural fat body

12.肋胸膜 costal pleura

13.肋膈隐窝 costodiaphragmatic recess

14.臂丛 brachial plexus

15.第一肋 first rib

16.锁骨下动、静脉 subclavian artery and vein

17.食管 esophagus

18.胸导管 thoracic duct

19.副半奇静脉 accessory hemiazygos vein

20.胸主动脉、主动脉丛 thoracic aorta, aortic plexus

21.肋间动、静脉、神经 intercostal artery, veins and nerve

22.胸交感神经节、胸交感干 thoracic sympathetic ganglion, thoracic sympathetic trunk

23.半奇静脉 hemiazygos vein

24.内脏大神经 greater splanchnic nerve

25.肺韧带 pulmonary ligament

26.膈胸膜 diaphragmatic pleura

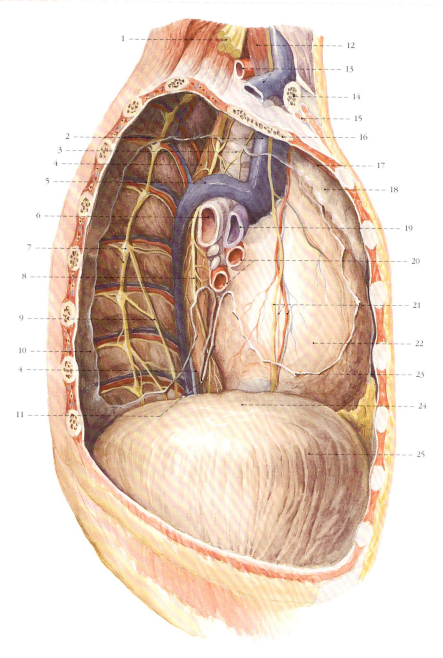

204. 纵隔（右外侧面观）

The mediastinum (right lateral aspect)

1.臂丛 brachial plexus

2.上腔静脉 superior vena cava

3.气管 trachea

4.食管 esophagus

5.奇静脉 azygos vein

6.右主支气管 right principal bronchus

7.胸交感神经节、胸交感干 thoracic
sympathetic ganglion and thoracic
sympathetic trunk

8.右迷走神经 right vagus nerve

9.内脏大神经 greater splanchnic nerve

10.肋胸膜 costal pleura

11.肺韧带 pulmonary ligament

12.前斜角肌 scalenus anterior

13.锁骨下动、静脉 subclavian artery
and vein

14.锁骨 clavicle

15.锁骨下肌 subclavius

16.第一肋 first rib

17.胸廓内动脉 internal thoracic artery

18.胸腺 thymus

19.肺动脉 pulmonary artery

20.肺静脉 pulmonary veins

21.膈神经，心包膈动、静脉 phrenic nerve,
pericardiacophrenic artery and vein

22.心包 pericardium

23.纵隔胸膜 mediastinal pleura

24.中心腱 central tendon

25.膈胸膜 diaphragm, diaphragmatic pleura

1.右肾 right kidney
2.输尿管 ureter
3.膀胱 urinary bladder
4.输精管 deferent duct
5.阴茎 penis
6.尿道 urethra
7.附睾 epididymis
8.睾丸 testis
9.肾盂 renal pelvis
10.左肾 left kidney
11.精囊 seminal vesicle
12.射精管 ejaculatory duct
13.前列腺 prostate
14.尿道球腺 bulbourethral gland

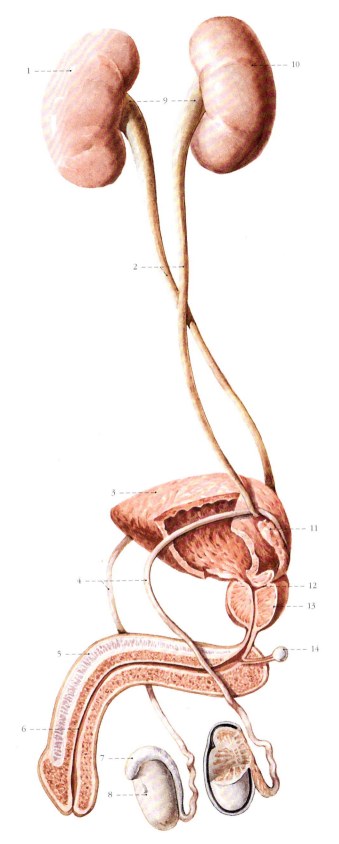

205. 男性泌尿生殖系统全貌
General arrangement of the male urogenital system

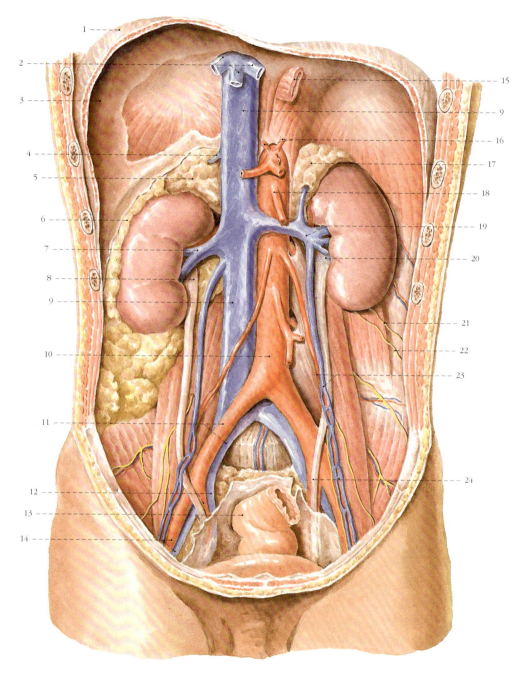

206. 腹后壁（示肾和输尿管）
Posterior abdominal wall (showing the kidneys and the ureters)

1.膈 diaphragm
2.肝静脉 hepatic veins
3.壁腹膜 parietal peritoneum
4.右肾上腺静脉 right adrenal vein
5.右肾上腺 right adrenal gland
6.肾脂肪囊 fatty capsule of kidney
7.右肾静脉 right renal vein
8.右肾盂 right renal pelvis

9.下腔静脉 inferior vena cava
10.腹主动脉 abdominal aorta
11.右髂总动、静脉 right common iliac artery, vein
12.右髂内动、静脉 right internal iliac artery, vein
13.直肠 rectum
14.右髂外动、静脉 right external iliac artery, vein
15.食管腹部 abdominal esophagus
16.膈下动脉 inferior phrenic artery

17.左肾上腺 left adrenal gland
18.肠系膜上动脉 superior mesenteric artery
19.左肾动、静脉 left renal artery, vein
20.左肾盂 left renal pelvis
21.髂腹下神经 iliohypogastric nerve
22.髂腹股沟神经 ilioinguinal nerve
23.睾丸动、静脉 testicular artery, vein
24.输尿管 ureter

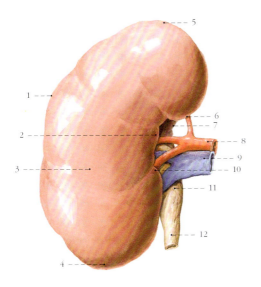

207. 右肾（前面观）
The right kidney (anterior aspect)

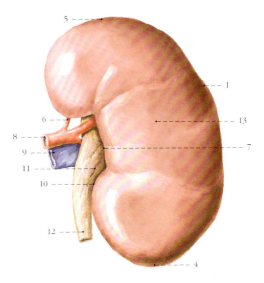

208. 右肾（后面观）
The right kidney (posterior aspect)

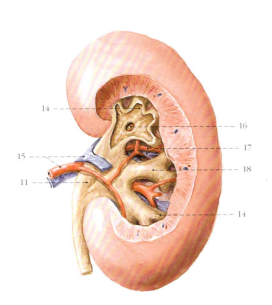

209. 肾窦及其结构
The renal sinus and its structures

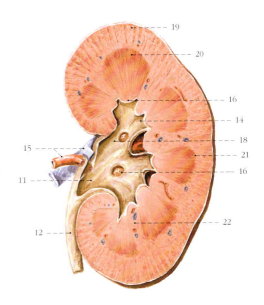

210. 肾的冠状切面（后面观）
The coronal section of the kidney (posterior aspect)

1.外侧缘 lateral border
2.肾前唇 anterior lip of kidney
3.前面 anterior surface
4.下端 inferior extremity
5.上端 superior extremity
6.上极动脉 superior polar artery
7.肾后唇 posterior lip of kidney
8.肾动脉 renal artery

9.肾静脉 renal vein
10.内侧缘 medial border
11.肾盂 renal pelvis
12.输尿管 ureter
13.后面 posterior surface
14.肾小盏 minor renal calices
15.肾动、静脉 renal artery and vein
16.肾乳头 renal papillae

17.肾动脉分支、静脉属支 branches of renal artery and tributaries of renal vein
18.肾大盏 major renal calices
19.肾皮质 renal cortex
20.肾锥体、肾髓质 renal pyramids and renal medulla
21.肾锥体底 base of renal pyramid
22.肾柱 renal columns

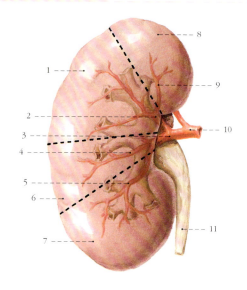

211. 肾段和肾段动脉（前面观）
The renal segments and the segmental arteries
(anterior aspect)

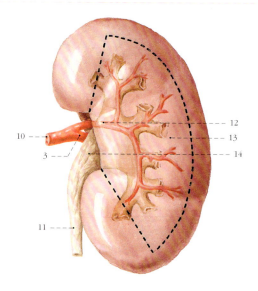

212. 肾段和肾段动脉（后面观）
The renal segments and the segmental arteries
(posterior aspect)

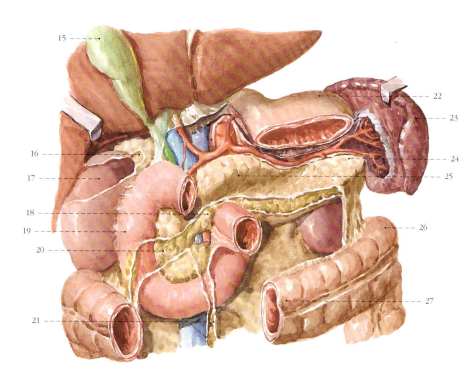

213. 肾的位置和毗邻（前面观）
The position of the kidneys and their relations (anterior aspect)

1. 上前段 anterior superior segment
2. 上前段动脉 superior anterior segmental artery
3. 肾动脉前支 anterior branch of renal artery
4. 下前段动脉 inferior anterior segmental artery
5. 下段动脉 inferior segmental artery
6. 下前段 anterior inferior segment
7. 下段 inferior segment
8. 上段 superior segment
9. 上段动脉 superior segmental artery
10. 肾动脉 renal artery
11. 输尿管 ureter
12. 肾动脉后支 posterior branch of renal artery
13. 后段 posterior segment
14. 肾盂 renal pelvis
15. 胆囊 gallbladder
16. 肾上腺 adrenal gland
17. 肾 kidney
18. 胰颈 neck of pancreas
19. 十二指肠 duodenum
20. 胰头 head of pancreas
21. 肠系膜根 radix of mesentery
22. 胃 stomach
23. 脾 spleen
24. 胰尾 tail of pancreas
25. 胰体 body of pancreas
26. 结肠左曲 left colic flexure
27. 横结肠 transverse colon

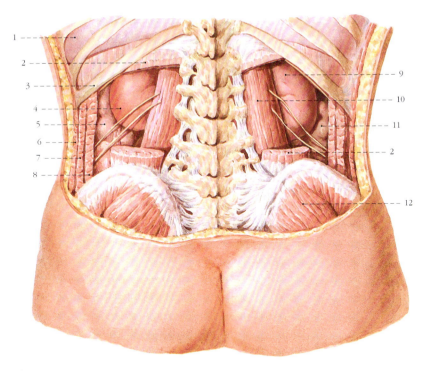

214. 肾的位置和毗邻（后面观）
The position of kidneys and their relations (posterior aspect)

1.壁胸膜 parietal pleura
2.腰方肌 quadratus lumborum
3.第十二肋 twelfth rib
4.左肾 left kidney
5.降结肠 descending colon
6.腹外斜肌 obliquus externus abdominis
7.腹内斜肌 obliquus internus abdominis
8.腹横肌 transversus abdominis
9.右肾 right kidney
10.腰大肌 psoas major
11.升结肠 ascending colon
12.臀大肌 gluteus maximus
13.第十一肋 eleventh rib
14.第一腰椎 first lumbar vertebra
15.第三腰椎 third lumbar vertebra
16.第十二胸椎 twelfth thoracic vertebra
17.肾盂 renal pelvis
18.右输尿管 right ureter

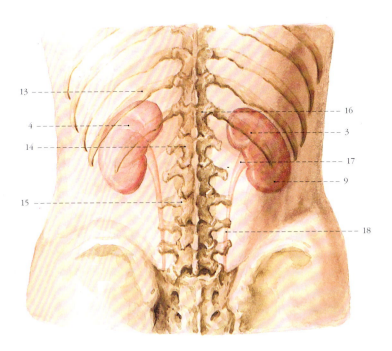

215. 肾和输尿管的体表投影
The surface projection of the kidneys and ureters

1.睾丸动脉 testicular artery
2.输精管 ductus deferents
3.精索外筋膜 external spermatic fascia
4.提睾肌 cremaster
5.精索内筋膜 internal spermatic fascia
6.睾丸鞘膜 tunica vaginalis of testis
7.附睾尾 tail of epididymis
8.蔓状静脉丛 pampiniform plexus
9.附睾附件 appendix of epididymis
10.附睾头 head of epididymis
11.附睾体 body of epididymis

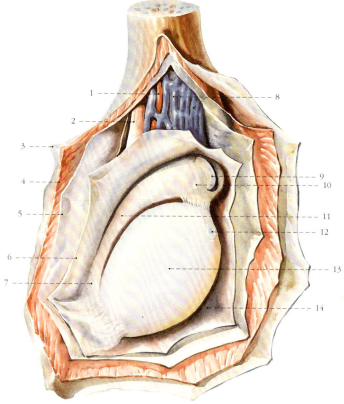

216. 睾丸、附睾及其被膜（外侧面观）
The testis, epididymis and their capsule (lateral aspect)

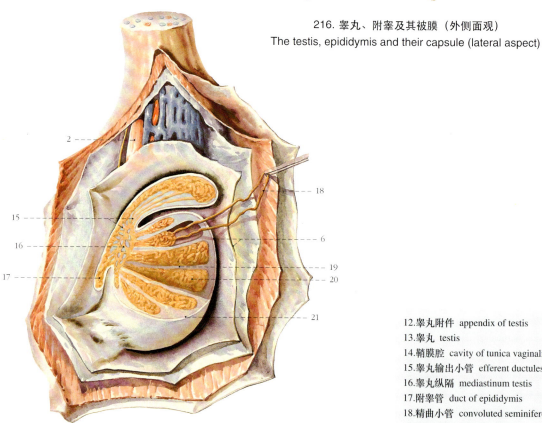

217. 睾丸、附睾的内部结构
Internal structures of the testis and the epididymis

12.睾丸附件 appendix of testis
13.睾丸 testis
14.鞘膜腔 cavity of tunica vaginalis
15.睾丸输出小管 efferent ductules testis
16.睾丸纵隔 mediastinum testis
17.附睾管 duct of epididymis
18.精曲小管 convoluted seminiferous tubules
19.睾丸小隔 septula testis
20.睾丸小叶 lobules of testis
21.白膜 tunica albuginea

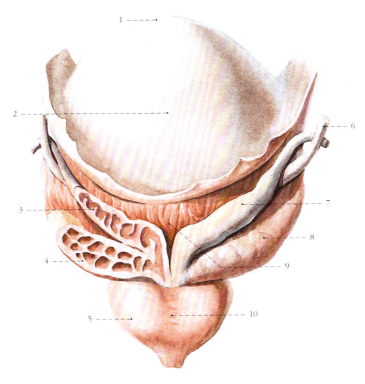

218. 膀胱、前列腺及精囊腺（后面观）
The urinary bladder, prostate and seminal vesicles
(posterior aspect)

1.膀胱顶 vesical vertex
2.膀胱体 body of bladder
3.输精管壶腹（断面）ampulla ductus
  deferentis（section）
4.精囊（断面）seminal vesicle（section）
5.前列腺 prostate
6.右输尿管 right ureter
7.输精管壶腹 ampulla ductus deferentis
8.精囊 seminal vesicle
9.膀胱底 fundus of bladder
10.前列腺沟 prostatic sulci
11.输尿管间襞 interureteric fold
12.前列腺小囊 prostatic utricle
13.输尿管口 ureteric orifice
14.膀胱三角 trigone of bladder
15.尿道嵴 urethral ridge
16.精阜 seminal colliculus

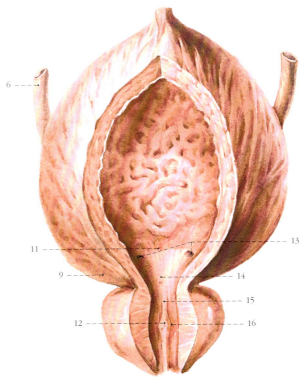

219. 膀胱底及男性尿道前列腺部（内面观）
The fundus of bladder and the prostatic part of the male
urethra (internal aspect)

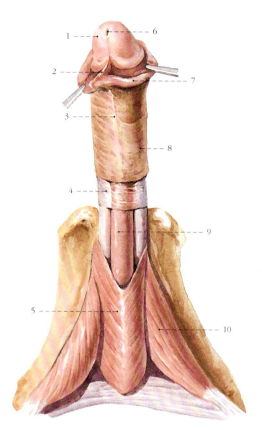

220. 阴茎的海绵体（1）
Cavernous bodies of the penis (1)

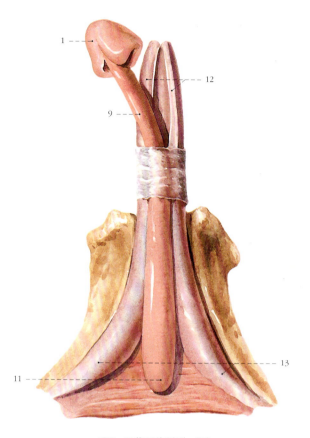

221. 阴茎的海绵体（2）
Cavernous bodies of the penis (2)

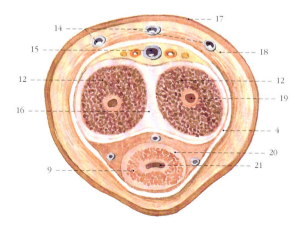

222. 阴茎体横切面
Transverse section through body of the penis

1.阴茎头 glans penis
2.包皮系带 frenulum of prepuce
3.阴茎缝 raphe penis
4.阴茎深筋膜 deep fascia of penis
5.球海绵体肌 bulbospongiosus
6.尿道外口 external orifice of urethra
7.阴茎包皮 prepuce of penis
8.阴茎体 body of penis
9.尿道海绵体 cavernous body of urethra
10.坐骨海绵体肌 ischiocavernosus
11.尿道球 bulb of urethra
12.阴茎海绵体 cavernous body of penis
13.阴茎脚 crus penis
14.阴茎背浅静脉 superficial dorsal veins of penis
15.阴茎背深静脉 deep dorsal vein of penis
16.阴茎中隔 septum of penis
17.皮肤 skin
18.阴茎浅筋膜 superficial fascia of penis
19.阴茎深动脉 deep artery of penis
20.尿道海绵体白膜 albuginea of cavernous body of urethra
21.男尿道 male urethra

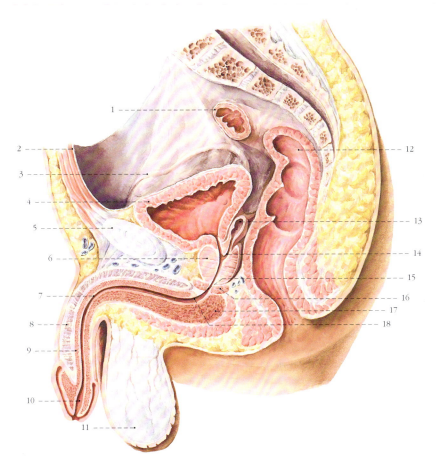

1.乙状结肠 sigmoid colon
2.壁腹膜 parietal peritoneum
3.输精管 ductus deferens
4.膀胱 urinary bladder
5.耻骨联合 pubic symphysis
6.前列腺 prostate
7.耻骨前弯 curvatura prepubica
  (prepubic curvature）
8.阴茎海绵体 cavernous body of
  penis
9.尿道海绵体 cavernous body of
  urethra
10.尿道舟状窝 navicular fossa of
  urethra
11.阴囊中隔 septum of scrotum
12.直肠 rectum
13.输精管壶腹 ampulla of deferent
  duct
14.射精管 ejaculatory duct
15.尿道膜部 membranous part of
  urethra
16.尿生殖膈 urogenital diaphragm
17.尿道球 bulb of urethra

223. 男性盆腔（正中矢状切面）
Male pelvic cavity (median sagittal section)

18.耻骨下弯 curvatura infrapubica
  (infrapubic curvature)
19.卵巢悬韧带 suspensory ligament
  of ovary
20.输卵管 uterine tube
21.卵巢 ovary
22.子宫圆韧带 round ligament of
  uterus
23.子宫 uterus
24.尿道 urethra
25.阴道口 vaginal orifice
26.小阴唇 lesser lip of pudendum
27.大阴唇 greater lip of pudendum
28.膀胱子宫陷凹 vesicouterine
  pouch
29.阴道穹（后部）fornix of vagina
  (posterior part)
30.直肠子宫陷凹 rectouterine
  pouch
31.阴道 vagina
32.肛门外括约肌 sphincter ani
  externus
33.肛门 anus

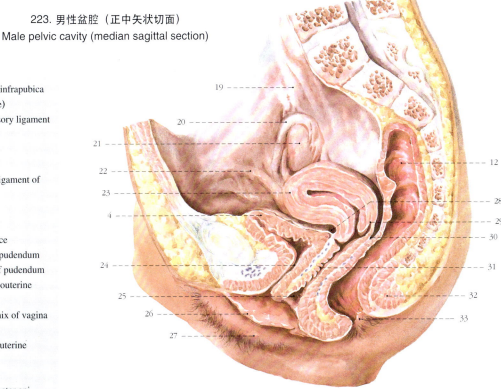

224. 女性盆腔（正中矢状切面）
Female pelvic cavity (median sagittal section)

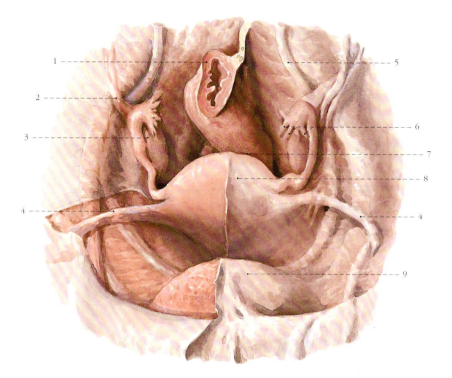

1.直肠 rectum
2.卵巢悬韧带 suspensory ligament of ovary
3.卵巢 ovary
4.子宫圆韧带 round ligament of uterus
5.输尿管 ureter
6.输卵管伞 fimbriae of uterine tube
7.直肠子宫陷凹 rectouterine pouch
8.子宫 uterus
9.膀胱 urinary bladder
10.输卵管壶腹 ampulla of uterine tube
11.输卵管漏斗 infundibulum of uterine tube
12.输卵管峡 isthmus of uterine tube
13.子宫腔 cavity of uterus
14.子宫体 body of uterus
15.子宫峡 isthmus of uterus
16.子宫颈 neck of uterus
17.阴道穹（侧部）fornix of vagina (lateral part)
18.阴道 vagina
19.子宫底 fundus of uterus
20.子宫部 uterine part
21.泡状卵泡 vesicular ovarian follicles
22.白体 corpus albicans
23.黄体 corpus luteum
24.子宫颈管 canal of cervix of uterus
25.子宫口 orifice of uterus

225. 女性盆腔器官（上面观）
Female pelvic organs (superior aspect)

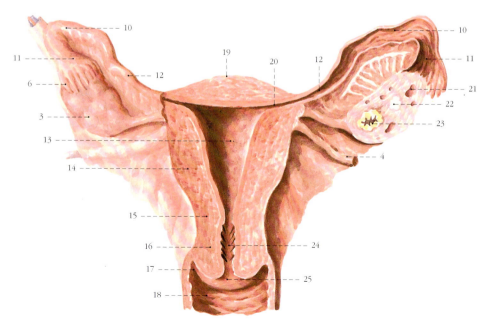

226. 女性内生殖器（冠状切面）
Female internal genital organs (coronal section)

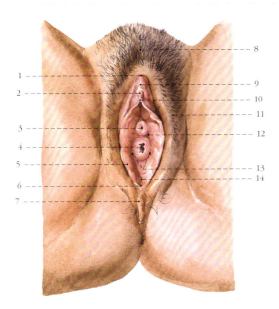

227. 女性外生殖器
Female external genital organs

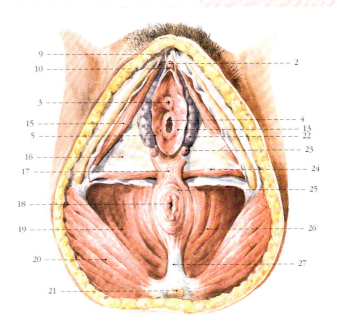

228. 前庭球和前庭大腺
The bulb of vestibule and the greater vestibular gland

1.唇前连合 anterior labial commissure
2.阴蒂头 glans of clitoris
3.尿道外口 external orifice of urethra
4.阴道口 vaginal orifice
5.小阴唇 lesser lip of pudendum
6.阴唇系带 frenulum of pudendal labia
7.唇后连合 posterior labial commissure
8.阴阜 mons pubis
9.阴蒂包皮 prepuce of clitoris
10.阴蒂系带 frenulum of clitoris
11.大阴唇 greater lip of pudendum
12.阴道前庭 vaginal vestibule
13.前庭大腺开口 opening of greater vestibular gland
14.阴道前庭窝 vestibular fossa of vagina
15.坐骨海绵体肌 ischiocavernosus
16.尿生殖膈下筋膜 inferior fascia of urogenital diaphragm
17.会阴中心腱 perineal central tendon
18.肛门 anus
19.坐骨肛门窝 ischioanal fossa
20.臀大肌 gluteus maximus
21.尾骨 coccyx
22.前庭球 bulb of vestibule
23.前庭大腺 greater vestibular gland
24.会阴浅横肌 superficial transverse muscle of perineum
25.肛门外括约肌 sphincter ani externus
26.肛提肌 levator ani
27.肛尾韧带 anococcygeal ligament
28.耻骨联合下缘 inferior margin of pubic symphysis
29.坐骨结节 ischial tuberosity
30.阴囊 scrotum
31.尿生殖区 urogenital region
32.肛区 anal region

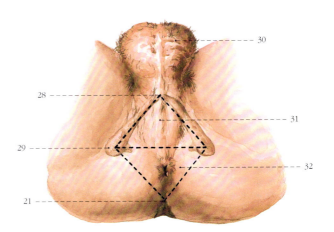

229. 男性会阴分区
The divisions of the male perineum

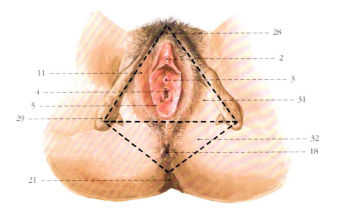

230. 女性会阴分区
The divisions of the female perineum

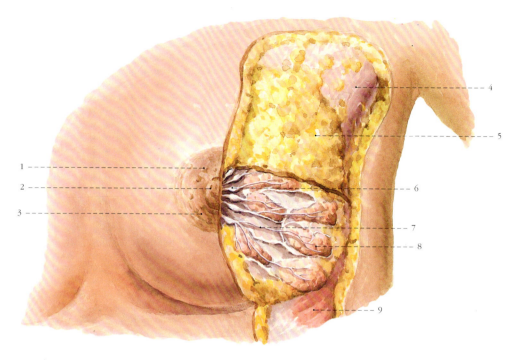

231. 女性乳房（前面观）
Female mamma (anterior aspect)

1.乳晕腺 areolar glands
2.乳头 nipple
3.乳晕 areola of breast
4.胸大肌 pectoralis major
5.乳房脂肪体 adipose body of mamma
6.输乳管窦 lactiferous sinuses
7.输乳管 lactiferous ducts
8.乳腺小叶 lobules of mammary gland
9.前锯肌 serratus anterior
10.第一肋 first rib
11.浅筋膜浅层 superficial layer of superficial fascia
12.皮肤 skin
13.乳房悬韧带 suspensory ligaments of breast
14.输乳孔 lactiferous orifice
15.锁骨 clavicle
16.胸肌筋膜 pectoral fascia
17.乳房后隙 retromammary space
18.肺 lung
19.浅筋膜深层 deep layer of superficial fascia
20.肋间肌 intercostal muscle

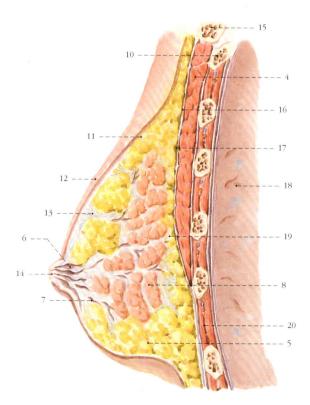

232. 女性乳房（矢状切面）
Female mamma (sagittal section)

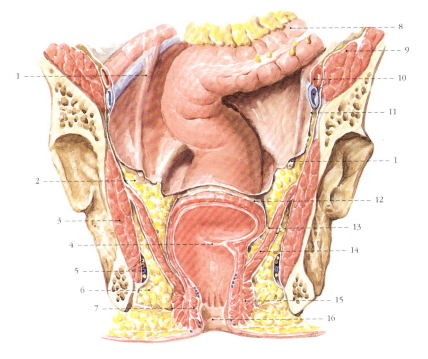

1.输尿管　ureter
2.腹膜外间隙　extraperitoneal space
3.闭孔内肌　obturator internus
4.直肠横襞　transverse fold of rectum
5.阴部内动、静脉和阴部神经　internal pudendal artery, vein and pudendal nerve
6.坐骨肛门窝　ischioanal fossa
7.肛门内括约肌　sphincter ani internus
8.乙状结肠　sigmoid colon
9.髂肌　iliacus
10.髂外动、静脉　external iliac artery and vein
11.腹膜　peritoneum
12.直肠筋膜　fascia of rectum
13.盆膈上、下筋膜　superior and inferior fascia of pelvic diaphragm
14.肛提肌　levator ani muscle
15.肛门外括约肌　sphincter ani externus
16.肛门　anus
17.输卵管伞　fimbriae of uterine tube

233. 男性盆腔（冠状切面）
Male pelvic cavity (coronal section)

18.子宫动、静脉　uterine artery and vein
19.阴道动脉　vaginal artery
20.闭孔膜　obturator membrane
21.闭孔筋膜　obturator fascia
22.尿生殖膈上、下筋膜　superior and inferior fascia of urogenital diaphragm
23.处女膜　hymen
24.子宫　uterus
25.子宫圆韧带　round ligament of uterus
26.子宫阔韧带　broad ligament of uterus
27.腹膜切缘　incisal edge of peritoneum
28.子宫主韧带　cardinal ligament of uterus
29.子宫颈阴道部　vaginal part of cervix
30.阴道　vagina
31.会阴深横肌　deep transverse muscle of perineum
32.耻骨下支　inferior ramus of pubis
33.阴蒂脚　crus of clitoris
34.坐骨海绵体肌　ischiocavernosus
35.球海绵体肌　bulbospongiosus

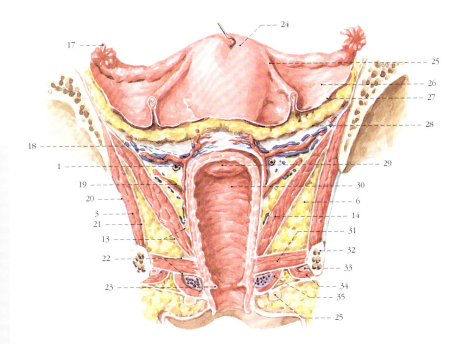

234. 女性盆腔（冠状切面）
Female pelvic cavity (coronal section)

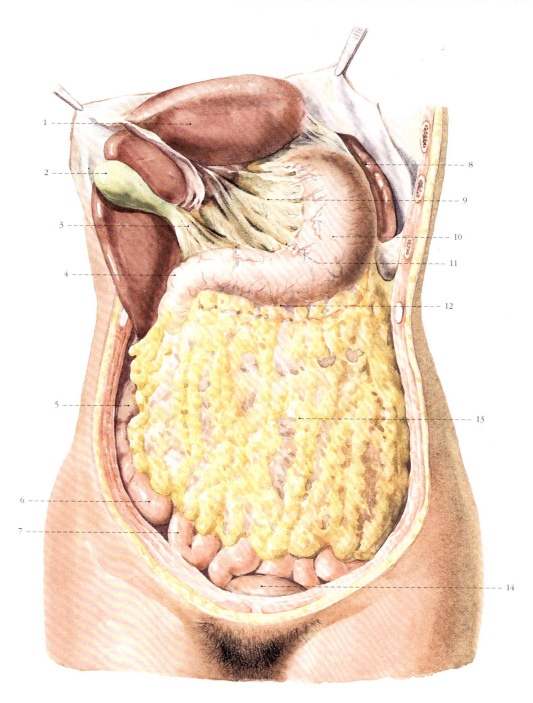

235. 小网膜和大网膜
Lesser omentum and greater omentum

1.肝 liver
2.胆囊 gallbladder
3.肝十二指肠韧带 hepatoduodenal ligament
4.十二指肠上部 superior part of duodenum
5.升结肠 ascending colon
6.盲肠 cecum
7.回肠 ileum

8.脾 spleen
9.肝胃韧带 hepatogastric ligament
10.胃 stomach
11.胃小弯 lesser curvature of stomach
12.胃大弯 greater curvature of stomach
13.大网膜 greater omentum
14.膀胱 urinary bladder

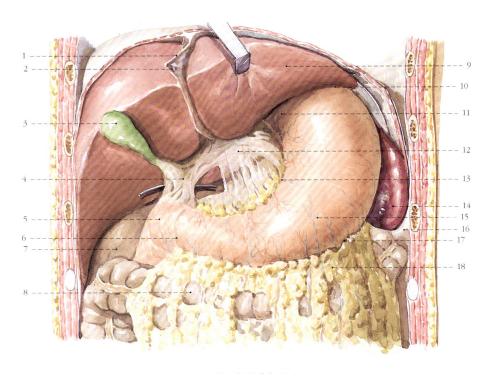

236. 小网膜和胃
The lesser omentum and stomach

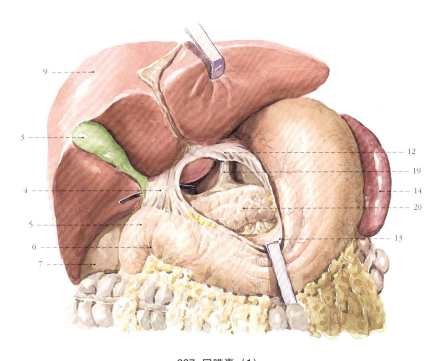

237. 网膜囊（1）
The omental bursa (1)

1.镰状韧带 falciform ligament of liver
2.肝圆韧带 ligamentum teres hepatis
3.胆囊 gallbladder
4.肝十二指肠韧带 hepatoduodenal ligament
5.十二指肠上部 superior part of duodenum
6.幽门 pyloric orifice
7.右肾 right kidney
8.横结肠 transverse colon
9.肝 liver
10.胃底 fundus of stomach
11.贲门部 cardiac part
12.肝胃韧带 hepatogastric ligament
13.胃小弯 lesser curvature of stomach
14.脾 spleen
15.胃体 body of stomach
16.膈结肠韧带 phrenicocolic ligament
17.胃大弯 greater curvature of stomach
18.胃结肠韧带 gastrocolic ligament
19.胃胰襞 gastropancreatic fold
20.胰 pancreas

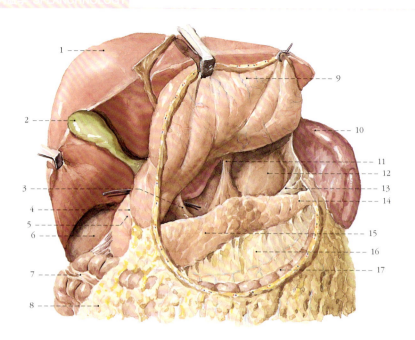

238. 网膜囊（2）
The omental bursa (2)

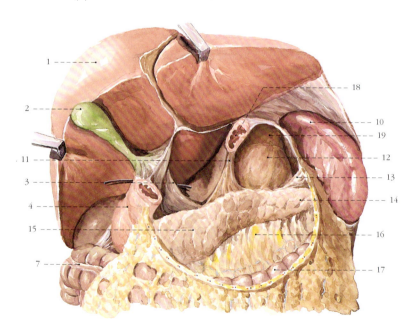

239. 网膜囊（3）
The omental bursa (3)

1.肝 liver	7.结肠右曲 right colic flexure	14.胰尾 tail of pancreas
2.胆囊 gallbladder	8.大网膜 greater omentum	15.胰体 body of pancreas
3.肝胰襞 hepatopancreatic fold	9.胃 stomach	16.横结肠系膜 transverse
4.幽门 pyloric orifice	10.脾 spleen	mesocolon
5.十二指肠上部 superior part of	11.胃胰襞 gastropancreatic fold	17.横结肠 transverse colon
duodenum	12.左肾 left kidney	18.贲门 cardiac orifice
6.右肾 right kidney	13.脾肾韧带 splenorenal ligament	19.左肾上腺 left suprarenal gland

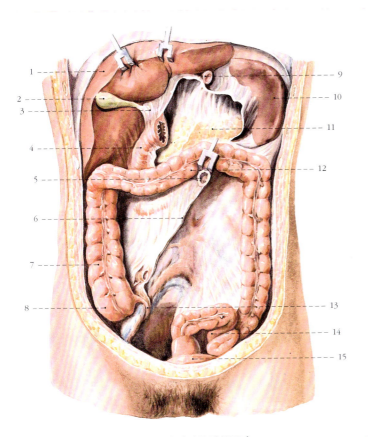

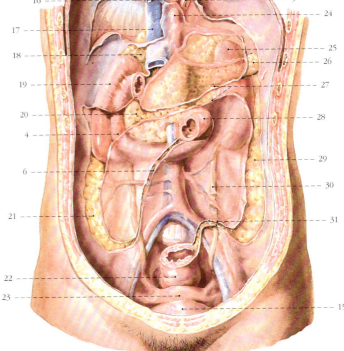

1.肝 liver
2.胆囊 gallbladder
3.肝十二指肠韧带 hepatoduodenal ligament
4.十二指肠 duodenum
5.空肠 jejunum
6.肠系膜根 radix of mesentery
7.升结肠 ascending colon
8.盲肠 cecum
9.食管 esophagus
10.脾 spleen
11.胰 pancreas
12.横结肠 transverse colon
13.阑尾 vermiform appendix
14.乙状结肠 sigmoid colon
15.膀胱 urinary bladder
16.肝静脉 hepatic veins
17.下腔静脉 inferior vena cava
18.肾上腺 suprarenal gland

240. 大肠及腹后壁腹膜的配布
The large intestine and distribution of the peritoneum
on the posterior abdominal wall

19.右肾 right kidney
20.胰头 head of pancreas
21.升结肠区 area of ascending colon
22.直肠 rectum
23.子宫 uterus
24.网膜囊上隐窝 superior omental recess
25.左肾 left kidney
26.胰尾 tail of pancreas
27.横结肠系膜根 radix of transverse mesocolon
28.十二指肠空肠曲 duodenojejunal flexure
29.降结肠区 area of descending colon
30.输尿管 ureter
31.乙状结肠系膜根 radix of sigmoid mesocolon

241. 腹后壁腹膜的配布（示系膜根）
Distribution of the peritoneum on the posterior abdominal wall
(showing the radix of mesentery)

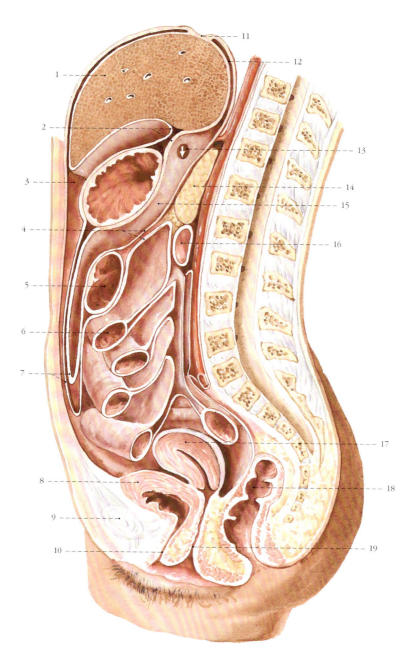

242. 女性腹腔（正中矢状切面）
Female abdominal cavity (median sagittal section)

1.肝 liver
2.肝胃韧带 hepatogastric ligament
3.腹膜腔 peritoneal cavity
4.横结肠系膜 transverse mesocolon
5.横结肠 transverse colon
6.空肠 jejunum
7.大网膜 greater omentum

8.膀胱 urinary bladder
9.耻骨联合 pubic symphysis
10.尿道 urethra
11.冠状韧带 coronary ligament
12.网膜囊上隐窝 superior omental recess
13.网膜孔 omental foramen

14.胰 pancreas
15.网膜囊 omental bursa
16.十二指肠 duodenum
17.子宫 uterus
18.直肠 rectum
19.阴道 vagina

VASCULAR SYSTEM
脉管系统

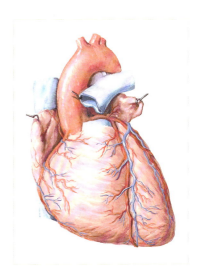

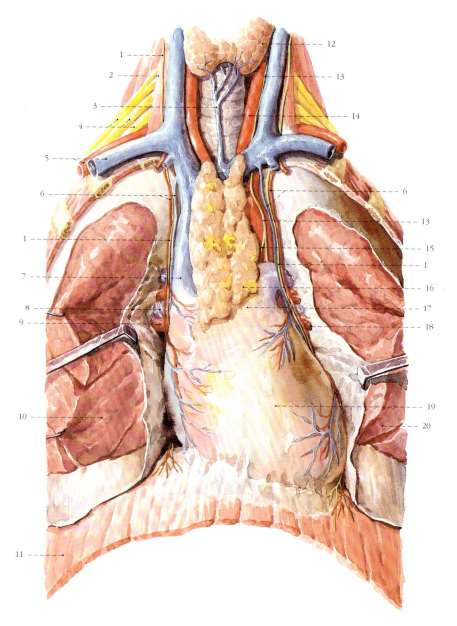

243. 心包及毗邻器官
Pericardium and its adjacent organs

1.膈神经 phrenic nerve
2.前斜角肌 scalenus anterior
3.甲状腺下静脉 inferior thyroid vein
4.臂丛 brachial plexus
5.锁骨下动、静脉 subclavian artery, vein
6.心包膈动、静脉 pericardiacophrenic artery, vein
7.上腔静脉 superior vena cava

8.右主支气管 right principal bronchus
9.右肺静脉 right pulmonary vein
10.右肺 right lung
11.膈 diaphragm
12.甲状腺 thyroid gland
13.迷走神经 vagus nerve
14.颈总动脉 common carotid artery

15.喉返神经 recurrent laryngeal nerve
16.胸腺 thymus
17.肺动脉 pulmonary artery
18.左肺静脉 left pulmonary vein
19.心包 pericardium
20.左肺 left lung

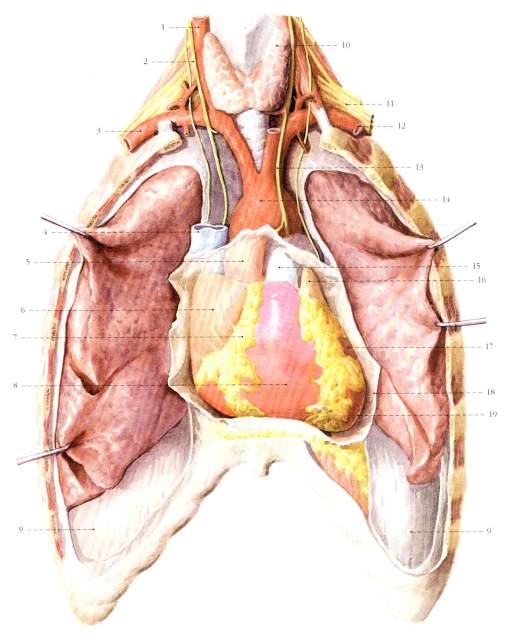

244. 心脏的位置和毗邻
Position and relations of the heart

1.右颈总动脉 right common carotid artery
2.右迷走神经 right vagus nerve
3.右锁骨下动脉 right subclavian artery
4.上腔静脉 superior vena cava
5.升主动脉 ascending aorta
6.右心耳 right auricle
7.冠状沟 coronary sulcus
8.右心室 right ventricle
9.膈 diaphragm
10.甲状腺 thyroid gland

11.臂丛 brachial plexus
12.左锁骨下动脉 left subclavian artery
13.左迷走神经 left vagus nerve
14.主动脉弓 aortic arch
15.肺动脉干 pulmonary trunk
16.左心耳 left auricle
17.左心室 left ventricle
18.心包 pericardium
19.心尖 cardiac apex

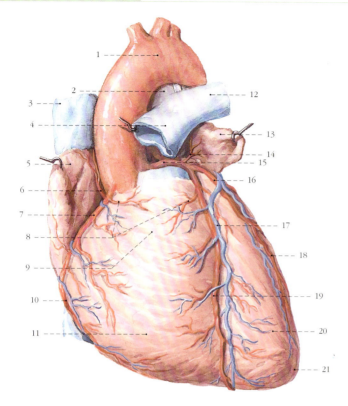

245. 心脏的外形和血管（前面观）
Outline form of the heart and its blood vessels (anterior aspect)

1.主动脉弓 aortic arch
2.右肺动脉 right pulmonary artery
3.上腔静脉 superior vena cava
4.肺动脉干 pulmonary trunk
5.右心耳 right auricle
6.窦房结支 branch of sinuatrial node
7.右冠状动脉 right coronary artery
8.动脉圆锥支 branch of arterial conus
9.动脉圆锥 conus arteriosus
10.右缘支 right marginal branch
11.右心室 right ventricle
12.左肺动脉 left pulmonary artery
13.左心耳 left auricle
14.左房支 left atrial branches
15.左冠状动脉 left coronary artery
16.旋支 circumflex branch
17.心大静脉 great cardiac vein
18.左缘支 left marginal branch
19.前室间支 anterior interventricular branch
20.左心室 left ventricle
21.心尖 cardiac apex
22.左肺静脉 left pulmonary vein
23.左房斜静脉 oblique vein of left atrium
24.冠状沟 coronary sulcus
25.冠状窦 coronary sinus
26.左室后支 posterior branch of left ventricle
27.左室后静脉 posterior vein of left ventricle
28.右肺静脉 right pulmonary vein
29.右心房 right atrium
30.下腔静脉 inferior vena cava
31.冠状窦口 orifice of coronary sinus
32.心小静脉 small cardiac vein
33.后室间支 posterior interventricular branch
34.心中静脉 middle cardiac vein

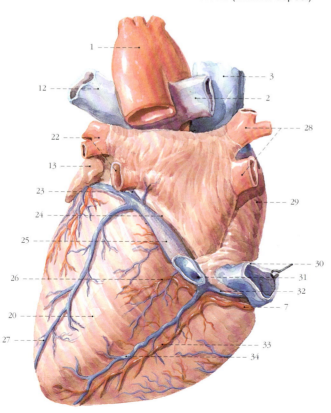

246. 心脏的外形和血管（后面观）
Outline form of the heart and its blood vessels (posterior aspect)

1.主动脉弓 aortic arch
2.上腔静脉 superior vena cava
3.右肺动脉 right pulmonary artery
4.界嵴 crista terminalis
5.房间隔 interatrial septum
6.卵圆窝 fossa ovalis
7.下腔静脉口、瓣 orifice and valve of inferior vena cava
8.肺动脉干 pulmonary trunk
9.右心耳 right auricle
10.梳状肌 pectinate muscles
11.右心室 right ventricle
12.三尖瓣隔侧尖 septal cusp of tricuspid valve
13.冠状窦口、瓣 orifice. valve of coronary sinus
14.三尖瓣前尖 anterior cusp of tricuspid valve
15.三尖瓣后尖 posterior cusp of tricuspid valve
16.前乳头肌 anterior papillary muscle
17.前半月瓣 anterior semilunar valve
18.左半月瓣 left semilunar valve
19.右半月瓣 right semilunar valve
20.动脉圆锥 conus arteriosus
21.室上嵴 supraventricular crest
22.隔侧乳头肌 septal papillary muscles
23.室间隔 interventricular septum
24.隔缘肉柱 septomarginal trabecula
25.后乳头肌 posterior papillary muscle

247. 右心房（内面观）
The right atrium (internal aspect)

248. 右心室（内面观）
The right ventricle (internal aspect)

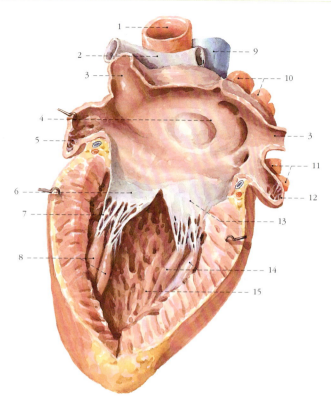

249. 左心房和左心室（内面观）
The left atrium and left ventricle (internal aspect)

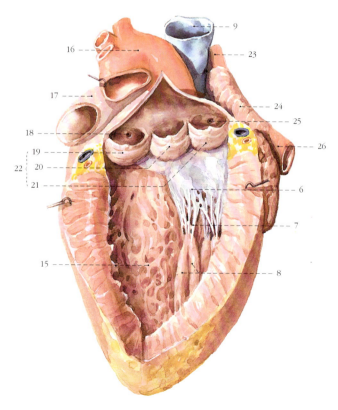

250. 左心室（内面观）
The left ventricle (internal aspect)

1.主动脉 aorta
2.肺动脉干 pulmonary trunk
3.左上肺静脉 left superior pulmonary vein
4.卵圆孔瓣 valve of foramen ovale
5.梳状肌 pectinate muscles
6.二尖瓣前尖 anterior cusp of mitral valve
7.腱索 chordae tendineae
8.前乳头肌 anterior papillary muscle
9.上腔静脉 superior vena cava
10.右肺静脉 right pulmonary vein
11.左下肺静脉 left inferior pulmonary vein
12.左心耳 left auricle
13.二尖瓣后尖 posterior cusp of mitral valve
14.后乳头肌 posterior papillary muscle
15.肉柱 trabeculae carneae
16.主动脉弓 aortic arch
17.肺动脉 pulmonary artery
18.右冠状动脉口 orifice of right coronary artery
19.右半月瓣 right semilunar valve
20.后半月瓣 posterior semilunar valve
21.左半月瓣 left semilunar valve
22.主动脉瓣 aortic valve
23.右上肺静脉 right superior pulmonarg vein
24.左心房 left atrium
25.左冠状动脉口 orifice of left coronary artery
26.左上肺静脉 left superior pulmonary vein

1.肺动脉瓣 valve of pulmonary trunk
2.前半月瓣 anterior semilunar valve
3.右半月瓣 right semilunar valve
4.左半月瓣 left semilunar valve
5.左冠状动脉 left coronary artery
6.左纤维三角 left fibrous trigone
7.右纤维三角 right fibrous trigone
8.二尖瓣 mitral valve
9.前尖 anterior cusp
10.后尖 posterior cusp
11.左纤维环 left fibrous ring
12.后半月瓣 posterior semilunar valve
13.主动脉瓣 aortic valve
14.右冠状动脉 right coronary artery
15.右纤维环 right fibrous ring
16.隔侧尖 septal cusp
17.三尖瓣 tricuspid valve
18.房室结支 branch of atrioventricular node
19.右心房 right atrum
20.卵圆窝 fossa ovalis
21.下腔静脉口 orifice of inferior vena cava
22.冠状窦口 orifice of coronary sinus
23.腱索 chordae tendineae
24.乳头肌 papillary muscles
25.肉柱 trabeculae carneae
26.右肺静脉 right pulmonary vein
27.左心房 left atrium
28.右肺静脉口 orifice of right pulmonary vein
29.左肺静脉口 orifice of left pulmonary vein
30.房间隔 interatrial septum
31.室间隔膜部 membranous part of interventricular septum

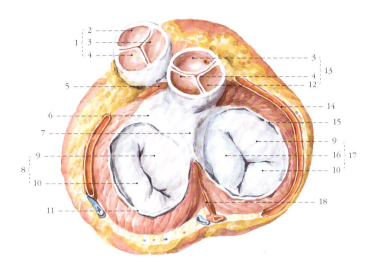

251. 心脏的瓣膜（上面观）
Cardiac valves (superior aspect)

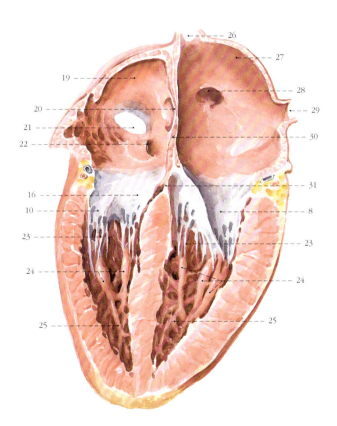

252. 房间隔和室间隔（切面）
Interatrial septum and interventricular septum (section)

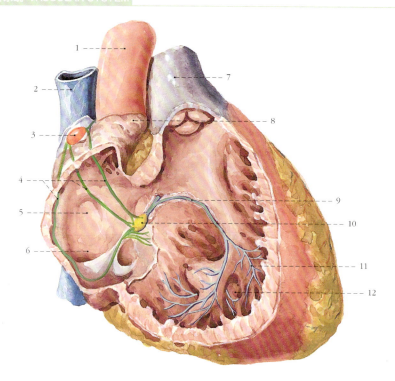

253. 心脏传导系统（右内面观）
Conducting system of the heart (right internal aspect)

1.主动脉 aorta
2.上腔静脉 superior vena cava
3.窦房结 sinuatrial node
4.前、中、后结间束 anterior, middle, posterior internodal tract
5.卵圆窝 fossa ovalis
6.右心房 right atrium
7.肺动脉干 pulmonary trunk
8.右心耳 right auricle
9.右束支 right bundle branch
10.房室结 atrioventricular node
11.心内膜下支 subendocardial branches
12.右心室 right ventricle
13.左束支 left bundle branch
14.左心室 left ventricle
15.左、右肺动脉 left, right pulmonary artery
16.肺静脉 pulmonary veins
17.左心房 left atrium

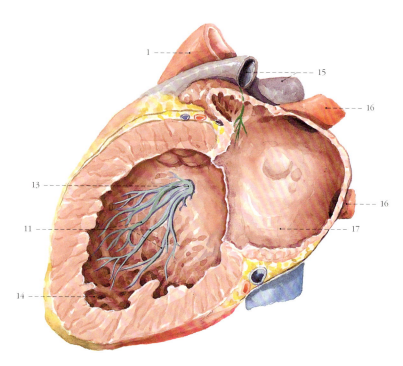

254. 心脏传导系统（左内面观）
Conducting system of the heart (left internal aspect)

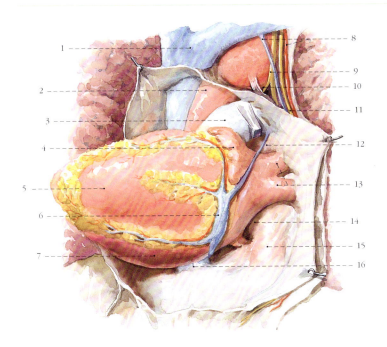

255. 心包腔（1）
The pericardial cavity (1)

1.上腔静脉 superior vena cava
2.升主动脉 ascending aorta
3.肺动脉干 pulmonary trunk
4.左心耳 left auricle
5.左心室 left ventricle
6.冠状窦 coronary sinus
7.右心室 right ventricle
8.心包膈动、静脉 pericardiacophrenic artery and veins
9.迷走神经 vagus nerve
10.喉返神经 recurrent laryngeal nerve
11.膈神经 phrenic nerve
12.心包横窦 transverse sinus of pericardium
13.左肺静脉 left pulmonary vein
14.心包斜窦 oblique sinus of pericardium
15.食管 esophagus
16.下腔静脉 inferior vena cava
17.右头臂静脉 right brachiocephalic vein
18.右肺静脉 right pulmonary vein
19.浆膜心包（壁层）serous pericardium (parietal layer)
20.膈 diaphragm
21.左锁骨下动脉 left subclavian artery
22.左头臂静脉 left brachiocephalic vein
23.纤维心包 fibrous pericardium

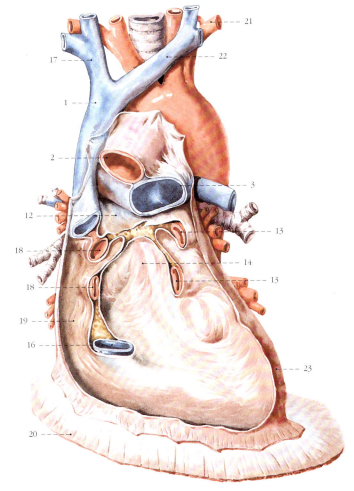

256. 心包腔（2）
The pericardial cavity (2)

1.气管　trachea
2.右肺　right lung
3.动脉韧带　arterial ligament
4.肺动脉干　pulmonary trunk
5.右肺动脉　right pulmonary artery
6.右肺中、下支气管　right middle inferior lobar bronchus
7.右下肺静脉　right inferior pulmonary vein
8.奇静脉　azygos vein
9.胸导管　thoracic duct
10.食管　esophagus
11.左肺　left lung
12.主动脉弓　aortic arch
13.左肺动脉　left pulmonary artery
14.左上肺静脉　left superior pulmonary vein
15.左下肺静脉　left inferior pulmonary vein
16.胸主动脉　thoracic aorta
17.左肺上叶　superior lobe of left lung
18.左主支气管　left principal bronchus
19.左肺下叶　inferior lobe of left lung
20.心包　pericardium
21.上腔静脉　superior vena cava
22.右肺上叶　superior lobe of right lung
23.右肺上叶支气管　right superior lobar bronchus
24.右肺中叶支气管　right middle lobar bronchus
25.右肺下叶支气管　right inferior lobar bronchus
26.右肺下叶　inferior lobe of right lung
27.膈　diaphragm
28.右心房　right atrium
29.右心室　right ventricle
30.下腔静脉　inferior vena cava
31.左心房　left atrium
32.左心室　left ventricle

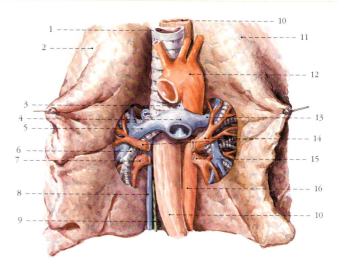

257. 肺根（前面观）
Root of the lung (anterior aspect)

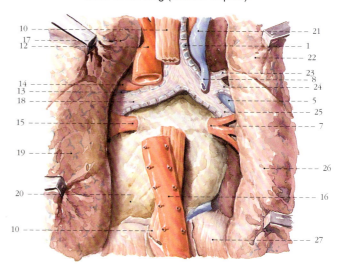

258. 肺根（后面观）
Roots of the lungs (posterior aspect)

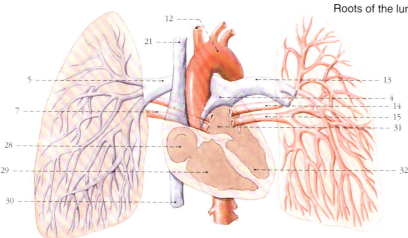

259. 肺循环的血管（模式图）
Vessels of pulmonary circulation (diagram)

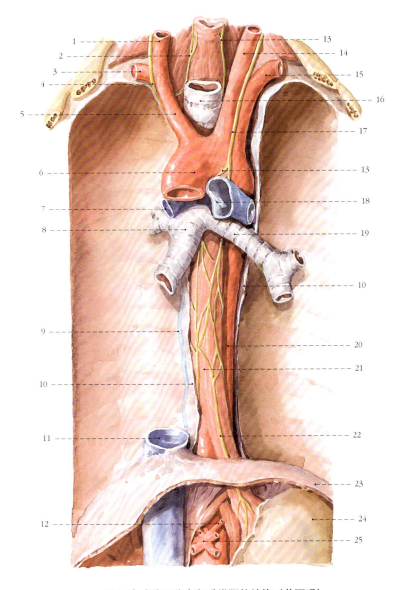

260. 主动脉弓分支和后纵隔的结构（前面观）

The branches of the aortic arch and structures of posterior mediastinum (anterior aspect)

1.右颈总动脉 right common carotid artery
2.右喉返神经 right recurrent laryngeal nerve
3.右锁骨下动脉 right subclavian artery
4.右迷走神经 right vagus nerve
5.头臂干 brachiocephalic trunk
6.主动脉弓 aortic arch
7.右肺动脉 right pulmonary artery
8.右主支气管 right principal bronchus
9.奇静脉 azygos vein

10.纵隔胸膜 mediastinal pleura
11.下腔静脉 inferior vena cava
12.膈下动脉 inferior phrenic artery
13.左喉返神经 left recurrent laryngeal nerve
14.左颈总动脉 left common carotid artery
15.锁骨下动脉 subclavian artery
16.气管 trachea
17.左迷走神经 left vagus nerve
18.肺动脉干 pulmonary trunk

19.左主支气管 left principal bronchus
20.胸主动脉 thoracic aorta
21.食管 esophagus
22.迷走神经前干 anterior vagal trunk
23.膈 diaphragm
24.胃 stomach
25.腹腔干 celiac trunk

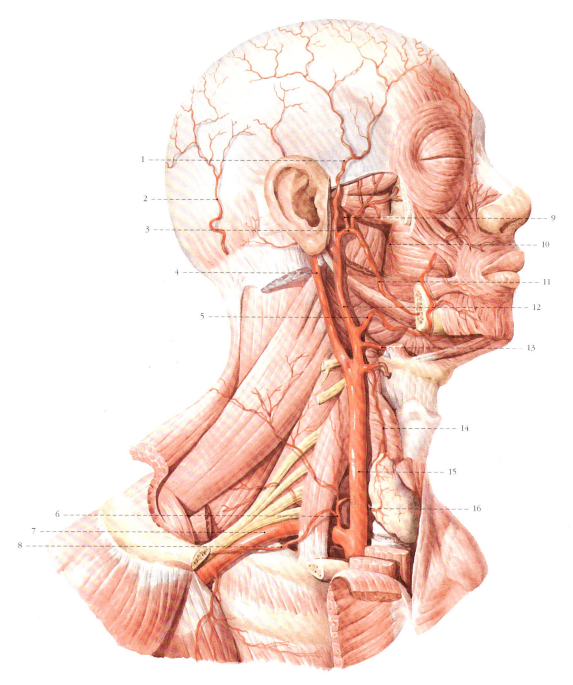

261. 头、颈部的动脉
Arteries of the head and neck

1.颞浅动脉 superficial temporal artery
2.枕动脉 occipital artery
3.上颌动脉 maxillary artery
4.颈内动脉 internal carotid artery
5.面动脉 facial artery
6.甲状颈干 thyrocervical trunk
7.锁骨下动脉 subclavian artery
8.肩胛上动脉 suprascapular artery

9.脑膜中动脉 middle meningeal artery
10.颊动脉 buccal artery
11.下牙槽动脉 inferior alveolar artery
12.颈外动脉 external carotid artery
13.舌动脉 lingual artery
14.甲状腺上动脉 superior thyroid artery
15.颈总动脉 common carotid artery
16.甲状腺下动脉 inferior thyroid artery

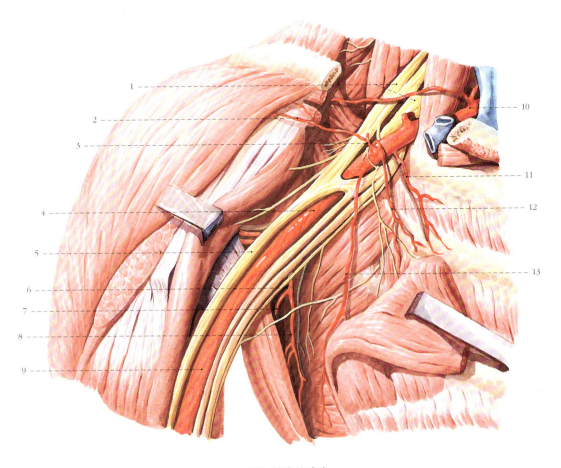

262. 腋窝的动脉
Arteries of the axillary fossa

1.臂丛 brachial plexus
2.三角肌支 deltoid branch
3.胸肩峰动脉 thoracoacromial artery
4.腋动脉 axillary artery
5.正中神经 median nerve
6.肩胛下动脉 subscapular artery
7.旋肩胛动脉 circumflex scapular artery
8.胸背动脉 thoracodorsal artery
9.肱动脉 brachial artery
10.锁骨下动脉 subclavian artery
11.胸上动脉 superior thoracic artery
12.胸肌支 pectoral branches
13.胸外侧动脉 lateral thoracic artery

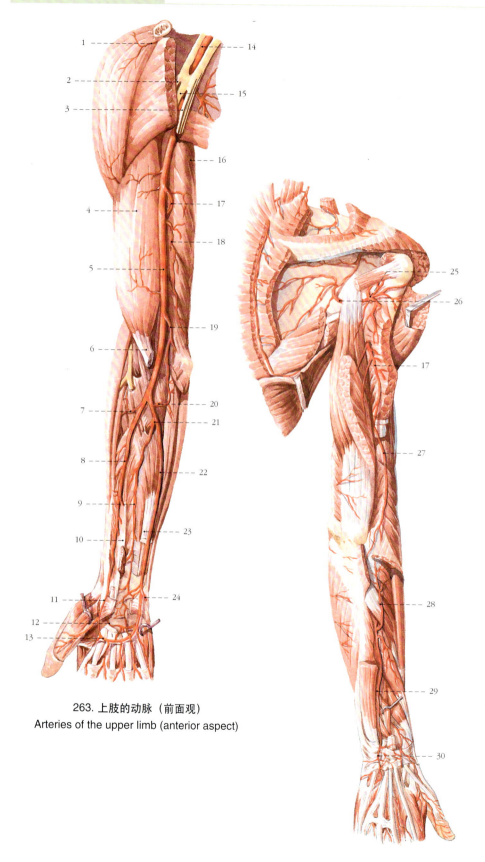

1. 肩峰支 acromial branch
2. 肌皮神经 musculocutaneous nerve
3. 尺神经 ulnar nerve
4. 肱二头肌 biceps brachii
5. 肱动脉 brachial artery
6. 肱二头肌腱 tendon of biceps brachii
7. 桡侧返动脉 radial recurrent artery
8. 桡动脉 radial artery
9. 骨间前动脉 anterior interosseous artery
10. 拇长屈肌 flexor pollicis longus
11. 掌浅支 superficial palmar branch
12. 掌深弓 deep palmar arch
13. 掌浅弓 superficial palmar arch
14. 腋动脉 axillary artery
15. 正中神经 median nerve
16. 肱三头肌 triceps brachii
17. 肱深动脉 deep brachial artery
18. 尺侧上副动脉 superior ulnar collateral artery
19. 尺侧下副动脉 inferior ulnar collateral artery
20. 尺侧返动脉 ulnar recurrent artery
21. 骨间总动脉 common interosseous artery
22. 尺动脉 ulnar artery
23. 指深屈肌 flexor digitorum profundus
24. 掌深支 deep palmar branch
25. 旋肱后动脉 posterior humeral circumflex artery
26. 旋肩胛动脉 circumflex scapular artery
27. 桡侧副动脉 radial collateral artery
28. 骨间返动脉 recurrent interosseous artery
29. 骨间后动脉 posterior interosseous artery
30. 腕背网 dorsal carpal rete

263. 上肢的动脉（前面观）
Arteries of the upper limb (anterior aspect)

264. 上肢的动脉（后面观）
Arteries of the upper limb (posterior aspect)

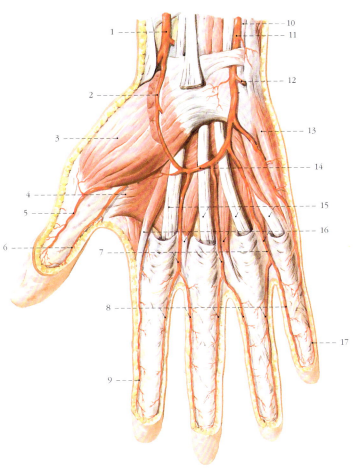

1. 桡动脉 radial artery
2. 掌浅支 superficial palmar branch
3. 拇短展肌 abductor pollicis brevis
4. 拇收肌 adductor pollicis
5. 拇指桡掌侧动脉 palmar radial artery of thumb
6. 拇指尺掌侧动脉 palmar ulnar artery of thumb
7. 指掌侧总动脉 common palmar digital arteries
8. 指掌侧固有动脉 proper palmar digital arteries
9. 示指桡侧动脉 radial artery of index
10. 尺神经 ulnar nerve
11. 尺动脉 ulnar artery
12. 掌深支 deep palmar branch

265. 右手掌面的动脉（浅层）
Arteries of the palm of right hand (superficial layer)

13. 小指展肌 abductor digiti minimi
14. 掌浅弓 superficial palmar arch
15. 指浅屈肌腱 tendon of flexor digitorum superficialis
16. 蚓状肌 lumbricales
17. 小指尺掌侧动脉 ulnar palmar artery of little finger
18. 拇主要动脉 principal artery of thumb
19. 腕掌支 palmar carpal branch
20. 掌深弓 deep palmar arch
21. 掌心动脉 palmar metacarpal arteries
22. 骨间掌侧肌 palmar interossei

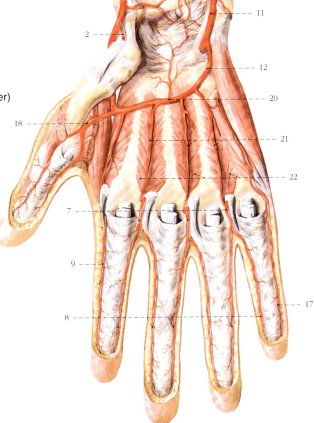

266. 右手掌面的动脉（深层）
Arteries of the palm of right hand (deep layer)

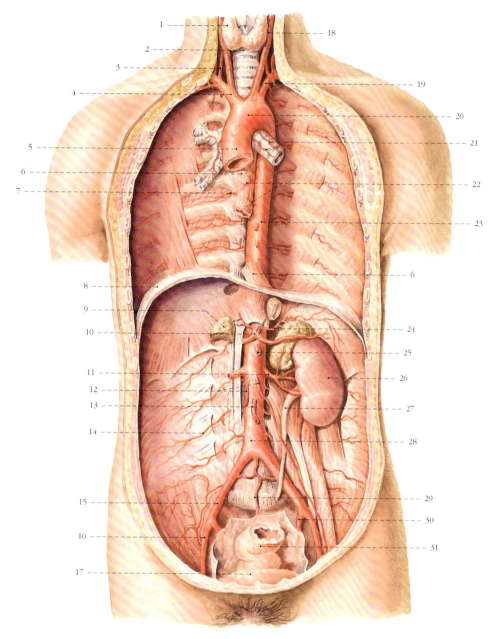

267. 胸主动脉、腹主动脉及其分支
Thoracic aorta and abdominal aorta and their branches

1.甲状腺 thyroid gland
2.气管 trachea
3.椎动脉 vertebral artery
4.头臂干 brachiocephalic trunk
5.升主动脉 ascending aorta
6.食管 esophagus
7.肋间后动脉 posterior intercostal arteries
8.膈 diaphragm
9.右肾上腺 right suprarenal gland
10.腹腔干 celiac trunk
11.左肾动脉 left renal artery

12.睾丸动脉 testicular artery
13.肠系膜下动脉 inferior mesenteric artery
14.腰动脉 lumbar arteries
15.髂总动脉 common iliac artery
16.髂外动脉 external iliac artery
17.膀胱 urinary bladder
18.左颈总动脉 left common carotid artery
19.左锁骨下动脉 left subclavian artery
20.主动脉弓 aortic arch
21.支气管支 bronchial branches
22.食管支 esophageal branches

23.胸主动脉 thoracic aorta
24.膈下动脉 inferior phrenic artery
25.肠系膜上动脉 superior mesenteric artery
26.左肾 left kidney
27.输尿管 ureter
28.腹主动脉 abdominal aorta
29.骶正中动脉 median sacral artery
30.髂内动脉 internal iliac artery
31.直肠 rectum

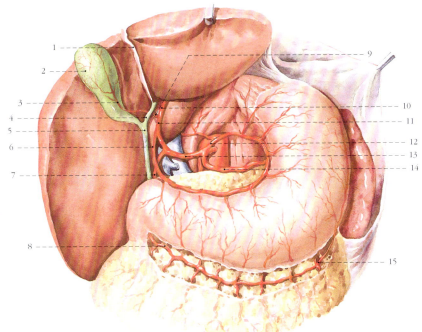

1.肝圆韧带 ligamentum teres hepatis

2.胆囊 gallbladder

3.胆囊动脉 cystic artery

4.肝总管 common hepatic duct

5.胆总管 common bile duct

6.胃右动脉 right gastric artery

7.胃十二指肠动脉 gastroduodenal artery

8.胃网膜右动脉 right gastroepiploic artery

9.右支 right branch

10.左支 left branch

11.肝固有动脉 proper hepatic artery

12.胃左动脉 left gastric artery

13.肝总动脉 common hepatic artery

14.脾动脉 splenic artery

15.胃网膜左动脉 left gastroepiploic artery

16.腹腔干 celiac trunk

17.胰 pancreas

18.胰十二指肠上前动脉 anterior superior pancreaticoduodenal artery

19.十二指肠 duodenum

20.肠系膜上动脉 superior mesenteric artery

21.胃短动脉 short gastric arteries

22.横结肠 transverse colon

268. 腹腔干及其分支（1）
Celiac trunk and its branches (1)

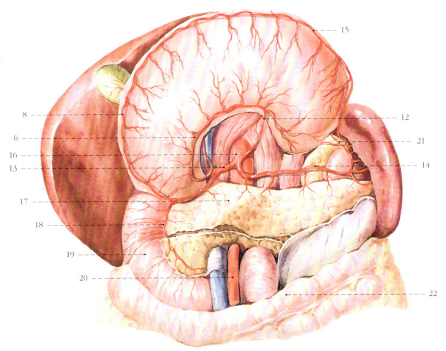

269. 腹腔干及其分支（2）
Celiac trunk and its branches (2)

1.横结肠 transverse colon
2.中结肠动脉 middle colic artery
3.右结肠动脉 right colic artery
4.升结肠 ascending colon
5.回结肠动脉 ileocolic artery
6.盲肠 cecum
7.阑尾 vermiform appendix
8.大网膜 greater omentum
9.横结肠系膜 transverse mesocolon
10.肠系膜上动脉 superior
   mesenteric artery
11.空肠动脉 jejunal arteries
12.空肠 jejunum
13.回肠动脉 ileal arteries

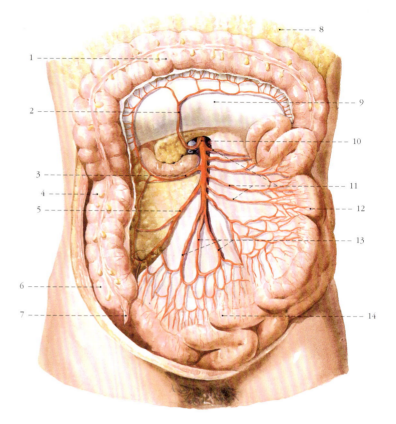

270. 肠系膜上动脉及其分支
The superior mesenteric artery and its branches

271. 肠系膜下动脉及其分支
The inferior mesenteric artery and its branches

14.回肠 ileum
15.腹主动脉 abdominal
   aorta
16. 肠系膜下动脉 inferior
   mesenteric artery
17.髂总动脉 common iliac
   artery
18.膀胱 urinary bladder
19.降结肠 descending colon
20.左结肠动脉 left colic
   artery
21.乙状结肠动脉 sigmoid
   arteries
22.直肠上动脉 superior
   rectal artery
23.乙状结肠 sigmoid colon

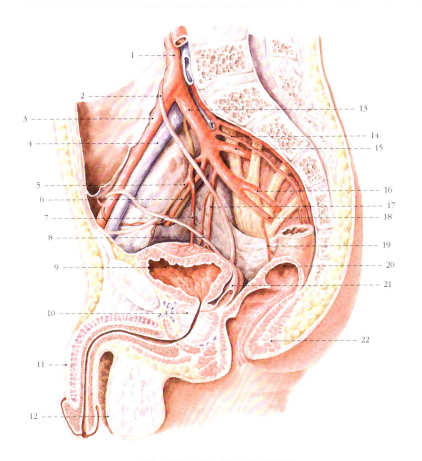

1.髂总动脉 common iliac artery
2.输尿管 ureter
3.髂外动脉 external iliac artery
4.髂外静脉 external iliac vein
5.脐动脉 umbilical artery
6.闭孔动脉 obturator artery
7.膀胱上动脉 superior vesical arteries
8.输精管 ductus deferents
9.膀胱 urinary bladder
10.前列腺 prostate
11.阴茎 penis
12.阴囊 scrotum
13.髂内动脉 internal iliac artery
14.骶外侧动脉 lateral sacral arteries
15.臀上动脉 superior gluteal artery
16.臀下动脉 inferior gluteal artery
17.膀胱下动脉 inferior vesical artery

272. 男性盆腔的动脉（正中矢状切面）
Arteries of the male pelvic cavity (median sagittal section)

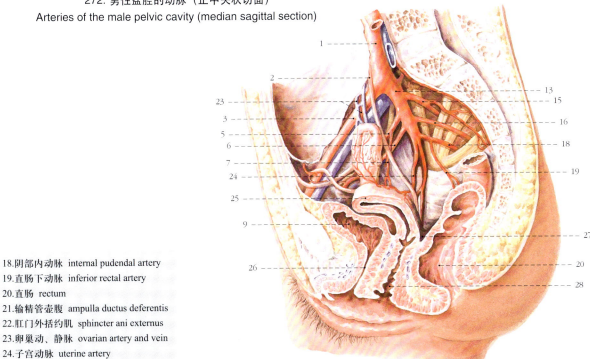

18.阴部内动脉 internal pudendal artery
19.直肠下动脉 inferior rectal artery
20.直肠 rectum
21.输精管壶腹 ampulla ductus deferentis
22.肛门外括约肌 sphincter ani externus
23.卵巢动、静脉 ovarian artery and vein
24.子宫动脉 uterine artery
25.子宫 uterus
26.尿道 urethra
27.直肠子宫陷凹 rectouterine pouch
28.阴道 vagina

273. 女性盆腔的动脉（正中矢状切面）
Arteries of the female pelvic cavity (median sagittal section)

125

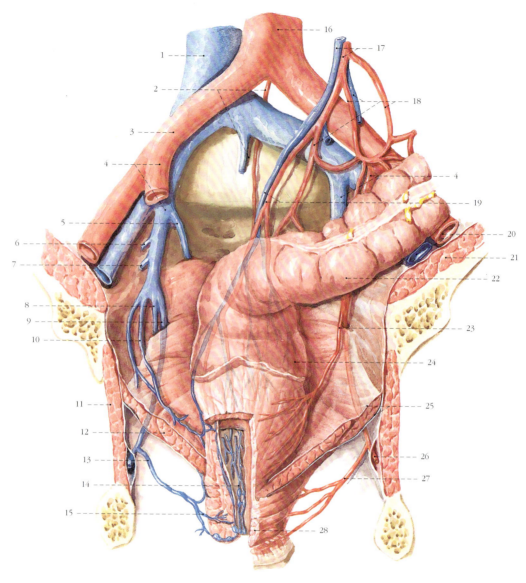

274. 直肠和肛管的血管
Blood vessels of rectum and anal canal

1.下腔静脉　inferior vena cava
2.骶正中动、静脉　median sacral artery and vein
3.髂总动脉　common iliac artery
4.髂内动、静脉　internal iliac artery and vein
5.臀上静脉　superior gluteal vein
6.闭孔静脉　obturator vein
7.膀胱上静脉　superior vesical vein
8.臀下静脉　inferior gluteal vein
9.阴部内静脉　internal pudendal vein
10.直肠下静脉　inferior rectal vein
11.闭孔内肌　obturator internus
12.肛提肌　levator ani muscle

13.肛静脉　anal vein
14.直肠内静脉丛　internal rectal venous plexus
15.直肠外静脉丛　external rectal venous plexus
16.腹主动脉　abdominal aorta
17.肠系膜下动、静脉　inferior mesenteric artery and vein
18.乙状结肠动、静脉　sigmoid arteries and veins
19.直肠上动、静脉　superior rectal artery and vein

20.髂外动、静脉　external iliac artery and vein
21.髂肌　iliacus
22.乙状结肠　sigmoid colon
23.直肠下动脉　inferior rectal artery
24.直肠　rectum
25.盆膈上、下筋膜　superior and inferior fascias of pelvic diaphragm
26.阴部内动脉　internal pudendal artery
27.肛动脉　anal artery
28.肛门外括约肌　external anal sphincter

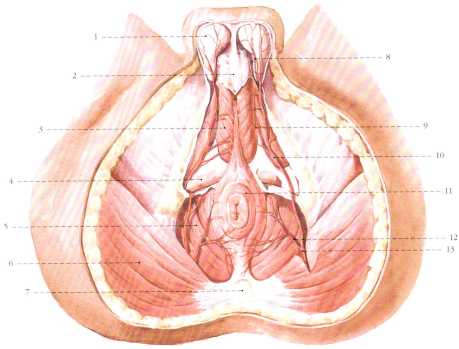

275. 男性会阴部的动脉
Arteries of the male perineum

1.睾丸 testis
2.尿道海绵体 cavernous body of urethra
3.球海绵体肌 bulbocavernosus muscle
4.会阴浅横肌 superficial transverse muscle of perineum
5.肛提肌 levator ani
6.臀大肌 gluteus maximus
7.尾骨 coccyx
8.阴囊后支 posterior scrotal branches
9.阴茎深动脉 deep artery of penis
10.会阴动脉 perineal artery
11.肛门外括约肌 external anal sphincter
12.肛动脉 anal artery
13.阴部内动脉 internal pudendal artery
14.阴蒂 clitoris
15.尿道外口 external orifice of urethra
16.前庭球 bulb of vestibule
17.前庭大腺 greater vestibular gland

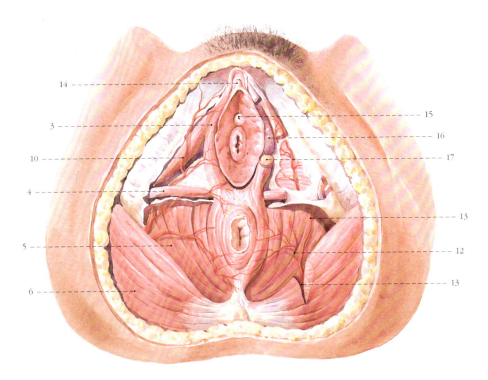

276. 女性会阴部的动脉
Arteries of the female perineum

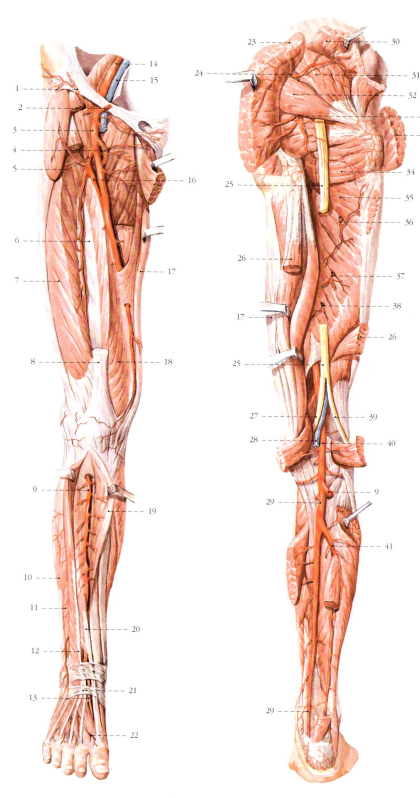

1.旋髂浅动脉 superficial iliac circumflex artery
2.腹壁浅动脉 superficial epigastric artery
3.股动脉 femoral artery
4.旋股内侧动脉 medial femoral circumflex artery
5.旋股外侧动脉 lateral femoral circumflex artery
6.股中间肌 vastus intermedius
7.股外侧肌 vastus lateralis
8.股直肌 rectus femoris
9.胫前动脉 anterior tibial artery
10.腓骨长肌 peroneus longus
11.腓骨短肌 peroneus brevis
12.趾长伸肌 extensor digitorum longus
13.足背动脉 dorsal artery of foot
14.髂外动脉 external iliac artery
15.髂外静脉 external iliac vein
16.股深动脉 deep femoral artery
17.股薄肌 gracilis
18.股内侧肌 vastus medialis
19.胫骨前肌 tibialis anterior
20.蹈长伸肌 extensor hallucis longus
21.伸肌下支持带 inferior extensor retinaculum
22.趾背动脉 dorsal digital arteries
23.臀大肌 gluteus maximus
24.臀上动脉 superior gluteal artery
25.坐骨神经 sciatic nerve
26.股二头肌（长头）biceps femoris (long head)
27.胫神经 tibial nerve
28.腘静脉 popliteal vein
29.胫后动脉 posterior tibial artery
30.臀中肌 gluteus medius
31.臀小肌 gluteus minimus
32.梨状肌 piriformis
33.臀下动脉 inferior gluteal artery
34.股方肌 quadratus femoris
35.小收肌 adductor minimus
36.第一穿动脉 first perforating artery
37.第二穿动脉 second perforating artery
38.第三穿动脉 third perforating artery
39.腓总神经 common peroneal nerve
40.腘动脉 popliteal artery
41.腓动脉 peroneal artery

277. 下肢的动脉（前面观）
Arteries of the lower limb
(anterior aspect)

278. 下肢的动脉（后面观）
Arteries of the lower limb
(posterior aspect)

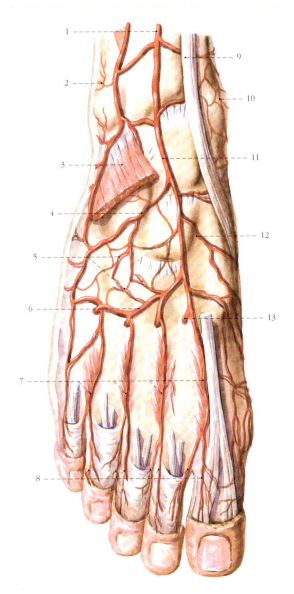

1.胫前动脉 anterior tibial artery
2.外踝网 lateral malleolar rete
3.趾短伸肌 extensor digitorum brevis
4.跗外侧动脉 lateral tarsal artery
5.足背动脉网 dorsal arterial rete of foot
6.弓状动脉 arcuate artery
7.跖背动脉 dorsal metatarsal arteries
8.趾背动脉 dorsal digital arteries
9.胫骨前肌腱 tendon of tibialis anterior
10.内踝网 medial malleolar rete
11.足背动脉 dorsal artery of foot
12.跗内侧动脉 medial tarsal arteries
13.足底深动脉 deep plantar artery

279. 足背的动脉
Arteries of the dorsum of foot

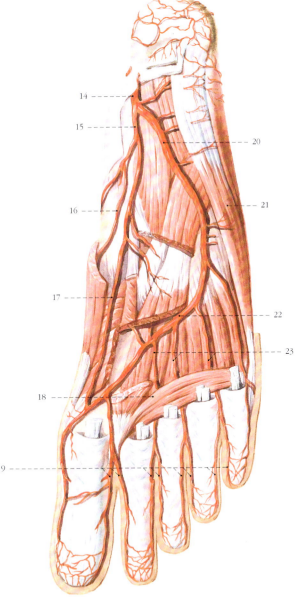

14.胫后动脉 posterior tibial artery
15.足底内侧动脉 medial plantar artery
16.浅支 superficial branch
17.深支 deep branch
18.踇收肌（横头）adductor hallucis (transverse head)
19.趾足底固有动脉 proper plantar digital arteries
20.足底外侧动脉 lateral plantar artery
21.小趾展肌 abductor digiti minimi
22.足底弓 plantar arch
23.趾足底总动脉 common plantar digital arteries

280. 足底的动脉
Plantar arteries

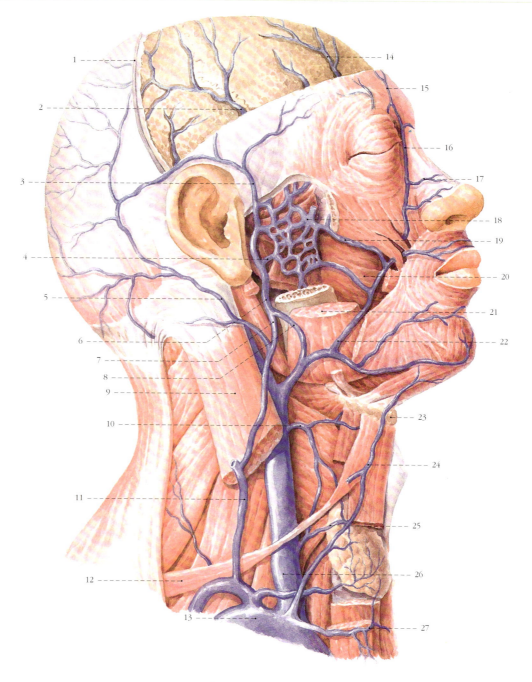

281. 头、颈部的静脉
Veins of head and neck

1.外板 outer plate
2.颞前板障静脉 anterior temporal diploic vein
3.颞浅静脉 superficial temporal veins
4.上颌静脉 maxillary veins
5.耳后静脉 posterior auricular vein
6.下颌后静脉 retromandibular vein
7.下颌后静脉（后支）retromandibular vein
　（posterior branch）
8.下颌后静脉（前支）retromandibular vein
　（anterior branch）

9.胸锁乳突肌 sternocleidomastoid
10.甲状腺上静脉 superior thyroid vein
11.颈外静脉 external jugular vein
12.肩胛舌骨肌 omohyoid
13.锁骨下静脉 subclavian vein
14.额板障静脉 frontal diploic vein
15.滑车上静脉 supratrochlear vein
16.内眦静脉 angular vein
17.鼻外静脉 external nasal vein
18.翼静脉丛 pterygoid venous plexus

19.面深静脉 deep facial vein
20.颊肌 buccinator
21.咬肌 masseter
22.面静脉 facial vein
23.舌骨 hyoid bone
24.颈前静脉 anterior jugular vein
25.甲状腺中静脉 middle thyroid
　vein
26.颈内静脉 internal jugular vein
27.颈静脉弓 jugular venous arch

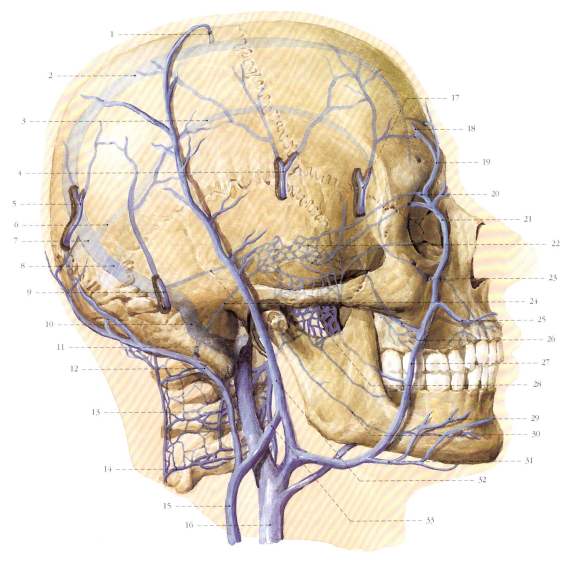

282. 颅内、外静脉的交通
Communications between intracranial and extracranial veins

1.顶导静脉 parietal emissary vein
2.上矢状窦 superior sagittal sinus
3.下矢状窦 inferior sagittal sinus
4.颞前板障静脉 anterior temporal diploic vein
5.枕板障静脉 occipital diploic vein
6.直窦 straight sinus
7.窦汇 confluence of sinuses
8.横窦 transverse sinus
9.颞后板障静脉 posterior temporal diploic vein
10.乙状窦 sigmoid sinus
11.乳突导静脉 mastoid emissary vein
12.枕静脉 occipital vein
13.髁导静脉 condylar emissary vein

14.椎静脉丛 vertebral venous plexus
15.颈外静脉 external jugular vein
16.颈内静脉 internal jugular vein
17.额板障静脉 frontal diploic vein
18.额导静脉 frontal emissary vein
19.眶上静脉 supraorbital vein
20.眼上静脉 superior ophthalmic vein
21.内眦静脉 angular vein
22.海绵窦 cavernous sinus
23.眶下静脉 infraorbital vein
24.岩上、下窦 superior and inferior petrosal sinus

25.上唇静脉 superior labial vein
26.面深静脉 deep facial vein
27.面静脉 facial vein
28.翼静脉丛 pterygoid venous plexus
29.下唇静脉 inferior labial veins
30.下牙槽静脉 inferior alveolar vein
31.颏下静脉 submental vein
32.下颌后静脉 retromandibular vein
33.下颌后静脉（后支）retromandibular vein（posterior branch）

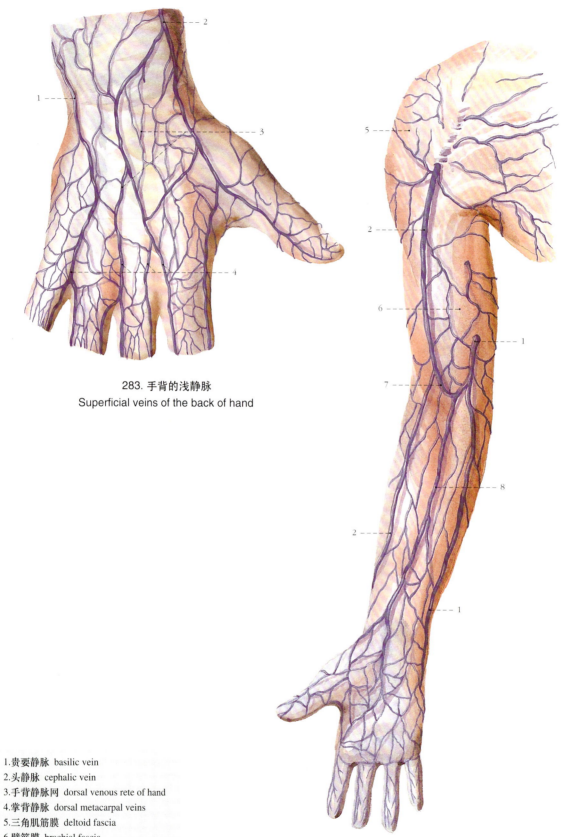

283. 手背的浅静脉
Superficial veins of the back of hand

1.贵要静脉 basilic vein
2.头静脉 cephalic vein
3.手背静脉网 dorsal venous rete of hand
4.掌背静脉 dorsal metacarpal veins
5.三角肌筋膜 deltoid fascia
6.臂筋膜 brachial fascia
7.肘正中静脉 median cubital vein
8.前臂正中静脉 median antebrachial vein

284. 上肢的浅静脉
Superficial veins of the upper limb

1.右头臂静脉 right brachiocephalic vein
2.上腔静脉 superior vena cava
3.奇静脉 azygos vein
4.膈下静脉 inferior phrenic veins
5.右肾上腺 right adrenal gland
6.左肾静脉 left renal vein
7.腰静脉 lumbar veins
8.髂总静脉 common iliac vein
9.髂内静脉 internal iliac vein
10.左头臂静脉 left brachiocephalic vein
11.副半奇静脉 accessory hemiazygos vein
12.半奇静脉 hemiazygos vein
13.下腔静脉 inferior vena cava
14.右肾上腺静脉 right suprarenal vein
15.腹主动脉 abdominal aorta
16.左睾丸静脉 left testicular vein
17.髂外静脉 external iliac vein

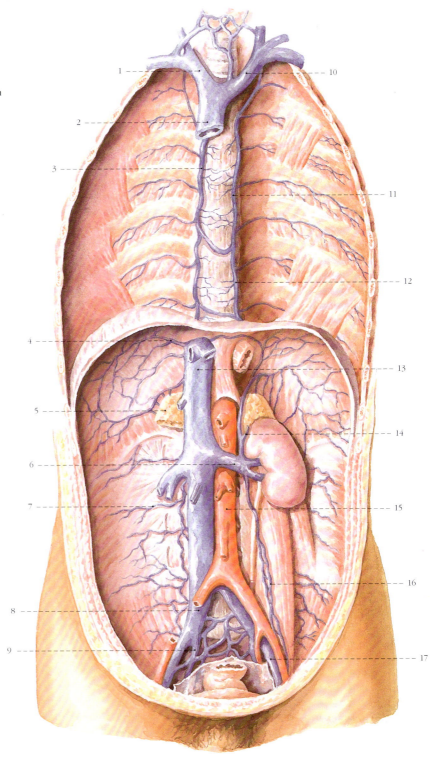

285. 上、下腔静脉及其属支
Superior vena cava, inferior vena cava and their tributaries

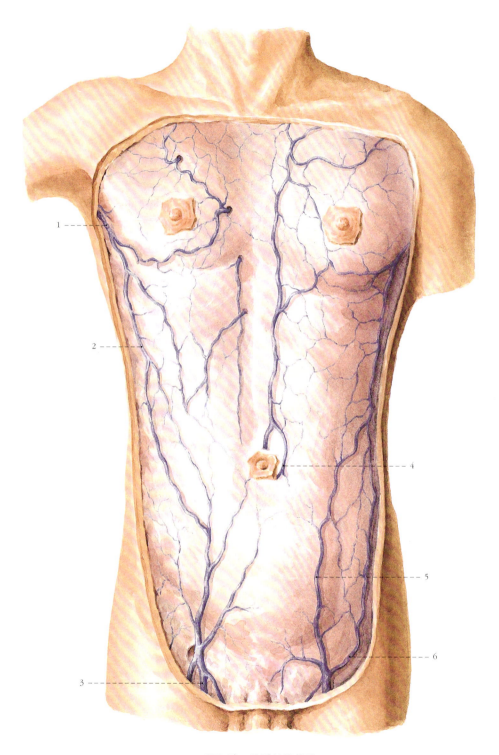

286. 胸、腹壁的浅静脉
Superficial veins of the thoracic and abdominal wall

1.胸外侧静脉 lateral thoracic vein
2.胸腹壁静脉 thoracoepigastric veins
3.大隐静脉 great saphenous vein
4.脐周围静脉网 periumbilical venous rete
5.腹壁浅静脉 superficial epigastric vein
6.旋髂浅静脉 superficial iliac circumflex vein

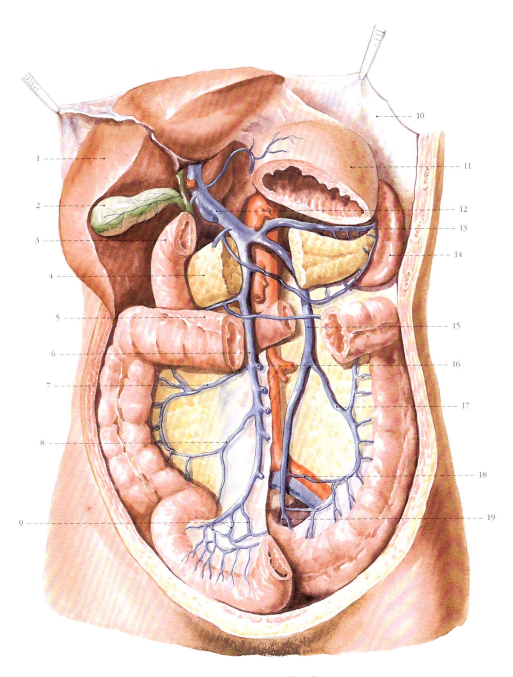

287. 肝门静脉及其属支
Hepatic portal vein and its tributaries

1.肝 liver
2.胆囊 gallbladder
3.十二指肠 duodenum
4.胰头 head of pancreas
5.横结肠 transverse colon
6.肠系膜上静脉 superior mesenteric vein
7.右结肠静脉 right colic vein

8.回结肠静脉 ileocolic vein
9.回肠静脉 ileal veins
10.膈 diaphragm
11.胃 stomach
12.肝门静脉 hepatic portal
  vein
13.脾静脉 splenic vein

14.脾 spleen
15.肠系膜下静脉 inferior mesenteric vein
16.空肠静脉（断端）jejunal veins
  (cutting end)
17.左结肠静脉 left colic vein
18.乙状结肠静脉 sigmoid veins
19.直肠上静脉 superior rectal vein

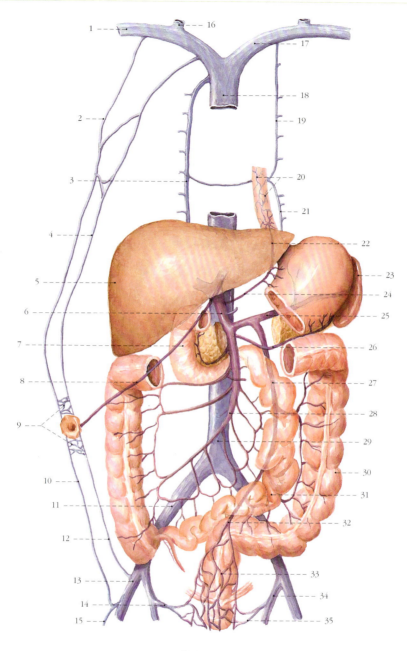

288. 肝门静脉和门腔静脉吻合
Hepatic portal vein and portacaval anastomosis

1.锁骨下静脉 subclavian vein
2.胸腹壁静脉 thoracoepigastric vein
3.奇静脉 azygos vein
4.腹壁上静脉 superior epigastric vein
5.肝 liver
6.肝门静脉 hepatic portal vein
7.十二指肠 duodenum
8.附脐静脉 paraumbilical vein
9.脐周静脉网 periumbilical venous rete
10.腹壁浅静脉 superficial epigastric vein
11.髂总静脉 common iliac vein
12.腹壁下静脉 inferior epigastric vein

13.髂外静脉 external iliac vein
14.直肠下静脉 inferior rectal vein
15.大隐静脉 great saphenous vein
16.颈内静脉 internal jugular vein
17.头臂静脉 brachiocephalic vein
18.上腔静脉 superior vena cava
19.副半奇静脉 accessory hemiazygos vein
20.食管静脉丛 esophageal venous plexus
21.半奇静脉 hemiazygos vein
22.食管支 esophageal branch
23.脾 spleen
24.胃左静脉 left gastric vein

25.脾静脉 splenic vein
26.胃网膜左、右静脉 left and right gastroepiploic veins
27.肠系膜下静脉 inferior mesenteric vein
28.肠系膜上静脉 superior mesenteric vein
29.下腔静脉 inferior vena cava
30.结肠 colon
31.小肠 small intestine
32.直肠上静脉 superior rectal vein
33.直肠静脉丛 rectal venous plexus
34.髂内静脉 internal iliac vein
35.肛静脉 anal vein

1.旋髂浅静脉 superficial iliac circumflex vein
2.股静脉 femoral vein
3.股外侧浅静脉 lateral superficial femoral vein
4.足背静脉网 dorsal venous rete of foot
5.腹壁浅静脉 superficial epigastric vein
6.阴部外浅静脉 external pudendal veins
7.大隐静脉 great saphenous vein
8.股内侧浅静脉 medial superficial femoral vein
9.内踝 medial malleolus
10.足背静脉弓 dorsal venous arch of foot
11.腘静脉 popliteal vein
12.小隐静脉 small saphenous vein
13.外踝 lateral malleolus

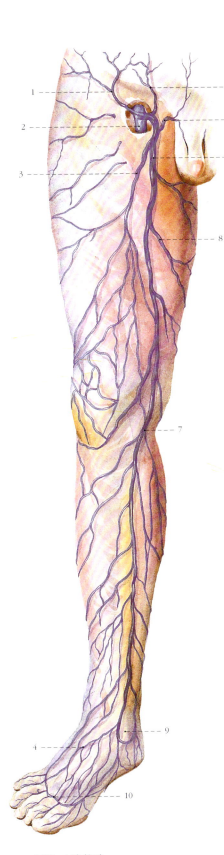

289. 大隐静脉
The great saphenous vein

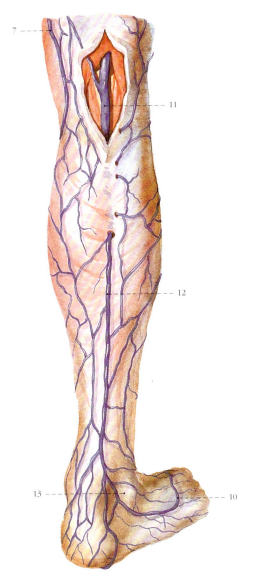

290. 小隐静脉
The small saphenous vein

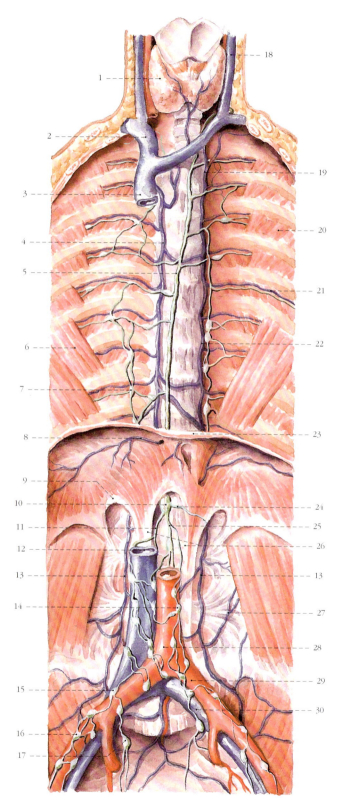

291. 体腔后壁淋巴结和淋巴导管

Lymph nodes and lymphatic ducts of the posterior wall of the coelom

1.甲状腺 thyroid gland

2.头臂静脉 brachiocephalic vein

3.上腔静脉 superior vena cava

4.奇静脉 azygos vein

5.胸导管 thoracic duct

6.肋下肌 subcostales

7.肋间淋巴结 intercostal lymph nodes

8.膈下静脉 inferior phrenic veins

9.内侧弓状韧带 medial arcuate ligament

10.乳糜池 cisterna chyli

11.右腰干 right lumbar trunk

12.下腔静脉 inferior vena cava

13.腰升静脉 ascending lumbar vein

14.腰淋巴结 lumbar lymph nodes

15.髂总淋巴结 common iliac lymph nodes

16.髂外淋巴结 external iliac lymph nodes

17.髂内淋巴结 internal iliac lymph nodes

18.颈内静脉 internal jugular vein

19.副半奇静脉 accessory hemiazygos vein

20.肋间内肌 intercostales interni

21.肋间后静脉 posterior intercostal veins

22.半奇静脉 hemiazygos vein

23.膈 diaphragm

24.肠干 intestinal trunks

25.左腰干 left lumbar trunk

26.右、左脚 right, left crus of diaphragm

27.腰静脉 lumbar veins

28.腹主动脉 abdominal aorta

29.髂总动脉 common iliac artery

30.髂总静脉 common iliac vein

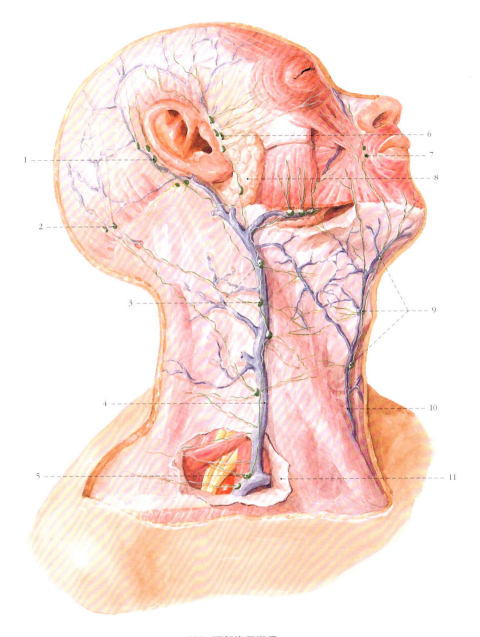

292. 颈部浅层淋巴
Superficial cervical lymph

1.耳后淋巴结 posterior auricular lymph nodes

2.枕淋巴结 occipital lymph nodes

3.颈外侧浅淋巴结 superficial lateral cervical lymph modes

4.颈外静脉 external jugular vein

5.锁骨上淋巴结 supraclavicular lymph nodes

6.腮腺浅淋巴结 superficial parotid lymph nodes

7.颊肌淋巴结 buccal lymph nodes

8.腮腺 parotid gland

9.颈前浅淋巴结 superficial anterior cervical lymph nodes

10.颈前静脉 anterior jugular vein

11.封套筋膜（颈深筋膜浅层）investing layer of cervical fascia（superficial layer of deep cervical fascia）

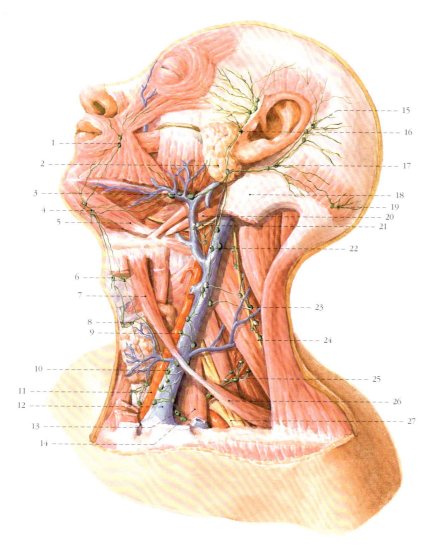

293. 颈部深层淋巴
Deep cervical lymph

1.颊肌淋巴结 buccal lymph nodes
2.腮腺 parotid gland
3.面静脉 facial vein
4.颏下淋巴结 submental lymph nodes
5.二腹肌前腹 anterior belly of digastric
6.喉前淋巴结 prelaryngeal lymph nodes
7.肩胛舌骨肌上腹 superior belly of omohyoid
8.甲状腺淋巴结 thyroid lymph nodes
9.颈内静脉肩胛舌骨肌淋巴结 juguloomohyoid lymph nodes
10.颈外侧下深淋巴结 inferior deep lateral cervical lymph nodes
11.颈总动脉 common carotid artery
12.颈内静脉 internal jugular vein
13.锁骨上淋巴结 supraclavicular lymph nodes
14.前斜角肌 anterior scalene muscle

15.耳后淋巴结 posterior auricular lymph nodes
16.腮腺浅淋巴结 superficial parotid lymph nodes
17.乳突淋巴结 mastoid lymph nodes
18.胸锁乳突肌 sternocleidomastoid
19.枕淋巴结 occipital lymph nodes
20.二腹肌后腹 posterior belly of digastric
21.舌下神经 hypoglossal nerve
22.颈内静脉二腹肌淋巴结 jugulodigastric lymph nodes
23.副神经淋巴结 lymph nodes along accessory nerve
24.副神经 accessory nerve
25.颈横动脉淋巴结 lymph nodes along transverse cervical artery
26.肩胛舌骨肌下腹 inferior belly of omohyoid
27.臂丛 brachial plexus

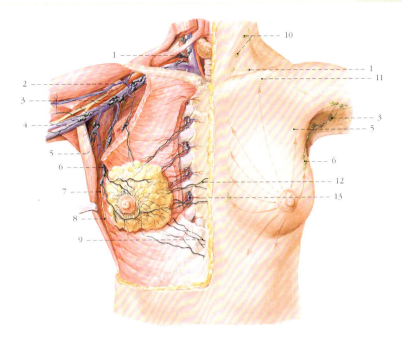

294. 腋窝、乳腺的淋巴管和淋巴结
The lymphatic vessels and the lymph nodes of the axilla and the mammary glands

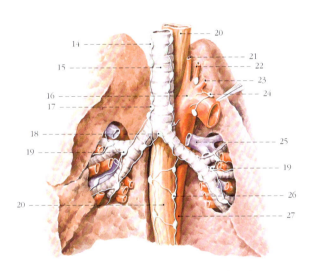

295. 气管、支气管和肺部的淋巴结
Lymph nodes of the trachea, the bronchi and the lungs

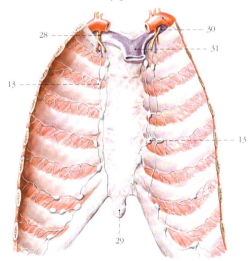

296. 胸骨旁淋巴结
The parasternal lymph nodes

1.锁骨上淋巴结 supraclavicular lymph nodes
2.尖淋巴结 apical lymph nodes
3.中央淋巴结 central lymph nodes
4.肩胛下淋巴结 subscapular lymph nodes
5.胸肌间淋巴结 interpectoral lymph nodes
6.胸肌淋巴结 pectoral lymph nodes
7.胸外侧动脉 lateral thoracic artery
8.胸长神经 long thoracic nerve
9.至肝的淋巴管 lymphatic vessels to liver
10.颈深淋巴结 deep cervical lymph nodes
11.锁骨下淋巴结 subclavicular lymph nodes
12.至对侧乳腺的淋巴管 lymphatic vessels to contralateral mammary gland

13.胸骨旁淋巴结 parasternal lymph nodes
14.气管旁淋巴结 paratracheal lymph nodes
15.气管 trachea
16.主动脉弓 aortic arch
17.气管、支气管上淋巴结 superior tracheobronchial lymph nodes
18.气管、支气管下淋巴结 inferior tracheobronchial lymph nodes
19.支气管肺门淋巴结 bronchopulmonary hilar lymph nodes
20.食管 esophagus
21.左锁骨下动脉 left subclavian artery

22.左颈总动脉 left common carotid artery
23.头臂干 brachiocephalic trunk
24.主动脉弓淋巴结 lymph nodes of aortic arch
25.左肺动脉 left pulmonary artery
26.纵隔后淋巴结 posterior mediastinal lymph nodes
27.胸主动脉 thoracic aorta
28.胸廓内动、静脉 internal thoracic artery and veins
29.剑突 xiphoid process
30.锁骨下动脉、静脉 subclavian artery and vein
31.上腔静脉 superior vena cava

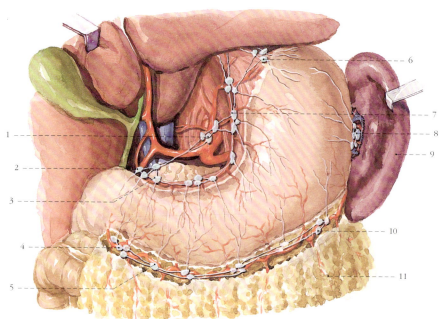

1

2

3

4

5

6

7

8

9

10

11

297. 胃的淋巴（前面观）
Lymph of stomach (anterior aspect)

1.腹腔淋巴结 celiac lymph nodes

2.幽门上淋巴结 suprapyloric lymph nodes

3.胃右淋巴结 right gastric lymph nodes

4.幽门下淋巴结 subpyloric lymph nodes

5.胃网膜右淋巴结 right gastroomental lymph nodes

6.贲门淋巴环 cardiac lymph ring

7.胃左淋巴结 left gastric lymph nodes

8.脾淋巴结 splenic lymph nodes

9.脾 spleen

10.胃网膜左淋巴结 left gastroomental lymph nodes

11.大网膜 greater omentum

12.肠系膜上淋巴结 superior mesenteric lymph nodes

13.胰上淋巴结 superior pancreatic lymph nodes

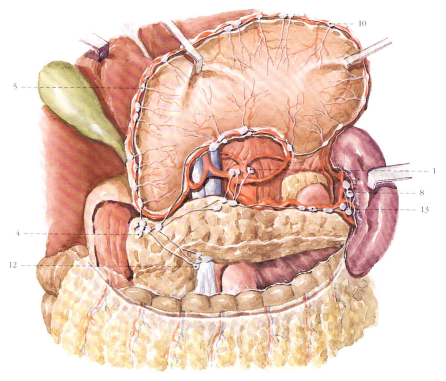

5

10

1

8

13

4

12

298. 胃的淋巴（后面观）
Lymph of stomach (posterior aspect)

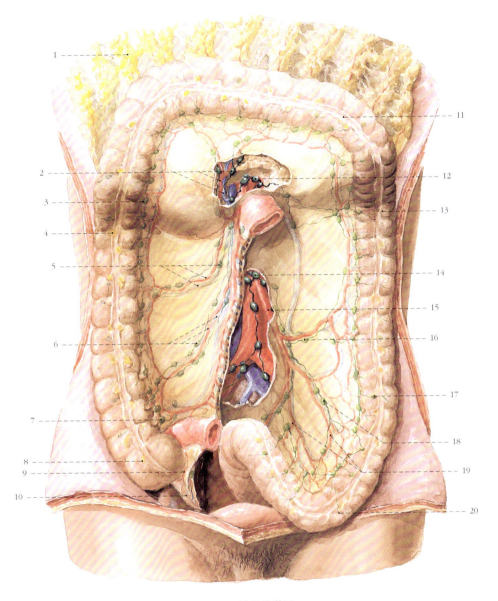

299. 结肠的淋巴
Lymph of colon

1.大网膜 greater omentum
2.中结肠动、静脉及淋巴结 middle colic artery, vein and lymph nodes
3.结肠旁淋巴结 paracolic lymph nodes
4.结肠右曲 right colic flexure
5.右结肠动、静脉及淋巴结 right colic artery, vein and lymph nodes
6.回结肠动、静脉及淋巴结 ileocolic artery, vein and lymph nodes
7.盲肠前淋巴结 prececal lymph nodes
8.盲肠 cecum
9.阑尾动脉 appendicular artery
10.阑尾 vermiform appendix

11.独立带 free band
12.肠系膜上淋巴结 superior mesenteric lymph nodes
13.结肠左曲 left colic flexure
14.肠系膜下淋巴结 inferior mesenteric lymph nodes
15.肠系膜下动脉 inferior mesenteric artery
16.左结肠动脉淋巴结 lymph nodes of left colic artery
17.结肠上淋巴结 superior colic lymph nodes
18.乙状结肠淋巴结 sigmoid lymph nodes
19.乙状结肠动脉 sigmoid artery
20.乙状结肠 sigmoid colon

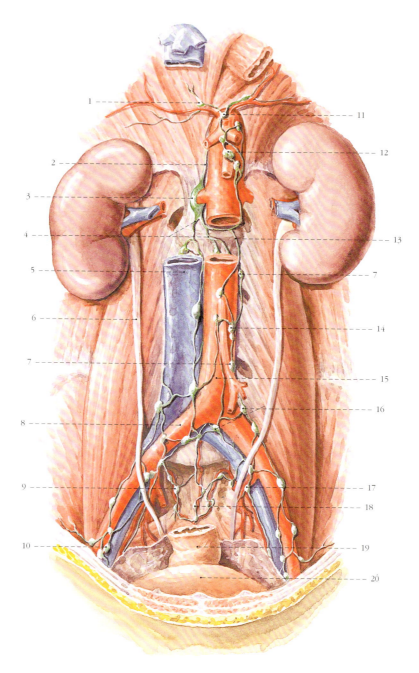

300. 腹膜后隙的淋巴
The lymph of the retroperitoneal space

1.膈下淋巴结 inferior phrenic lymph nodes
2.胸导管 thoracic duct
3.乳糜池 cisterna chyli
4.左、右腰干 left and right lumbar trunk
5.下腔静脉 inferior vena cava
6.右输尿管 right ureter
7.腰淋巴结 lumbar lymph node
8.髂总动脉 common iliac artery

9.骶外侧淋巴结 laterat sacral lymph nodes
10.髂外淋巴结 external iliac lymph nodes
11.腹腔淋巴结 celiac lymph nodes
12.肠系膜上淋巴结 superior mesenteric lymph nodes
13.肠干 intestinal trunks
14.肠系膜下淋巴结 inferior mesenteric lymph nodes

15.腹主动脉 abdominal aorta
16.髂总淋巴结 common iliac lymph nodes
17.髂内淋巴结 internal iliac lymph nodes
18.骶正中淋巴结 median sacral lymph nodes
19.直肠 rectum
20 膀胱 urinary bladder

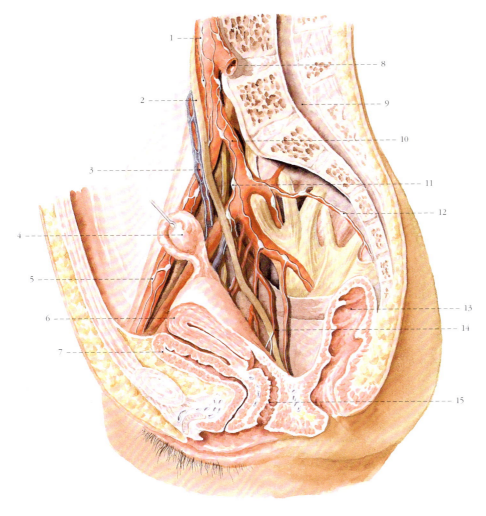

301. 女性生殖器的淋巴管和淋巴结（1）
The lymphatic vessels and lymph nodes of the female genital organs (1)

1.髂总淋巴结 common iliac lymph nodes
2.输尿管 ureter
3.卵巢动脉 ovarian artery
4.卵巢 ovary
5.髂外淋巴结 external iliac lymph nodes
6.子宫 uterus
7.膀胱 urinary bladder
8.左髂总动脉 left common iliac artery
9.骶管 sacral canal
10.髂内动脉 internal iliac artery
11.髂内淋巴结 internal iliac lymph nodes
12.骶淋巴结 sacral lymph nodes
13.直肠 rectum
14.子宫动脉 uterine artery
15.阴道 vagina
16.腰淋巴结 lumbar lymph nodes
17.髂外动脉 external iliac artery
18.闭孔淋巴结 obturator lymph nodes

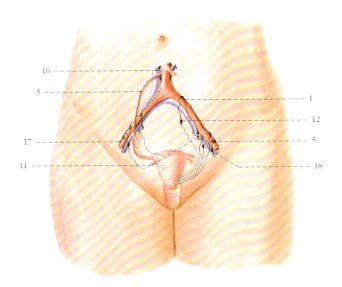

302. 女性生殖器的淋巴管和淋巴结（2）
The lymphatic vessels and lymph nodes of the female genital organs (2)

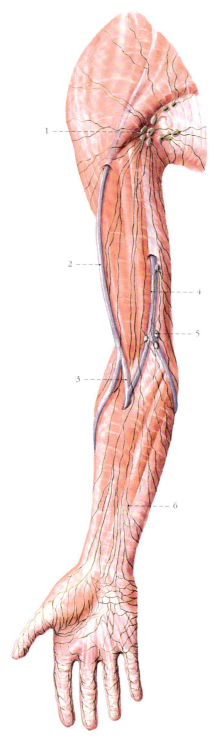

303. 上肢浅部淋巴管和淋巴结
Superficial lymphatic vessels and lymph nodes of upper limb

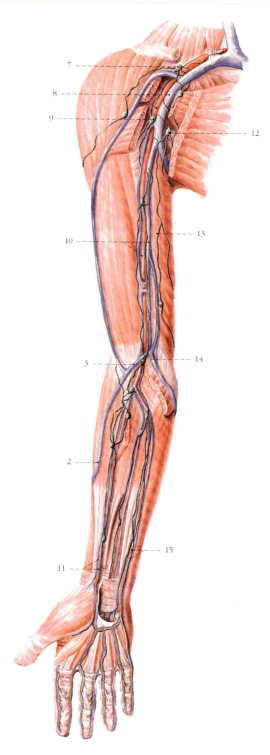

304. 上肢深部淋巴管和淋巴结
Deep lymphatic vessels and lymph nodes of upper limb

1.腋淋巴结 axillary lymph nodes
2.头静脉 cephalic vein
3.肘正中静脉 median cubital vein
4.贵要静脉 basilic vein
5.肘浅淋巴结 superficial cubital lymph nodes

6.淋巴管 lymphatic vessel
7.尖淋巴结 apical lymph nodes
8.腋动、静脉 axillary artery and vein
9.外侧淋巴结 lateral lymph nodes
10.肱动、静脉 brachial artery and veins

11.桡动、静脉 radial artery and veins
12.中央淋巴结 central lymph nodes
13.深淋巴管 deep lymphatic vessels
14.肘深淋巴结 deep cubital lymph nodes
15.尺动、静脉 ulnar artery and veins

1.腹股沟上浅淋巴结 superior superficial inguinal lymph nodes
2.大隐静脉 great saphenous vein
3.浅淋巴管 superficial lymphatic vessel
4.腹股沟下浅淋巴结 inferior superficial inguinal lymph nodes
5.内踝 medial malleolus
6.输尿管 ureter
7.髂总淋巴结 common iliac lymph nodes
8.髂外淋巴结 external iliac lymph nodes
9.腹股沟深淋巴结 deep inguinal lymph nodes
10.股动、静脉 femoral artery and vein
11.腹主动脉 abdominal aorta
12.髂内淋巴结 internal iliac lymph nodes
13.腹股沟浅淋巴结 superficial inguinal lymph nodes

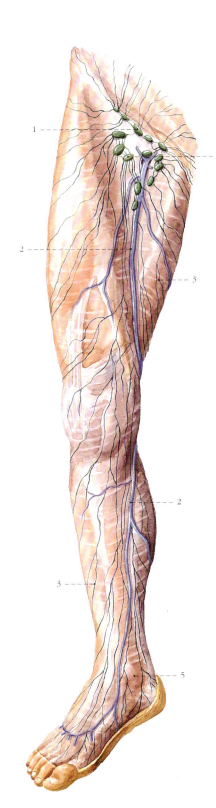

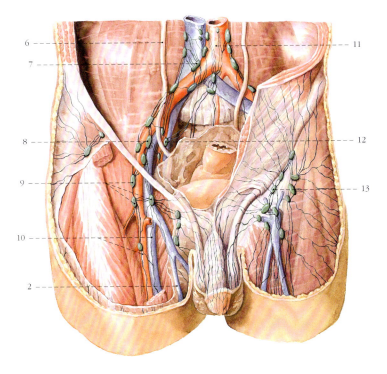

306. 腹股沟深部淋巴结
Deep inguinal lymph nodes

305. 下肢浅部淋巴管和淋巴结
Superficial lymphatic vessels and lymph nodes of lower limb

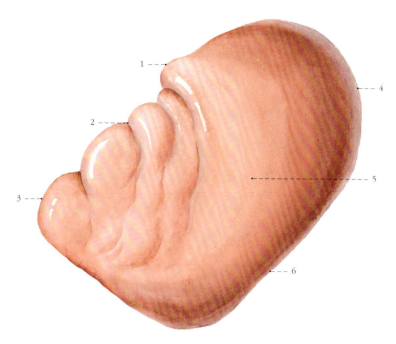

307. 脾（膈面）
Spleen (diaphragmatic surface)

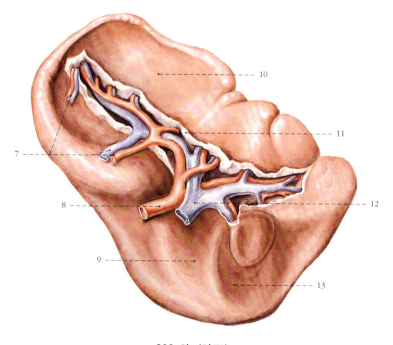

308. 脾（脏面）
Spleen (visceral surface)

1.上缘 superior border
2.脾切迹 splenic notch
3.前端 anterior extremity
4.后端 posterior extremity
5.膈面 diaphragmatic surface
6.下缘 inferior border
7.胃短动、静脉 short gastric artery and vein
8.脾动脉 splenic artery
9.肾面 renal surface
10.胃面 gastric surface
11.脾门 hilum of spleen
12.脾静脉 splenic vein
13.结肠面 colic surface

SENSATIVE ORGANS
感觉器官

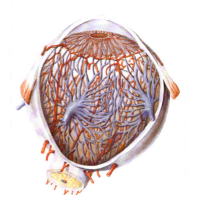

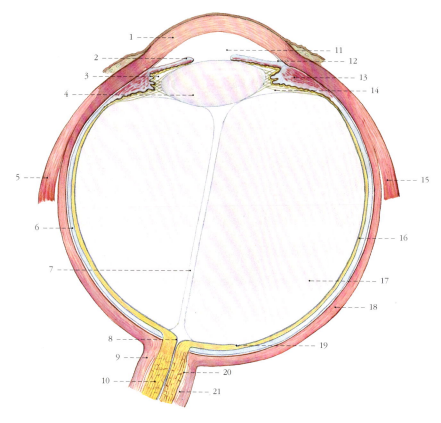

309. 眼球水平切面（模式图）
Horizontal section of the eyeball (diagram)

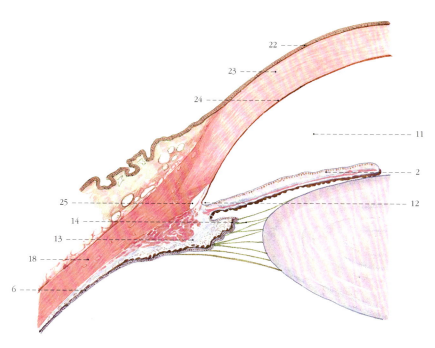

310. 眼球前部水平切面（虹膜、睫状体、晶状体切面）
Horizontal section of the anterior part of the eyeball
(section through iris, ciliary body and lens)

1.角膜 cornea
2.虹膜 iris
3.眼后房 posterior chamber
4.晶状体 lens
5.内直肌 medial rectus
6.脉络膜 choroid
7.玻璃体管 hyaloid canal
8.视神经盘 optic disc
9.硬脑膜 cerebral dura mater
10.视神经 optic nerve
11.眼前房 anterior chamber
12.虹膜角膜角 iridocorneal angle
13.睫状体 ciliary body
14.睫状小带 ciliary zonule
15.外直肌 lateral rectus
16.视网膜 retina
17.玻璃体 vitreous body
18.巩膜 sclera
19.中央凹 fovea centralis
20.软脑膜 cerebral pia mater
21.蛛网膜下腔 subarachoid space
22.前上皮 anterior epithelium
23.角膜固有层 lamina propria of cornea
24.后上皮 posterior epithelium
25.巩膜静脉窦 sinus venosus sclerae

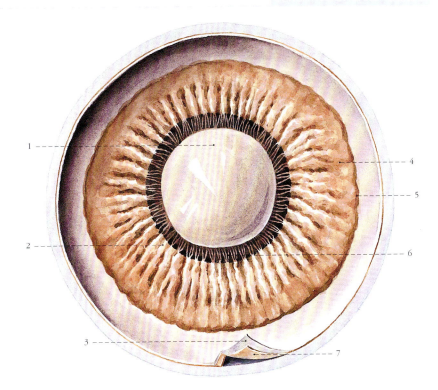

311. 眼球前部（内面观）
Anterior part of the eyeball (internal aspect)

1.晶状体　lens
2.睫状突　ciliary processes
3.视网膜　retina
4.睫状环　ciliary ring
5.锯状缘　ora serrata
6.睫状小带　ciliary zonule
7.脉络膜　choroid
8.视网膜颞侧上小动脉　superior temporal arteriole of retina
9.黄斑　macula lutea
10.视网膜颞侧下小动脉　inferior temporal arteriole of retina
11.视网膜鼻侧上小动脉　superior nasal arteriole of retina
12.视神经盘　optic disc
13.视网膜鼻侧下小动脉　inferior nasal arteriole of retina
14.巩膜　sclera

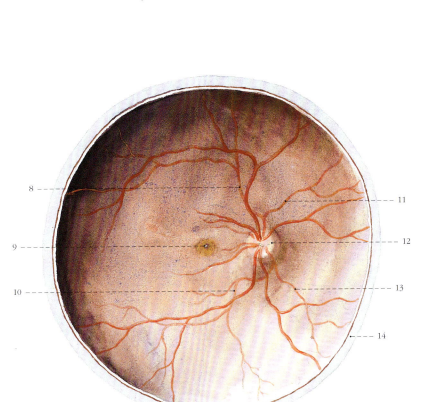

312. 眼球后部（内面观）
Posterior part of the eyeball (internal aspect)

151

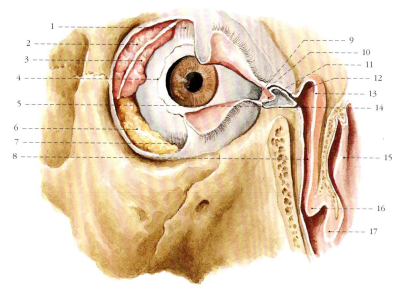

313. 右侧泪器（前面观）
Right lacrimal apparatus (anterior aspect)

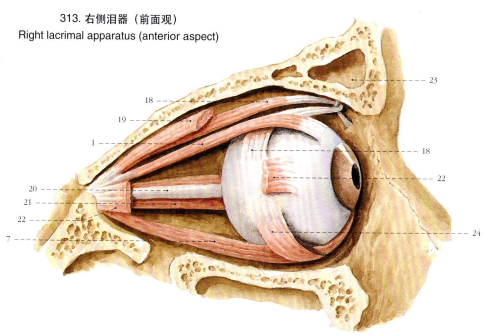

314.眼球外肌（外侧面观）
The ocular muscles (lateral aspect)

1.上直肌 superior rectus
2.泪腺眶部 orbital part of lacrimal gland
3.泪腺睑部 palpebral part of lacrimal gland
4.球结膜 bulbar conjunctiva
5.下泪点 lower lacrimal punctum
6.眶脂体 adipose body of orbit
7.下直肌 inferior rectus
8.鼻泪管 nasolacrimal duct

9.结膜半月襞 conjunctival semilunar fold
10.上泪点 upper lacrimal punctum
11.泪阜 lacrimal caruncle
12.上泪小管 upper lacrimal ductule
13.泪囊 lacrimal sac
14.下泪小管 lower lacrimal ductule
15.中鼻甲 middle nasal concha
16.泪襞 lacrimal fold

17.下鼻甲 inferior nasal concha
18.上斜肌 superior obliquus
19.上睑提肌 levator palpebrae superioris
20.视神经 optic nerve
21.内直肌 medial rectus
22.外直肌 lateral rectus
23.额窦 frontal sinus
24.下斜肌 inferior obliquus

1.上睑提肌 levator palpebrae superioris
2.角膜 cornea
3.视神经 optic nerve
4.眼球鞘 sheath of eyeball
5.结膜上穹 superior conjunctival fornix
6.睑结膜 palpebral conjunctiva
7.睑板腺 tarsal glands
8.眼轮匝肌 orbicularis oculi
9.上睑板 superior tarsus
10.晶状体 lens
11.下睑板 inferior tarsus
12.球结膜 bulbar conjunctiva
13.结膜下穹 inferior conjunctival fornix
14.上斜肌 superior obliquus
15.内直肌 medial rectus
16.上睑提肌（断端）levator palpebrae superioris
   (cutting end)
17.眼球 eyebll
18.上直肌 superior rectus
19.下直肌 inferior rectus
20.外直肌 lateral rectus
21.视交叉 optic chiasma
22.眶上动脉 supraorbital artery
23.泪腺 lacrimal gland
24.泪腺动脉 lacrimal artery
25.睫后长、短动脉 long and short posterior
   ciliary arteries
26.眼动脉 ophthalmic artery
27.颈内动脉 internal carotid artery

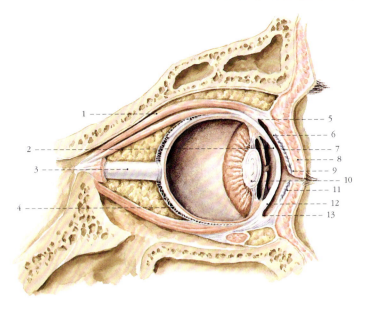

315. 右侧眼球及眶矢状切面
Sagittal section through the right eyeball and orbital cavity

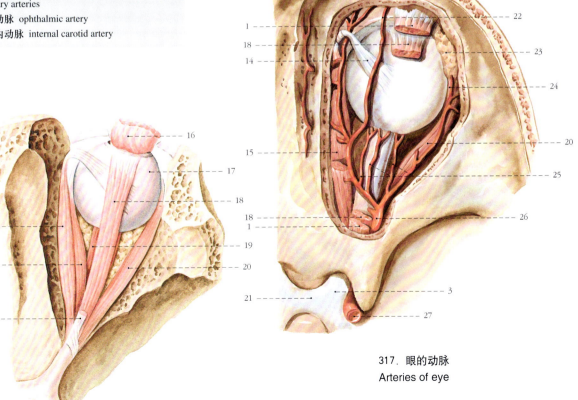

316. 眼球外肌（上面观）
Extraocular muscles (superior aspect)

317. 眼的动脉
Arteries of eye

153

1.角膜 cornea
2.虹膜大环 greater ring of iris
3.脉络膜 choroid
4.涡静脉 vorticose veins
5.睫后长动脉 long posterior ciliary arteries
6.睫后短动脉 short posterior ciliary arteries
7.瞳孔 pupil
8.虹膜小环 lesser ring of iris
9.巩膜 sclera

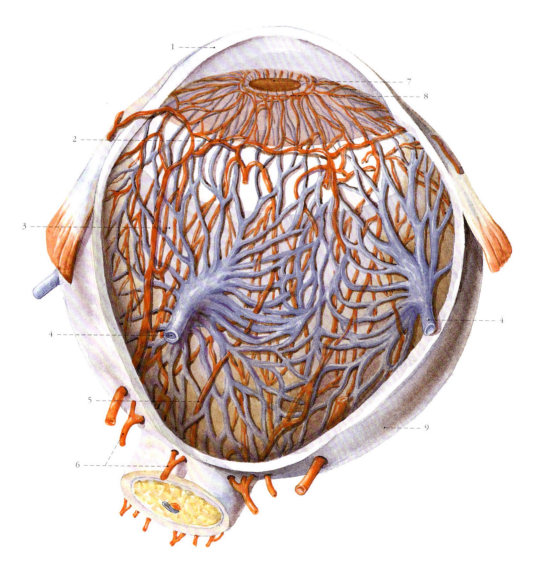

318. 眼球的血管
Blood vessels of eyeball

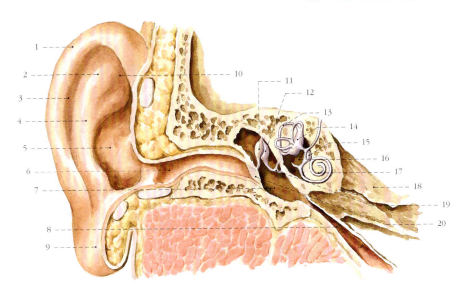

319. 前庭蜗器（切面）
Vestibulocochlear organ (section)

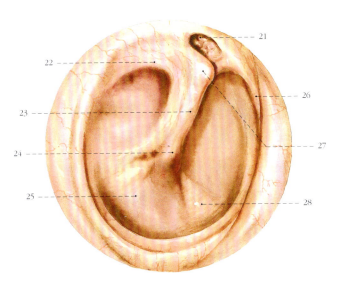

320. 右侧鼓膜（外侧面观）
Right tympanic membrane (lateral aspect)

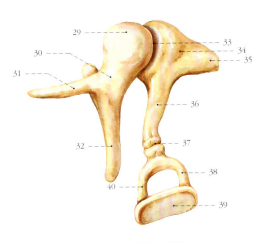

321. 右侧听小骨
Right auditory ossicles

1.耳轮 helix
2.对耳轮脚 crura of antihelix
3.耳舟 scapha
4.对耳轮 antihelix
5.耳甲 auricular concha
6.外耳道 external acoustic meatus
7.鼓室 tympanic cavity
8.咽鼓管 auditory tube
9.耳垂 auricular lobule
10.三角窝 triangular fossa
11.锤骨 malleus
12.砧骨 incus
13.骨半规管 bony semicircular canals

14.椭圆囊 utricle
15.球囊 saccule
16.前庭 vestibule
17.耳蜗 cochlea
18.岩部（锥体） petrous part
19.镫骨 stapes
20.鼓膜 tympanic membrane
21.松弛部 flaccid part
22.锤骨后襞 posterior malleolar fold
23.锤纹 malleolar stria
24.鼓膜脐 umbo of tympanic membrane
25.紧张部 tense part
26.锤骨前襞 anterior malleolar fold
27.锤凸 malleolar prominence

28.反射光锥 reflective cone of light
29.锤骨头 head of malleus
30.锤骨颈 neck of malleus
31.前突 anterior process
32.锤骨柄 manubrium of malleus
33.砧锤关节 incudomalleal joint
34.砧骨体 body of incus
35.短脚 short crus
36.长脚 long crus
37.砧镫关节 incudostapedial joint
38.后脚 posterior crus
39.镫骨底 base of stapes
40.前脚 anterior crus

155

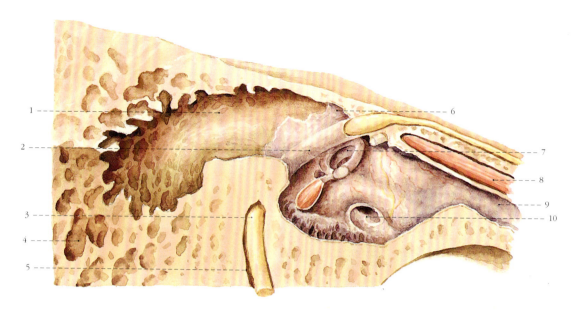

322. 右侧鼓室（内侧壁）
Right tympanic cavity (medial walls)

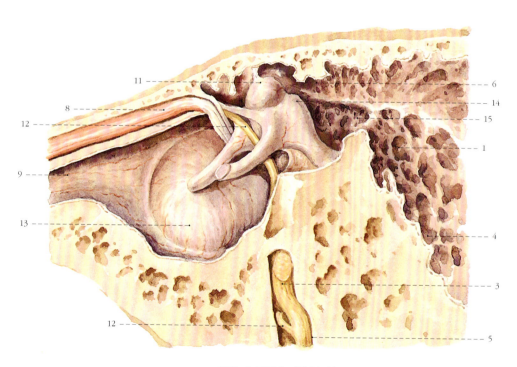

323. 右侧鼓室（外侧壁）
Right tympanic cavity (lateral walls)

1.乳突窦 mastoid antrum
2.面神经管凸 prominence of facial canal
3.面神经 facial nerve
4.乳突小房 mastoid cells
5.面神经管 facial canal
6.鼓室上隐窝 epitympanic recess
7.前庭窗 fenestra vestibuli
8.鼓膜张肌 tensor tympani
9.咽鼓管 auditory tube
10.蜗窗 fenestra cochleae
11.锤骨 malleus
12.鼓索 chorda tympani
13.鼓膜 tympanic membrane
14.砧骨 incus
15.乳突窦入口 entrance to mastoid antrum

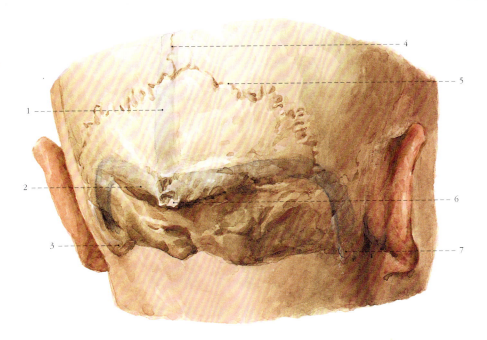

324. 矢状窦、横窦和乙状窦的体表投影
The surface projection of the sagittal sinus, transverse sinus
and the sigmoid sinus

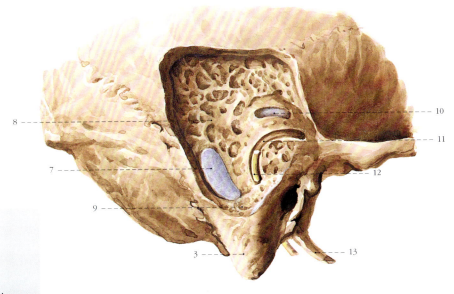

1.上矢状窦 superior sagittal sinus
2.横窦 transverse sinus
3.乳突 mastoid process
4.矢状缝 sagittal suture
5.人字缝 lambdoid suture
6.枕外隆凸 external occipital protuberance
7.乙状窦 sigmoid sinus
8.颞骨 temporal bone
9.乳突小房 mastoid cells
10.外膜半规管 lateral semicircular duct
11.面神经管 facial canal
12.面神经 facial nerve
13.茎突 styloid process

325. 乳突、乙状窦和面神经的关系
Relations among the mastoid process, sigmoid sinus
and the facial nerve

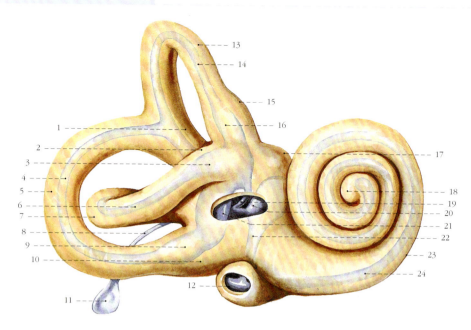

326. 右侧骨迷路和膜迷路（前外侧面观）
Right bony labyrinth and membranous labyrinth (anterior lateral aspect)

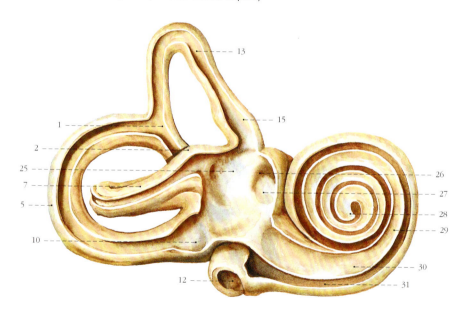

327. 右侧骨迷路内腔
Internal cavity of the right osseous labyrinth

1.总骨脚 common bony crus
2.外骨壶腹 lateral bony ampulla
3.外膜壶腹 lateral membranous ampulla
4.后膜半规管 posterior semicircular duct
5.后骨半规管 posterior semicircular canal
6.外膜半规管 lateral semicircular duct
7.外骨半规管 laternal semicircular canal
8.内淋巴管 endolymphatic duct
9.后膜壶腹 posterior membranous ampulla
10.后骨壶腹 posterior bony ampulla

11.内淋巴囊 endolymphatic sac
12.蜗窗 fenestra cochleae
13.前骨半规管 anterior semicircular canal
14.前膜半规管 anterior semicircular ducts
15.前骨壶腹 anterior bony ampulla
16.前膜壶腹 anterior membranous ampulla
17.前庭 vestibule
18.蜗顶 cupula of cochlea
19.椭圆球囊管 utriculosaccular duct
20.球囊 saccule

21.椭圆囊 utricle
22.连合管 ductus reuniens
23.耳蜗 cochlea
24.蜗管 cochlear duct
25.椭圆囊隐窝 elliptical recess
26.前庭嵴 vestibular crest
27.球囊隐窝 spherical recess
28.螺旋板沟 hamulus of spiral lamina
29.骨螺旋板 osseous spiral lamina
30.前庭阶 scala vestibuli
31.鼓阶 scala tympani

NERVOUS AND ENDOCRINE SYSTEMS

神经和内分泌系统

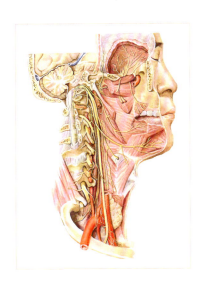

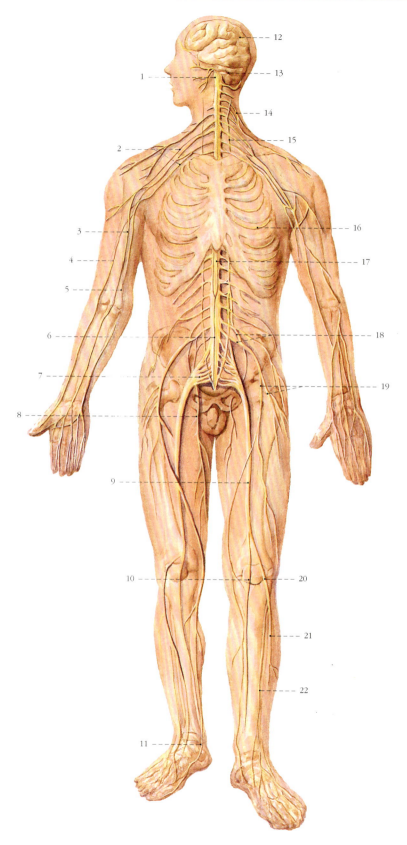

1.脑干 brain stem
2.臂丛 brachial plexus
3.正中神经 median nerve
4.桡神经 radial nerve
5.尺神经 ulnar nerve
6.终丝 filum terminale
7.骶丛 sacral plexus
8.闭孔神经 obturator nerve
9.坐骨神经 sciatic nerve
10.胫神经 tibial nerve
11.隐神经 saphenous nerve
12.大脑 cerebrum
13.小脑 cerebellum
14.颈丛 cervical plexus
15.交感干 sympathetic trunk
16.肋间神经 intercostal nerve
17.脊髓 spinal cord
18.腰丛 lumbar plexus
19.股神经 femoral nerve
20.腓总神经 common peroneal nerve
21.腓浅神经 superficial peroneal nerve
22.腓深神经 deep peroneal nerve

328. 神经系统概观
General view of the nervous system

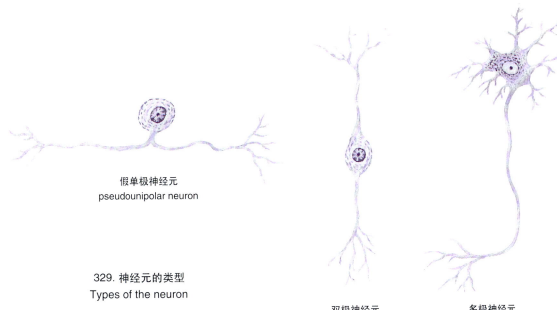

假单极神经元
pseudounipolar neuron

329. 神经元的类型
Types of the neuron

双极神经元
bipolar neuron

多极神经元
multipolar neuron

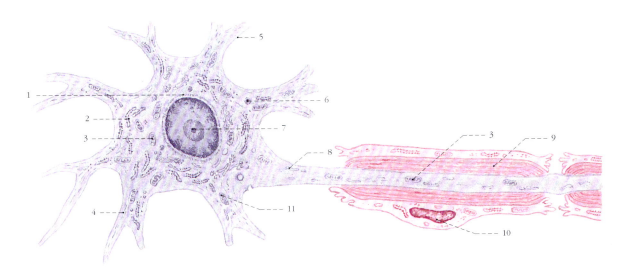

330. 神经元的结构（电镜模式图）
Structure of the neuron (electron microscopic diagram)

1.核膜 nuclear membrane
2.粗面内质网 rough endoplasmic reticulum
3.线粒体 mitochondrion
4.微丝 microfilament
5.树突 dendrite
6.溶酶体 lysosome
7.核仁 nucleolus
8.滑面内质网 smooth endoplasmic reticulum
9.髓鞘 myelin sheath
10.施万细胞核 nucleus of Schwann cell
11.小泡 vesicle

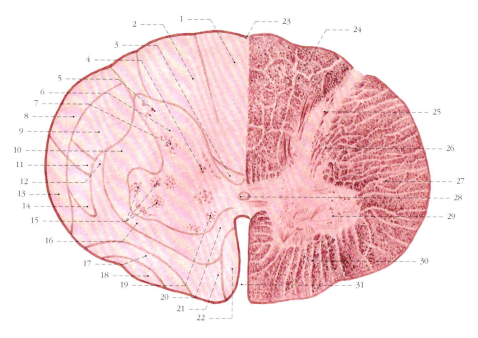

331. 脊髓颈段横切面
Transverse section through cervical segment of spinal cord

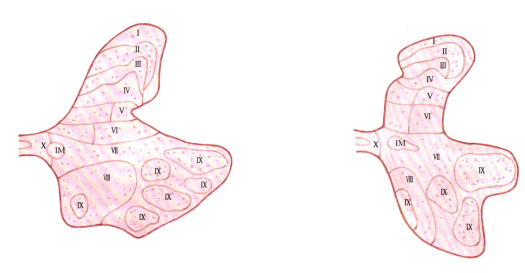

332. 脊髓的细胞构筑分层
Cytoarchitectonic layers of the spinal cord

1.薄束 fasciculus gracilis
2.楔束 fasciculus cuneatus
3.后固有束 posterior fasciculus proprius
4.胸核 nucleus thoracicus
5.后角边缘核 marginal nucleus
6.胶状质 substantia gelatinosa
7.后角固有核 nucleus proprius
8.脊髓小脑后束 posterior spinocerebellar tract
9.皮质脊髓侧束 lateral corticospinal tract
10.外侧固有束 lateral fasciculus proprius
11.红核脊髓束 rubrospinal tract

12.网状脊髓束 reticulospinal tract
13.脊髓小脑前束 arterior spinocerebellar tract
14.脊髓丘脑侧束 lateral spinothalamic tract
15.外侧运动核 lateral motor nucleus
16.前固有束 anterior fasciculus proprius
17.前庭脊髓束 vestibulospinal tract
18.脊髓丘脑前束 anterior spinothalamic tract
19.内侧运动核 medial motor nucleus
20.内侧纵束 medial longitudinal fasciculus
21.顶盖脊髓束 tectospinal tract
22.皮质脊髓前束 anterior corticospinal tract

23.后正中沟 posterior median sulcus
24.后索 posterior funiculus
25.后角 posterior horn
26.网状结构 reticular formation
27.外侧索 lateral funiculus
28.中央管 central canal
29.前角 anterior horn
30.前索 anterior funiculus
31.前正中裂 anterior median fissure

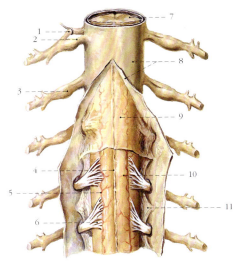

333. 脊髓的被膜（后面观）
Capsules of spinal cord
(posterior aspect)

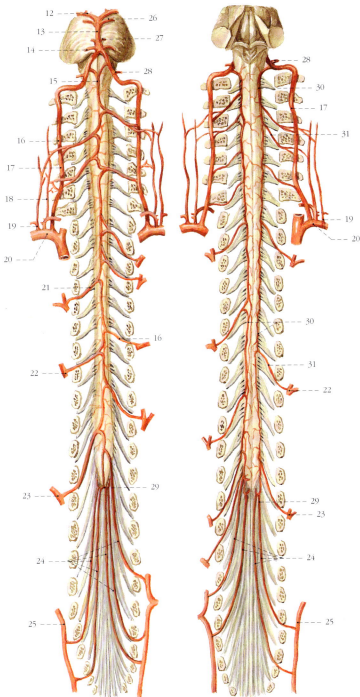

334. 脊髓的动脉
Arteries of spinal cord

1.前根　anterior root
2.后根　posterior root
3.脊神经节　spinal ganglia
4.后正中沟　posterior median sulcus
5.后外侧沟　posterolateral sulcus
6.后根纤维　posterior radicular fibers
7.脊髓　spinal cord
8.硬脊膜　spinal dura mater
9.蛛网膜　arachnoid mater
10.软脊膜　spinal pia mater
11.齿状韧带　denticulate ligament
12.大脑后动脉　posterior cerebral artery
13.基底动脉　basilar artery
14.小脑下前动脉　anterior inferior cerebellar artery
15.脊髓前动脉　anterior spinal artery
16.前根动脉　anterior radicular artery
17.椎动脉　vertebral artery
18.颈升动脉　ascending cervical artery
19.颈深动脉　deep cervical artery
20.锁骨下动脉　subclavian artery
21.大前根动脉　great anterior radicular artery
22.肋间后动脉　posterior intercostal artery
23.腰动脉　lumbar artery
24.马尾动脉　caudal artery
25.骶外侧动脉　lateral sacral artery
26.小脑上动脉　superior cerebellar artery
27.迷路动脉　labyrinthine artery
28.小脑下后动脉　posterior inferior cerebellar artery
29.吻合袢（与脊髓前动脉）anastomotic ansa
30.脊髓后动脉　posterior spinal artery
31.后根动脉　posterior radicular artery

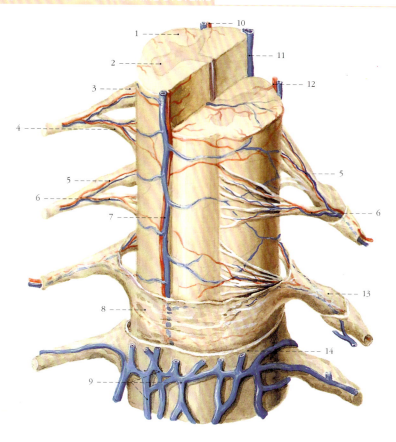

335. 脊髓的血管
Blood vessels of spinal cord

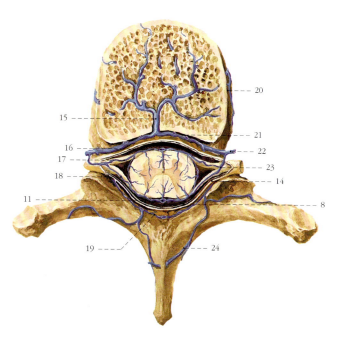

336. 脊髓的静脉
Veins of spinal cord

1.白质 white matter
2.灰质 gray matter
3.后根 posterior root
4.前根 anterior root
5.后根动、静脉 posterior radicular artery and vein
6.前根动、静脉 anterior radicular artery and vein
7.脊髓前动、静脉 anterior spinal artery and vein
8.蛛网膜 arachnoid mater
9.椎内静脉丛 internal vertebral venous plexus
10.右脊髓后动、静脉 right posterior spinal artery and vein
11.脊髓后静脉 posterior spinal vein
12.左脊髓后动、静脉 left posterior spinal artery and vein
13.脊神经节 spinal ganglia
14.硬脊膜 spinal dura mater
15.椎体静脉 basivertebral veins
16.脊髓前静脉 anterior spinal veins
17.前根静脉 anterior radicular vein
18.后根静脉 posterior radicular vein
19.椎内后静脉丛 posterior internal vertebral venous plexus
20.椎外前静脉丛 anterior external vertebral venous plexus
21.椎内前静脉丛 anterior internal vertebral venous plexus
22.椎间静脉 intervertebral vein
23.根静脉 radicular vein
24.椎外后静脉丛 posterior external vertebral venous plexus

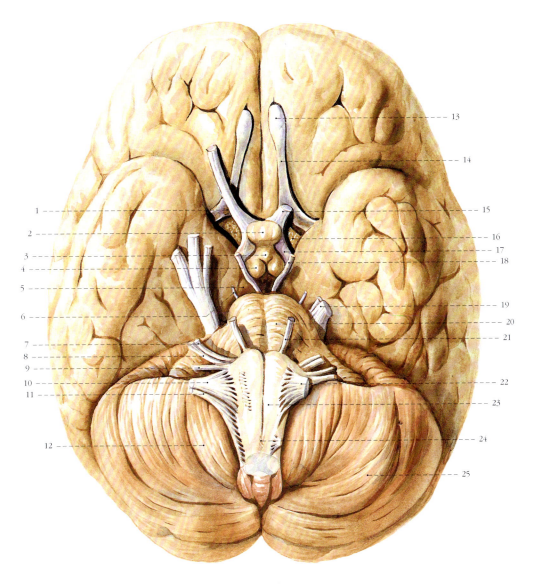

337. 脑底面
Basal surface of the brain

1.嗅三角 olfactory trigone
2.脑垂体 hypophysis
3.灰结节 tuber cinereum
4.乳头体 mamillary body
5.大脑脚 cerebral peduncle
6.滑车神经 trochlear nerve
7.面神经 facial nerve
8.前庭蜗神经 vestibulocochlear nerve
9.舌咽神经 glossopharyngeal nerve

10.迷走神经 vagus nerve
11.副神经 accessory nerve
12.小脑扁桃体 tonsil of cerebellum
13.嗅球 olfactory bulb
14.嗅束 olfactory tract
15.视神经 optic nerve
16.前穿质 anterior perforated substance
17.视束 optic tract
18.动眼神经 oculomotor nerve

19.三叉神经 trigeminal nerve
20.脑桥 pons
21.展神经 abducent nerve
22.舌下神经 hypoglossal nerve
23.锥体 pyramid
24.锥体交叉 decussation of pyramid
25.小脑 cerebellum

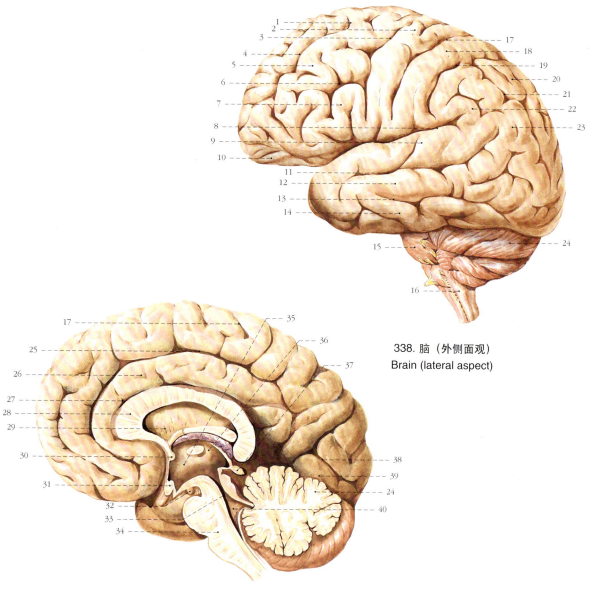

338. 脑（外侧面观）
Brain (lateral aspect)

339. 脑（内侧面观）
Brain (medial aspect)

1.额上回 superior frontal gyrus
2.中央前回 precentral gyrus
3.中央前沟 precentral sulcus
4.额上沟 superior frontal sulcus
5.额中回 middle frontal gyrus
6.额下沟 inferior frontal sulcus
7.额下回 inferior frontal gyrus
8.外侧沟 lateral sulcus
9.颞上回 superior temporal gyrus
10.眶回 orbital gyri
11.颞上沟 superior temporal sulcus
12.颞中回 middle temporal gyrus
13.颞下沟 inferior temporal sulcus
14.颞下回 inferior temporal gyrus

15.脑桥 pons
16.延髓 medulla oblongata
17.中央沟 central sulcus
18.中央后回 central gyrus
19.中央后沟 postcentral sulcus
20.顶上小叶 superior parietal lobule
21.顶内沟 intraparietal sulcus
22.缘上回 supramarginal gyrus
23.角回 angular gyrus
24.小脑 cerebellum
25.扣带沟 cingulate sulcus
26.扣带回 cingulate gyrus
27.胼胝体沟 callosal sulcus
28.胼胝体 corpus callosum

29.透明隔 septum pellucidum
30.前连合 anterior commissure
31.视交叉 optic chiasma
32.乳头体 mamillary body
33.中脑水管 mesencephalic duct
34.脑干 brain stem
35.第三脑室 third ventricle
36.背侧丘脑 dorsal thalamus
37.松果体 pineal body
38.距状沟 calcarine sulcus
39.舌回 lingual gyrus
40.第四脑室 fourth ventricle

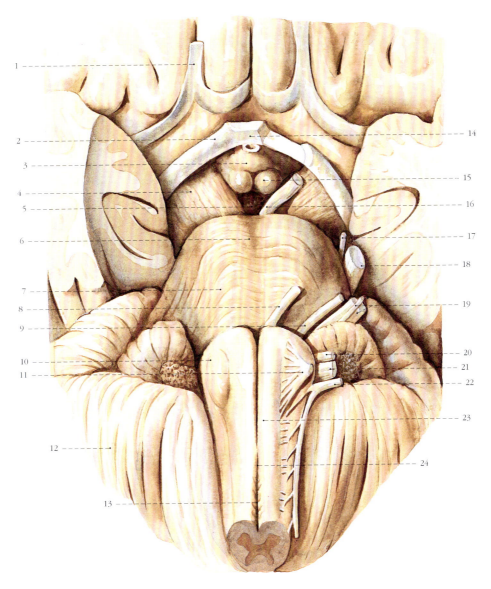

340. 脑干（腹侧面观）
Brain stem (ventral aspect)

1.嗅束 olfactory tract
2.视束 optic tract
3.灰结节 tuber cinereum
4.大脑脚 cerebral peduncle
5.脚间窝 interpeduncle fossa
6.基底沟 basilar sulcus
7.脑桥 pons
8.展神经 abducent nerve

9.面神经 facial nerve
10.橄榄 olive
11.舌下神经 hypoglossal nerve
12.小脑 cerebellum
13.锥体交叉 decussation of pyramid
14.视交叉 optic chiasma
15.乳头体 mamillary body
16.动眼神经 oculomotor nerve

17.滑车神经 trochlear nerve
18.三叉神经 trigeminal nerve
19.前庭蜗神经 vestibulocochlear nerve
20.舌咽神经 glossopharyngeal nerve
21.迷走神经 vagus nerve
22.副神经 accessory nerve
23.锥体 pyramid
24.前正中裂 anterior median fissure

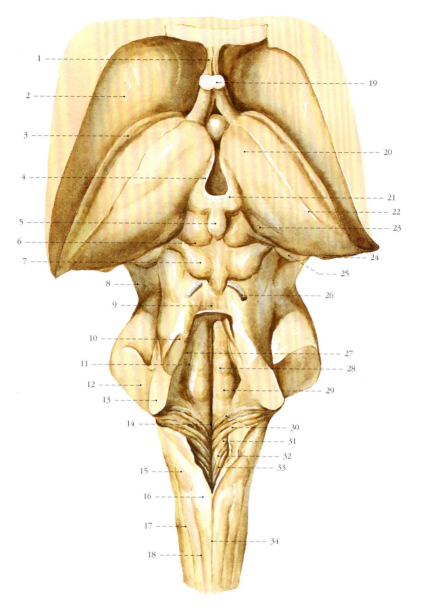

341. 脑干（背面观）
Brain stem (dorsal aspect)

1.透明隔 septum pellucidum
2.尾状核 caudate nucleus
3.终纹 terminal stria
4.丘脑髓纹 thalamic medullary stria
5.松果体 pineal body
6.上丘 superior colliculus
7.下丘 inferior colliculus
8.大脑脚 cerebral peduncle
9.前髓帆 anterior medullary velum
10.小脑上脚 superior cerebellar peduncle
11.界沟 sulcus limitans
12.小脑中脚 middle cerebellar peduncle

13.小脑下脚 inferior cerebellar peduncle
14.正中沟 median sulcus
15.楔束结节 cuneate tubercle
16.薄束结节 gracile tubercle
17.后外侧沟 posterolateral sulcus
18.后中间沟 posterior intermediate sulcus
19.穹窿 fornix
20.背侧丘脑 dorsal thalamus
21.缰三角 habenular trigone
22.脉络带 tenia choroidea
23.枕 pulvinar
24.外侧膝状体 lateral geniculate body

25.内侧膝状体 medial geniculate body
26.滑车神经 trochlear nerve
27.蓝斑 locus cerulens
28.内侧隆起 medial eminence
29.面神经丘 facial colliculus
30.髓纹 medullary stria
31.舌下神经三角 hypoglossal triangle
32.迷走神经三角 vagal triangle
33.最后区 area postrema
34.后正中沟 posterior median sulcus

1.薄束核 gracile nucleus

2.楔束核 cuneate nucleus

3.边缘带 limbic zone

4.胶状质 gelatinous substance

5.大细胞核 magnocellular nucleus

6.三叉神经脊束核尾侧部 caudal part of the spinal nucleus of the trigeminal nerve

7.红核脊髓束 rubrospinal tract

8.脊髓小脑后束 posterior spinocerebellar tract

9.脊髓丘脑束 spinothalamic tract

10.脊髓小脑前束 anterior spinocerebellar tract

11.副神经核 accessory nucleus

12.前角运动神经元内侧群 motor neuron of anterior horn medial group

13.锥体束 pyramidal tract

14.薄束 fasciculus gracilis

15.楔束 fasciculus cuneatus

16.中央灰质 central gray matter

17.三叉神经脊束 spinal tract of trigeminal nerve

18.三叉神经脊束核 spinal nucleus of trigeminal nerve

19.中央管 central canal

20.锥体交叉 decussation of pyramid

21.前庭脊髓内侧束（内侧纵束降部）medial cord of the vestibulospinal tract（descending part of the medial longitudinal fasciculus）

22.前庭脊髓外侧束和网状脊髓束 lateral vestibulospinal tract and reticulospinal tract

23.顶盖脊髓束 tectospinal tract

24.孤束核 nucleus of solitary tract

25.迷走神经背核 dorsal nucleus of vagus nerve

26.舌下神经核 hypoglossal nucleus

27.疑核 nucleus ambiguus

28.网状结构 reticular formation

29.外侧网状核 lateral reticular nucleus

30.下橄榄主核 chief inferior olivary nucleus

31.内侧副橄榄核 medial accessory oilvary nucleus

32.弓状核 arcuate nucleus

33.内弓状纤维 internal arcuate fibers

34.舌下神经纤维 hypoglossal nerve fibers

35.内侧丘系和内侧丘系交叉 medial lemniscus and decussation of medial lemniscus

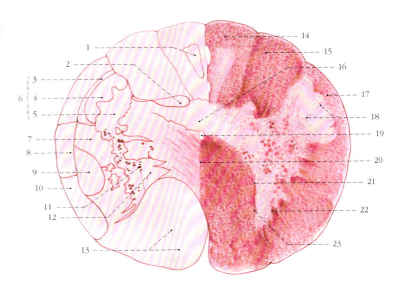

342. 延髓尾侧部水平切面（经锥体交叉）

Horizontal section of the caudal part of the medulla oblongata (through the pyramidal decussation)

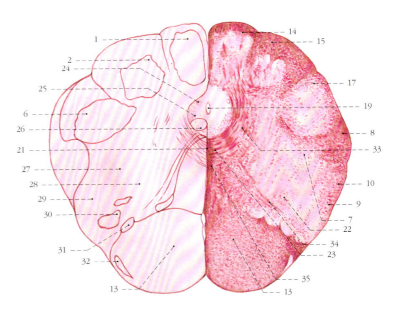

343. 延髓水平切面（经内侧丘系交叉）

Horizontal section of the medulla oblongata (through the decussation of the medial lemniscus)

1.迷走神经背核 dorsal nucleus of vagus nerve
2.前庭内侧核 medial vestibular nucleus
3.前庭下核 inferior vestibular nucleus
4.前庭神经核 vestibular nuclei
5.楔束副核 accessory nucleus of cuneate tract
6.孤束核 solitary tract nucleus
7.舌下神经核 hypoglossal nucleus
8.三叉神经脊束核极间部 interpolar part of the
  spinal nucleus of trigeminal nerve
9.疑核 nucleus ambiguus
10.网状结构 reticular formation
11.外侧网状核 lateral reticular nucleus
12.背侧副橄榄核 dorsal accessory olivary nucleus
13.下橄榄主核 chief inferior olivary nucleus
14.内侧副橄榄核 medial accessory oilvary nucleus
15.下橄榄核 inferior olivary nucleus
16.背侧纵束 dorsal longitudinal fasciculus
17.孤束 solitary tract
18.小脑下脚 inferior cerebellar peduncle
19.内侧纵束 medial longitudinal fasciculus

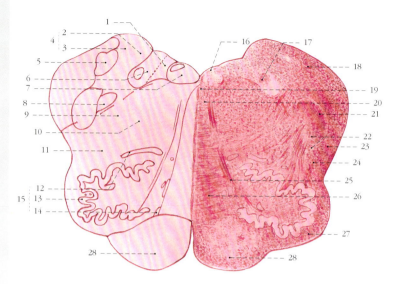

344. 延髓水平切面（经橄榄中部）
Horizontal section of the medulla oblongata
(through the middle part of the olive)

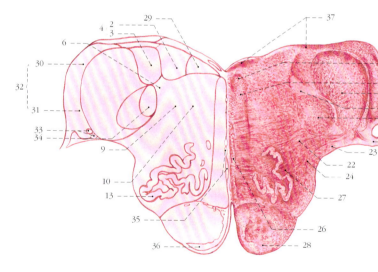

345. 延髓水平切面（经橄榄上部）
Horizontal section of the medulla oblongata
(through the superior part of the olive)

20.顶盖脊髓束 tectospinal tract
21.三叉神经脊束 spinal tract of trigeminal nerve
22.红核脊髓束 rubrospinal tract
23.脊髓小脑前束 anterior spinocerebellar tract
24.脊髓丘脑束 spinothalamic tract
25.舌下神经纤维 hypoglossal nerve fibers
26.内侧丘系 medial lemniscus
27.被盖中央束 central tract of tegmentum
28.锥体束 pyramidal tract
29.舌下前置核 nucleus prepositus hypoglossi
30.蜗背侧核 dorsal cochlear nueleus
31.蜗腹侧核 ventral cochlear nucleus
32.蜗神经核 cochlear nuclei
33.桥延体核 pontobulbar nucleus
34.三叉神经脊束核颅侧部 cranial part of the spinal
  nucleus of the trigeminal nerve
35.中缝大核 nucleus raphes magnus
36.弓状核 arcuate nucleus
37.髓纹 striae medullares
38.舌咽神经 glossopharyngeal nerve

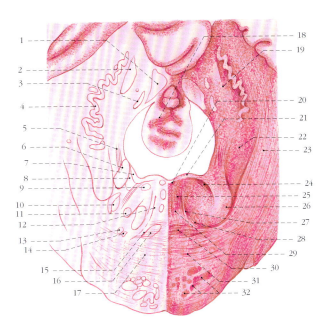

346. 脑桥水平切面（经脑桥中、下部）
Horizontal section of the pons (through the middle、inferior part of the pons)

1.顶核　fastigial nucleus
2.栓状核　emboliform nucleus
3.球状核　globose nucleus
4.齿状核　dentate nucleus
5.旁绳状体　pararestiform body
6.前庭上核　superior vestibular nucleus
7.前庭内侧核　medial vestibular nucleus
8.前庭外侧核　lateral vestibular nucleus
9.展神经核　nucleus of abducent nerve
10.三叉神经脊束核颅侧部　cranial part of the spinal
　　nucleus of the torigeminal nerve
11.面神经核　facial nucleus
12.网状结构　reticular formation
13.外侧丘系　lateral lemniscus
14.上橄榄核　superior olivary nucleus
15.三叉丘系　trigeminal lemniscus
16.内侧丘系　medial lemniscus
17.脑桥核　pontine nucleus
18.小结　nodule
19.小脑上脚　superior cerebellar peduncle
20.面神经膝　genu of facial nerve
21.背侧纵束　dorsal longitudinal fasciculus
22.小脑下脚　inferior cerebellar peduncle
23.小脑中脚　middle cerebellar peduncle
24.面神经纤维　facial nerve fibers
25.内侧纵束　medial longitudinal fasciculus
26.三叉神经脊束　spinal tract of trigeminal nerve
27.展神经纤维　abducent nerve fibers
28.被盖中央束　central tract of tegmentum
29.顶盖脊髓束　tectospinal tract
30.斜方体　trapezoid body
31.脑桥小脑纤维　pontocerebellar filbers
32.皮质脊髓束及皮质核束　corticospinal tract and
　　corticobulbar tract
33.第四脑室　fourth ventricle
34.室周灰质　periventricular gray matter
35.三叉神经中脑核　mesencephalic nucleus of trigeminal
　　nerve
36.三叉神经脑桥核　pontine nucleus of trigeminal nerve
37.三叉神经运动核　motor nucleus of trigeminal nerve
38.三叉神经中脑束　mesencephalic tract of trigeminal nerve
39.三叉神经纤维　trigeminal nerve fivers
40.被盖中央束　central tegmental tract
41.脊髓丘脑束　spinothalamic tract
42.红核脊髓束　rubrospinal tract
43.皮质脊髓束、皮质核束及皮质脑桥束　corticospinal
　　tract, corticobulbar tract and corticopontine tract

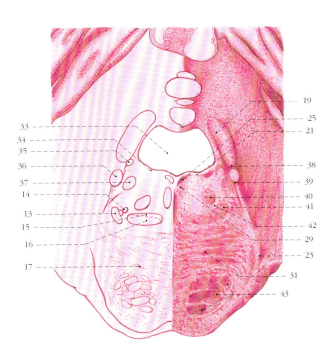

347. 脑桥水平切面（经脑桥中部）
Horizontal section of the pons (through the middle part of the pons)

1.上髓帆 superior medullary velum

2.第四脑室 fourth ventricle

3.室周灰质 periventricular gray matter

4.三叉神经中脑核 mesencephalic nucleus of trigeminal nerve

5.外侧丘系核 nucleus of lateral lemniscus

6.蓝斑 locus ceruleus

7.臂旁核 parabrachial nuclei

8.被盖背核 dorsal tegmental nucleus

9.网状结构 reticular formation

10.中央上核 superior central nucleus

11.脚桥被盖网状核 pedunculopontine reticular tegmental nucleus

12.脑桥核 pontine nucleus

13.滑车神经交叉 decussation of trochlear nerve

14.浅出的滑车神经纤维 trochlear nerve fibers

15.从同侧中脑下行的滑车神经纤维 trochlear nerve fibers descending from the unilateral midbrain

16.背侧纵束 dorsal longitudinal fasciculus

17.外侧丘系 lateral lemniscus

18.被盖中央束 central tegmental tract

19.内侧纵束 medial longitudinal fasciculus

20.脊髓丘系束 spinothalamic tract

21.顶盖脊髓束 tectospinal tract

22.小脑上脚及其交叉 superior cerebellar peduncle and its decussation

23.三叉丘系 trigeminal lemniscus

24.内侧丘系 medial lemniscus

25.皮质脊髓束、皮质核束及皮质脑桥束 corticospinal tract、corticobulbar tract and corticopontine tract

26.小脑中脚 middle cerebellar peduncle

27.脑桥小脑纤维 pontocerebellar fibers

28.下丘连合 commissure of inferior colliculus

29.下丘（中央核）inferior colliculus（central nucleus）

30.导水管周围灰质 periaqueductal gray matter

31.二叠体旁核 parabigeminal nucleus

32.中缝背核 nucleus raphes dorsalis

33.滑车神经核 nucleus of trochlear nerve

34.脚桥被盖核 pedunculopontine tegmental nucleus

35.黑质 substantia nigra

36.脚间核 interpeduncular nucleus

37.中脑水管 cerebral aqueduct

38.下丘臂 brachium of inferior colliculus

39.三叉神经中脑束 mesencephalic tract of trigeminal nerve

40.滑车神经纤维 trochlear nerve fibers

41.大脑脚底 base of cerebral peduncle

42.红核脊髓束 rubrospinal tract

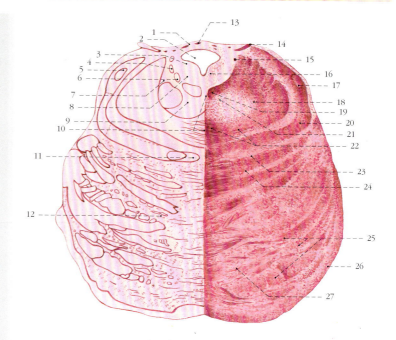

348. 脑桥水平切面（经脑桥上部）
The horizontal section of the pons (through the superior part of pons)

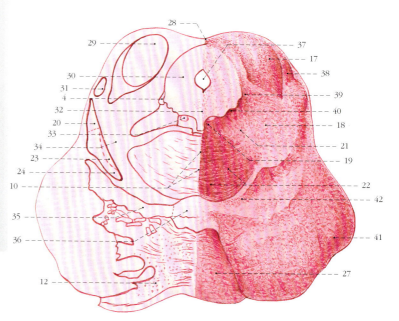

349. 中脑水平切面（经下丘）
The horizontal section of midbrain (through the inferior colliculus)

1.上丘 superior colliculus

2.导水管周围灰质 periaqueductal gray matter

3.三叉神经中脑核 mesencephalic nucleus of trigeminal nerve

4.动眼神经副核 accessory nucleus of oculomotor nerve

5.网状结构 reticular formation

6.内侧膝状体核 medial geniculate nucleus

7.脑脚周核 peripeduncular nucleus

8.外侧膝状体核 lateral geniculate nucleus

9.内侧纵束颅侧中介核 cranial intercalatus nucleus of medial longitudinal fasciculus

10.顶枕颞桥束 parietooccipito-temporopontine tract

11.红核（小细胞部） red nucleus (parvocellular part)

12.皮质脊髓束 corticospinal tract

13.皮质核束 corticobulbar tract

14.额桥束 frontal pontine tract

15.动眼神经核 nucleus of oculomotor nerve

16.中脑水管 cerebral aqueduct

17.三叉神经中脑束 mesencephalic tract of trigeminal nerve

18.背侧纵束 dorsal longitudinal fasciculus

19.内侧纵束 medial longitudinal fasciculus

20.下丘臂 brachium of inferior colliculus

21.上丘臂 brachium of superior colliculus

22.脊髓丘脑束 spinothalamic tract

23.被盖中央束 central tegmental tract

24.三叉丘系 trigeminal lemniscus

25.视束 optic tract

26.内侧丘系 medial lemniscus

27.小脑丘脑纤维 fibers of cerebellum and thalamus

28.黑质 substantia nigra

29.缰核脚间束 habenulointerpeduncular tract

30.动眼神经纤维 oculomotor nerve fiber

31.Darkschewitsch核 nucleus of Darkschewitsch

32.顶盖前区 pretectal area

33.背核 dorsal nucleus

34.腹核 ventral nucleus

35.未定带 zona incerta

36.底丘脑核 subthalamic nucleus

37.Cajal中介核 Cajal intercalatus nucleus

38.动眼神经副核 accessory nucleus of oculomotor nerve

39.腹侧被盖区 venrtal tegmental area

40.后连合 posterior commissure

41.尾状核尾 tail of caudate nucleus

42.终纹 terminal stria

43.丘脑枕 pulvinar

44.视辐射 optic radiation

45.大脑脚底 base of cerebral peduncle

46.乳头体 mamillary bodies

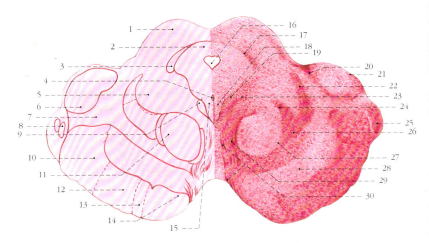

350. 中脑水平切面（经上丘颅侧部）
The horizontal section of midbrain (through the cranial part of superior colliculus)

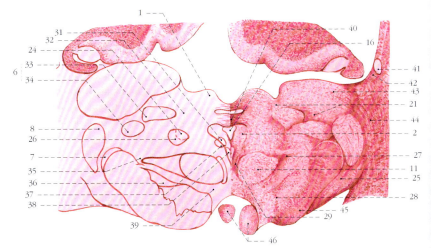

351. 中脑上端与间脑之间水平切面（经后连合）
The horizontal section between mesencephalic superior extremity and diencephalon (through posterior commissure)

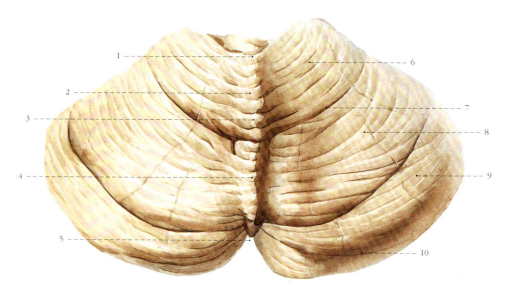

352. 小脑（上面观）
Cerebellum (superior aspect)

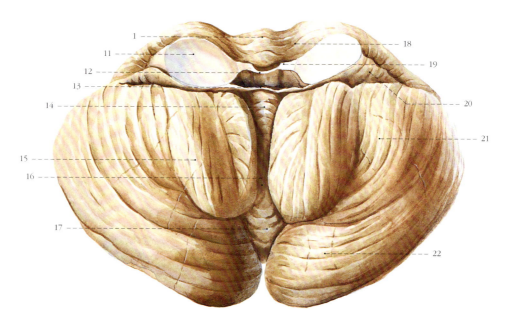

353. 小脑（下面观）
Cerebellum (inferior aspect)

1.中央小叶 central lobule
2.山顶 culmen
3.小脑蚓 vermis
4.山坡 declive
5.小脑后切迹 posterior cerebellar notch
6.方形小叶前部 anterior quadrangular lobule
7.原裂 primary fissure
8.方形小叶后部 posterior quadrangular lobule

9.上半月小叶 superior semilunar lobule
10.水平裂 horizontal fissure
11.小脑中脚 middle cerebellar peduncle
12.前髓帆 anterior medullary velum
13.后髓帆 posterior medullary velum
14.小结 nodule
15.小脑扁桃体 tonsil of cerebellum
16.蚓垂 uvula of vermis

17.蚓锥体 pyramid of vermis
18.中央小叶翼 ala of central lobule
19.小脑上脚 superior cerebellar
   peduncle
20.绒球 flocculus
21.二腹小叶 biventral lobule
22.下半月小叶 inferior semilunar
   lobule

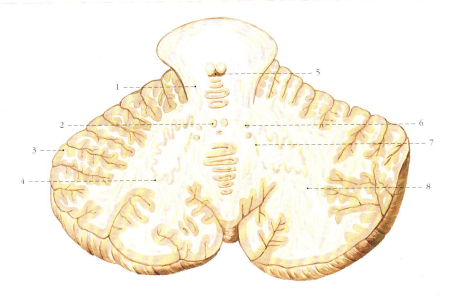

354. 小脑深核
Deep cerebellar nucleus

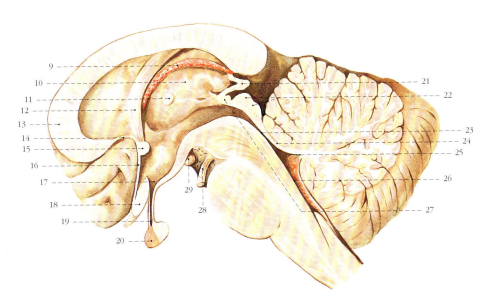

355. 间脑（内侧面观）
Diencephalon (medial aspect)

1.小脑上脚 superior cerebellar
　peduncle
2.顶核 fastigial nucleus
3.皮质 cortex
4.齿状核 dentate nucleus
5.菱形窝 rhomboid fossa
6.球状核 globose nucleus
7.栓状核 emboliform nucleus
8.髓质 medullary substance
9.第三脑室脉络丛 choroid plexus of
　third ventricle

10.背侧丘脑 dorsal thalamus
11.丘脑间粘合 interthalamic adhesion
12.穹窿体 body of fornix
13.胼胝体膝 genu of corpus callosum
14.胼胝体嘴 rostrum of corpus
　callosum
15.前连合 anterior commissure
16.终板 lamina terminalis
17.漏斗隐窝 infundibular recess
18.视交叉 optic chiasma
19.漏斗 infundibulum

20.垂体 hypophysis
21.松果体 pineal body
22.上丘、下丘 superior colliculus, inferior
　colliculus
23.中脑水管 mesencephalic aqueduct
24.前髓帆 anterior medullary velum
25.第四脑室盖 tegmen of fourth ventricle
26.第四脑室 fourth ventricle
27.后连合 posterior commissure
28.动眼神经 oculomotor nerve
29.乳头体 mamillary body

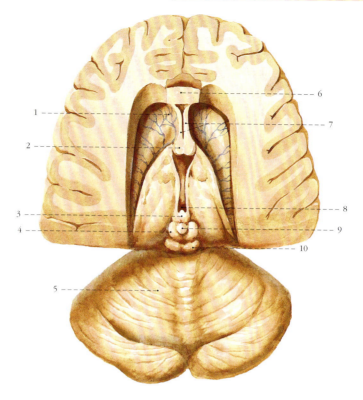

356. 间脑（后上面观）
Diencephalon (posterosuperior aspect)

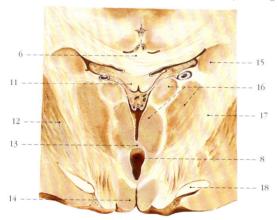

357. 间脑冠状切面（乳头体平面）
Coronal section of diencephalon (level of the
mammilary body)

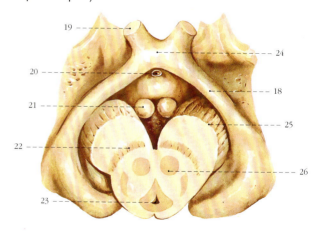

358. 下丘脑（下面观）
Hypothalamus (inferior aspect)

1.尾状核头 head of caudate nucleus
2.穹窿柱 collumn of fornix
3.缰连合 habenular commissure
4.上丘 superior colliculus
5.小脑 cerebellum
6.胼胝体 corpus callosum
7.透明隔 septum pellucidum
8.第三脑室 third ventricle
9.松果体 pineal body
10.下丘 inferior colliculus
11.穹窿体 body of fornix
12.豆状核 lentiform nucleus
13.丘脑间粘合 interthalamic adhesion
14.乳头体核 mamillary nucleus
15.尾状核 caudate nucleus
16.背侧丘脑 dorsal thalamus
17.内囊 internal capsule
18.视束 optic tract
19.视神经 optic nerve
20.漏斗 infundibulum
21.乳头体 mamillary body
22.黑质 substantia nigra
23.中脑水管 mesencephalic aqueduct
24.视交叉 optic chiasma
25.大脑脚 cerebral peduncle
26.红核 red nucleus

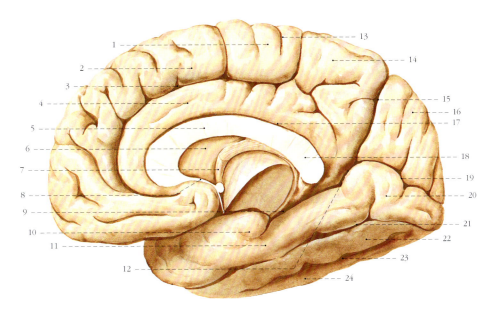

359. 大脑半球内面的沟回

Gyruses and sulcuses of medial surface of the cerebral hemisphere

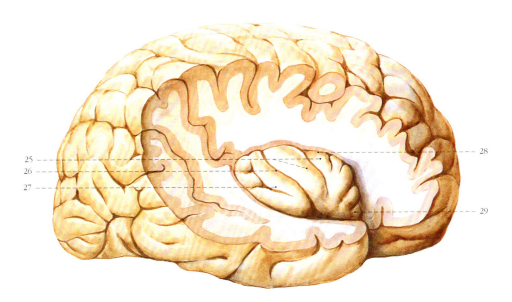

360. 大脑岛叶的沟回

Sulcuses and gyri of cerebral insula

1.旁中央小叶 paracentral lobule

2.额上回 superior frontal gyrus

3.扣带沟 cingulate sulcus

4.扣带回 cingulate gyrus

5.胼胝体干 trunk of corpus callosum

6.透明隔 septum pellucidum

7.穹窿 fornix

8.胼胝体嘴 rostrum of corpus callosum

9.海马沟 hippocampal sulcus

10.钩 uncus

11.海马旁回 parahippocampal gyrus

12.弓状沟 arcuate sulcus

13.中央沟 central sulcus

14.楔前叶 precuneus

15.顶枕沟 parietooccipital sulcus

16.楔叶 cuneus

17.胼胝体沟 callosal sulcus

18.胼胝体（压部）corpus callosum
　（splenium）

19.距状沟 calcarine sulcus

20.舌回 lingual gyrus

21.侧副沟 collateral sulcus

22.枕颞内侧回 medial occipitotemporal gyrus

23.枕颞沟 occipitotemporal sulcus

24.枕颞外侧回 lateral occipitotemporal gyrus

25.岛短回 short gyri of insula

26.岛中央沟 central sulcus of insula

27.岛长回 long gyrus of insula

28.岛环状沟 circular sulcus of insula

29.岛阈 limen of insula

1.尾状核头 head of caudate nucleus

2.屏状核 claustrum

3.透明隔 septum pellucidum

4.穹窿柱 column of fornix

5.壳 putamen

6.苍白球 globus pallidus

7.豆状核 lentiform nucleus

8.外囊 external capsule

9.最外囊 extreme capsule

10.穹窿脚 crus of fornix

11.胼胝体压部 splenium of corpus callosum

12.前角 anterior horn

13.内囊前肢 anterior limb of internal capsule

14.内囊膝 genu of internal capsule

15.前核群 anterior nuclear group

16.内髓板 internal medullary lamina

17.外侧核群 lateral nuclear group

18.内囊后肢 posterior limb of internal capsule

19.内侧核群 medial nuclear group

20.侧副三角 collateral trigone

21.禽距 calcar avis

22.后角 posterior horn

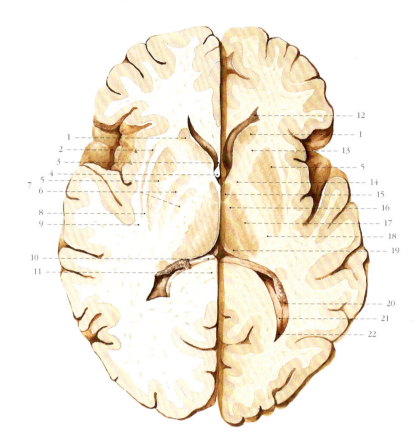

361. 脑的水平切面
Horizontal section of the brain

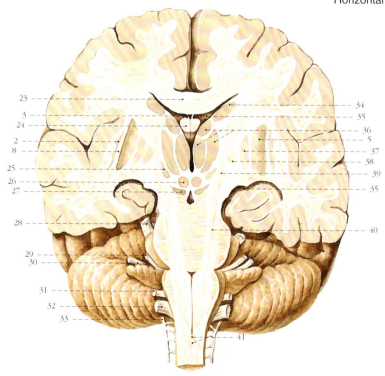

362. 脑的冠状切面
Coronal section of the brain

23.胼胝体膝 genu of corpus callosum

24.穹窿 fornix

25.底丘脑核 subthalamic nucleus

26.红核 red nucleus

27.黑质 substantia nigra

28.三叉神经 trigeminal nerve

29.面神经 facial nerve

30.前庭蜗神经 vestibulocochlear nerve

31.舌咽神经 glossopharyngeal nerve

32.迷走神经 vagus nerve

33.副神经 accessory nerve

34.尾状核 caudate nucleus

35.侧脑室脉络丛 choroid plexus of lateral ventricle

36.背侧丘脑 dorsal thalamus

37.外侧苍白球 lateral globus pallidus

38.内侧苍白球 medial globus pallidus

39.内囊 internal capsule

40.锥体束 pyramidal tract

41.锥体交叉 decussation of pyramid

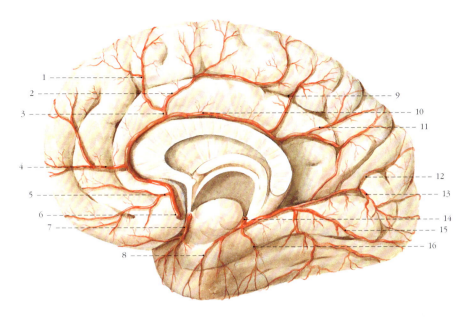

363. 大脑的动脉（内侧面观）
Cerebral arteries (medial aspect)

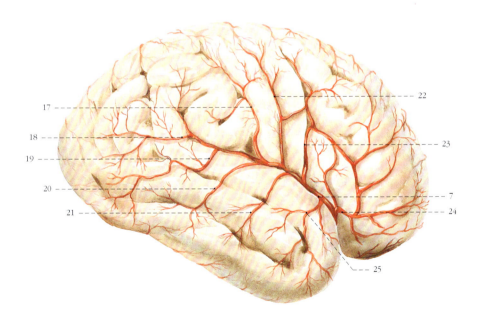

364. 大脑的动脉（外侧面观）
Cerebral arteries (lateral aspect)

1.额中间内侧支 frontal intermediomedial branch
2.额后内侧支 frontal posteromedial branch
3.胼胝体缘动脉 callosomarginal artery
4.额前内侧支 frontal anteromedial branch
5.额底内侧动脉 medial frontobasal artery
6.大脑前动脉 anterior cerebral artery
7.大脑中动脉 middle cerebral artery
8.颞前支 anterior temporal branches

9.中央旁动脉 paracentral artery
10.胼胝体周围动脉 pericallosal artery
11.楔前动脉 precuneal artery
12.顶枕支 parietooccipital branch
13.距状沟支 calcarine branch
14.大脑后动脉 posterior cerebral artery
15.颞后支 posterior temporal branches
16.颞中间的内侧支 intermediomedial temporal branch

17.中央后沟动脉 artery of postcentral sulcus
18.顶后动脉 posterior parietal artery
19.角回动脉 artery of angular gyrus
20.颞后动脉 posterior temporal artery
21.颞中间动脉 middle temporal artery
22.中央沟动脉 artery of central sulcus
23.中央前沟动脉 artery of precentral sulcus
24.额底外侧动脉 lateral frontobasal artery
25.颞前动脉 anterior temporal artery

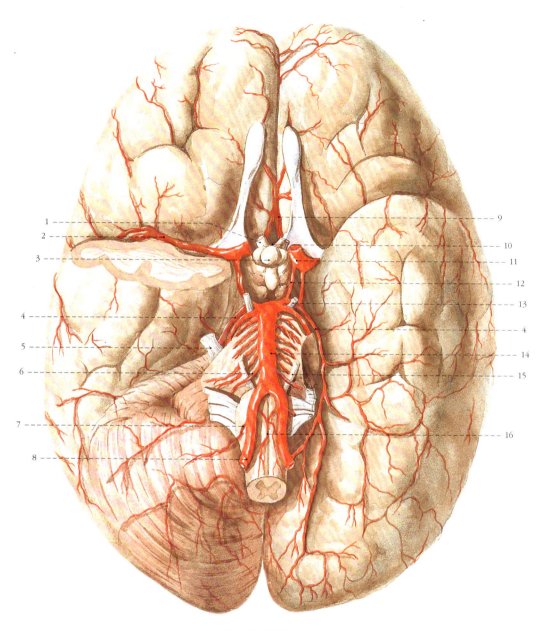

365. 脑底部的动脉

Arteries at the base of the brain

1.视神经 optic nerve
2.大脑中动脉 middle cerebral artery
3.脑垂体 hypophysis
4.大脑后动脉 posterior cerebral artery
5.三叉神经 trigeminal nerve
6.小脑下前动脉 anterior inferior cerebellar artery
7.小脑下后动脉 posterior inferior cerebellar artery
8.椎动脉 vertebral artery

9.大脑前动脉 anterior cerebral artery
10.前交通支 anterior communicating artery
11.颈内动脉 internal carotid artery
12.后交通支 posterior communicating artery
13.动眼神经 oculomotor nerve
14.基底动脉 basilar artery
15.展神经 abducent nerve
16.脊髓前动脉 anterior spinal artery

1.胼胝体 corpus callosum
2.尾状核 caudate nucleus
3.内囊 internal capsule
4.静脉中央支 central branches of vein
5.大脑中深静脉 deep middle cerebral vein
6.大脑前动脉皮质支 cortical branches of anterior cerebral artery
7.纹状体 corpus striatum
8.前外侧中央动脉（外侧支）anteriolateral central arteries (lateral branches)
9.前外侧中央动脉（内侧支）anteriolateral central arteries (medial branches)
10.大脑中动脉 middle cerebral artery
11.丘脑纹静脉 thalamostriate vein
12.丘脑 thalamus
13.大脑内静脉 internal cerebral vein
14.侧脑室静脉 lateral ventricular vein
15.透明隔前静脉 septum pellucidium vein
16.脉络丛静脉 vein of choroid plexus
17.大脑大静脉 great cerebral vein

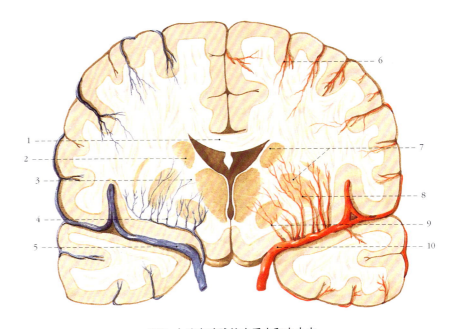

366. 大脑中动脉的皮质支和中央支
The cortical and median branches of the middle cerebral artery

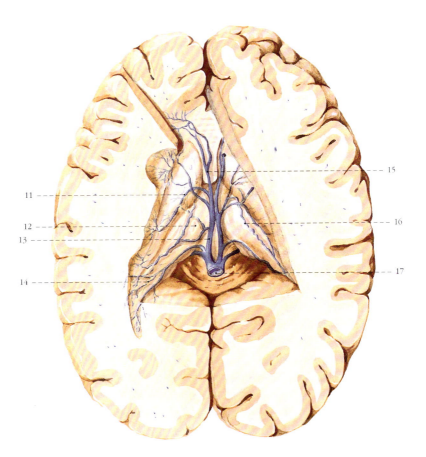

367. 大脑的深静脉（上面观）
The deep cerebral veins (superior aspect)

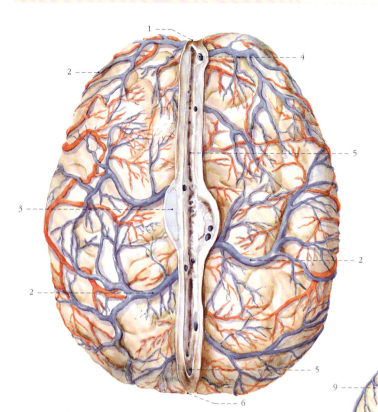

368. 大脑表面的静脉和上矢状窦
Veins of cerebral surface and superior sagittal sinus

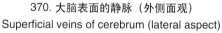

370. 大脑表面的静脉（外侧面观）
Superficial veins of cerebrum (lateral aspect)

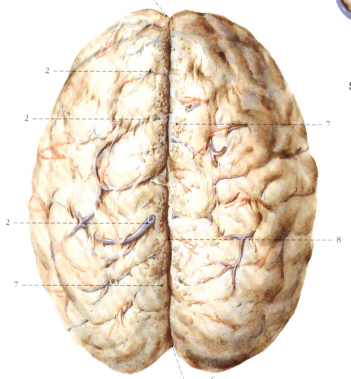

369. 蛛网膜及蛛网膜粒（上面观）
Arachnoid mater and granulations (superior aspect)

1.额侧 frontal side
2.大脑上静脉 superior cerebral vein
3.硬膜 dura mater
4.大脑上静脉开口 orifice of superior
　cerebral vein
5.上矢状窦 superior sagittal sinus
6.枕侧 occipital side
7.蛛网膜粒 arachnoid granulations
8.大脑纵裂 cerebral longitudinal fissure
9.上吻合静脉 superior anastomotic vein
10.下吻合静脉 inferior anastomotic vein
11.大脑中浅静脉 superficial middle
　cerebral veins
12.大脑下静脉 inferior cerebral vein

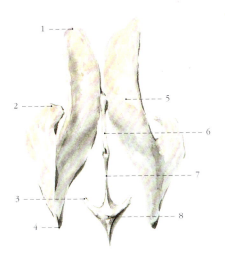

371. 脑室铸型（上面观）
Cast form of the cerebral ventricle
(superior aspect)

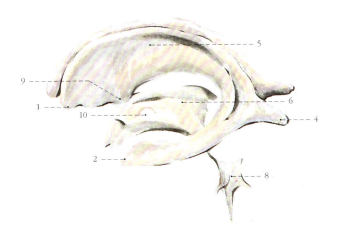

372. 脑室铸型（侧面观）
Cast form of the cerebral ventricle (lateral aspect)

1.侧脑室前角 anterior horn of lateral ventricle
2.侧脑室下角 inferior horn of lateral ventricle
3.外侧隐窝 lateral recess
4.侧脑室后角 posterior horn of lateral ventricle
5.中央部 central part
6.第三脑室 third ventricle
7.中脑水管 mesencephalic aqueduct
8.第四脑室 fourth ventricle
9.室间孔 interventricular foramen
10.丘脑间粘合 interthalamic adhesion
11.终纹 stria terminalis
12.背侧丘脑 dorsal thalamus
13.内侧纵纹 medial longitudinal stria
14.胼胝体 corpus callosum
15.禽距 calcar
16.尾状核头 head of caudate nucleus
17.尾状核体 body of caudate nucleus
18.海马 hippocampus
19.侧脑室脉络丛 choroid plexus of lateral ventricle
20.侧副三角 collateral trigone

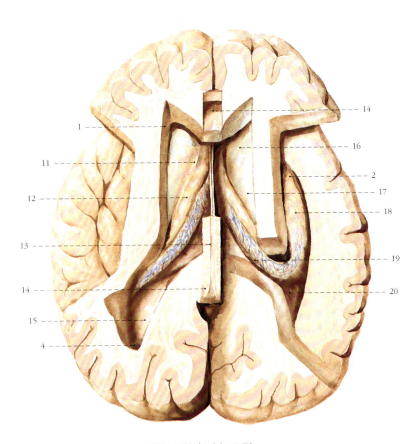

373. 侧脑室（上面观）
Lateral ventricle (superior aspect)

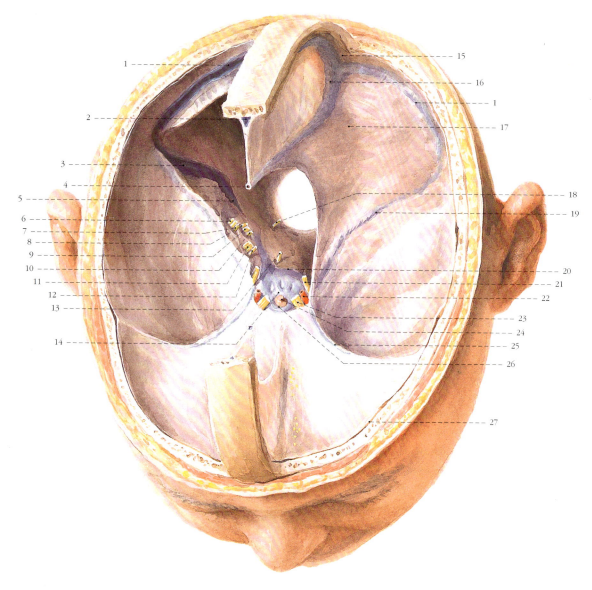

374. 硬脑膜、硬脑膜窦和脑神经

Cerebral dura mater, sinuses of dura mater and cranial nerves

1.横窦　transverse sinus
2.上矢状窦　superior sagittal sinus
3.乙状窦　sigmoid sinus
4.下矢状窦　inferior sagittal sinus
5.岩下窦　inferior petrosal sinus
6.前庭蜗神经　vestibulocochlear nerve
7.面神经　facial nerve
8.副神经　accessory nerve
9.迷走神经　vagus nerve

10.舌咽神经　glossopharyngeal nerve
11.三叉神经　trigeminal nerve
12.滑车神经　trochlear nerve
13.展神经　abducent nerve
14.海绵间后窦　posterior intercavernous sinuses
15.窦汇　confluence of sinuses
16.直窦　straight sinus
17.小脑幕　tentorium of cerebellum
18.舌下神经　hypoglossal nerve

19.岩上窦　superior petrosal sinus
20.基底丛　basal plexus
21.动眼神经　oculomotor nerve
22.眼动脉　ophthalmic artery
23.视神经　optic nerve
24.垂体　pituitary gland
25.蝶顶窦　sphenoparietal sinus
26.海绵间前窦　anterior intercavernous sinuses
27.硬膜　dura mater

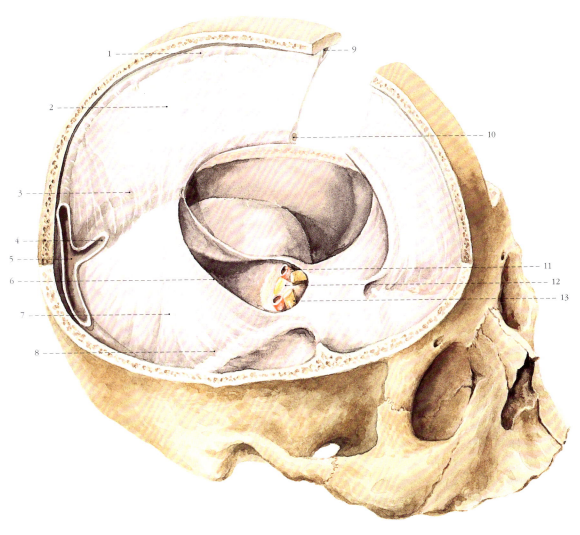

375. 硬脑膜及硬脑膜静脉窦
Cerebral dura mater and venous sinuses of cerebral dura mater

1.上矢状窦 superior sagittal sinus
2.大脑镰 cerebral falx
3.横窦 transverse sinus
4.直窦 straight sinus
5.窦汇 confluence of sinuses
6.幕切迹 tentorial incisure
7.小脑幕 tentorium of cerebellum

8.岩上窦 superior petrosal sinus
9.上矢状窦（断面）superior sagittal sinus（section）
10.下矢状窦（断面）inferior sagittal sinus（section）
11.颈内动脉 internal carotid artery
12.漏斗 infundibulum
13.视神经 optic nerve

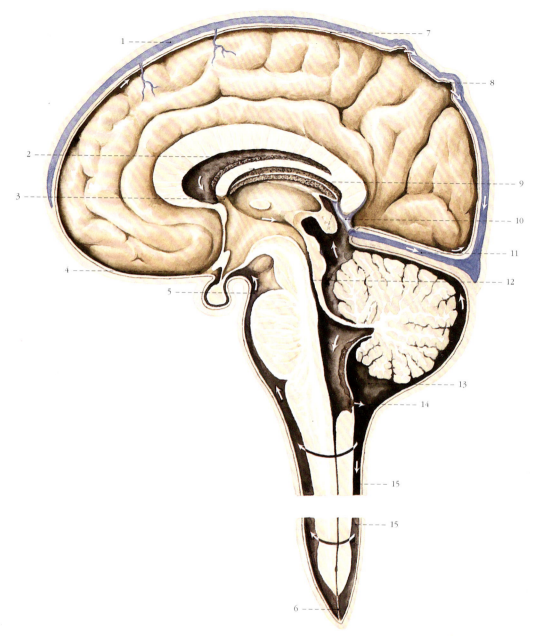

376. 脑脊液循环（模式图）
Cerebrospinal fluid circulation (diagram)

1.上矢状窦 superior sagittal sinus
2.侧脑室脉络丛 choroid plexus of lateral ventricle
3.室间孔 interventricular foramen
4.交叉池 chiasmatic cistern
5.脚间池 interpeduncular cistern
6.终池 terminal cistern
7.脑蛛网膜 cerebral arachnoid mater
8.蛛网膜粒 arachnoid granulations
9.第三脑室脉络丛 choroid plexus of third ventricle
10.大脑大静脉 great cerebral vein
11.直窦 straight sinus
12.中脑水管 mesencephalic aqueduct
13.小脑延髓池 cerebellomedullary cistern
14.第四脑室正中孔 median aperture of fourth ventricle
15.蛛网膜下隙 subarachnoid space

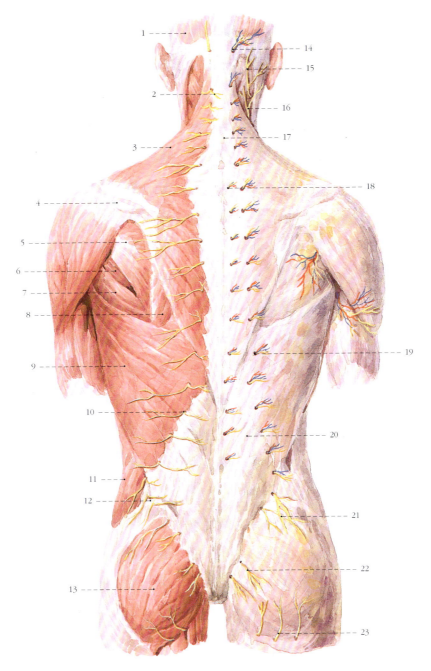

377. 脊神经的后支
Posterior branches of spinal nerves

1.枕额肌枕腹 occipital belly of
　occipitofrontalis
2.第三颈神经 third cervical nerve
3.斜方肌 trapezius
4.肩胛冈 spine of scapula
5.冈下肌 infraspinatus
6.小圆肌 teres minor
7.大圆肌 teres major
8.菱形肌 rhomboideus

9.背阔肌 latissimus dorsi
10.胸神经后支 posterior branch of thoracic nerves
11.腹外斜肌 obliquus externus abdominis
12.髂嵴 iliac crest
13.臀大肌 gluteus maximus
14.枕大神经和枕动、静脉 greater occipital nerve
　and occipital artery and vein
15.枕小神经 lesser occipital nerve
16.耳大神经 great auricular nerve

17.项筋膜 nuchal fascia
18.胸神经后支的内侧支 medial branch
　of posterior branches of thoracic nerve
19.胸神经后支的外侧支 lateral branch
　of posterior branches of thoracic nerve
20.胸腰筋膜 thoracolumbar fascia
21.臀上皮神经 superior gluteal nerves
22.臀中皮神经 middle gluteal nerves
23.臀下皮神经 inferior gluteal nerves

1.颈外（浅）静脉 external jugular vein
2.封套筋膜 lnvesting layer of cervical fascia
3.颈横神经上支 superior branches of transverse nerve of neck
4.颈阔肌 platysma
5.颈横神经下支 inferior branches of transverse nerve of neck
6.锁骨上神经 supraclavicular nerves
7.枕小神经 lesser occipital nerve
8.头夹肌 splenius capitis
9.肩胛提肌 levator scapulae
10.副神经 accessory nerve
11.后斜角肌 scalenus posterior
12.颈内静脉 internal jugular vein
13.肩胛舌骨肌 omohyoid
14.臂丛 brachial plexus
15.胸锁乳突肌 sternocleidomastoid
16.耳大神经 great auricular nerve
17.颈横神经 transverse nerve of neck
18.中斜角肌 scalenus medius
19.膈神经 phrenic nerve
20.颈横动、静脉 transverse cervical artery and vein
21.前斜角肌 scalenus anterior
22.锁骨 clavicle
23.锁骨下动脉 subclavian artery

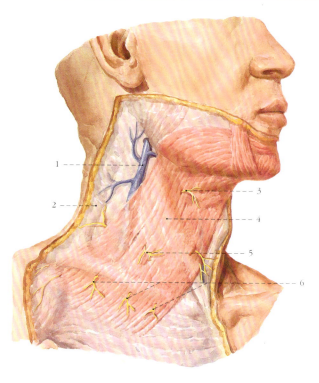

378. 颈神经丛的皮支
Cutaneous branches of cervical plexus

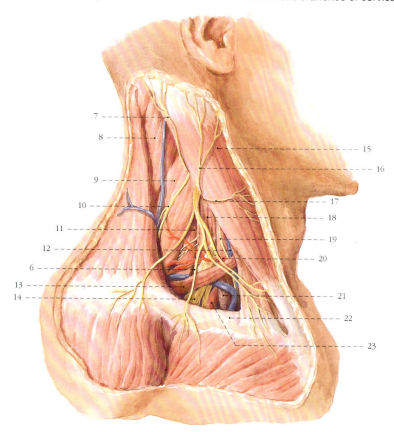

379. 颈部浅层神经
Nerves of the superficial layer of the neck

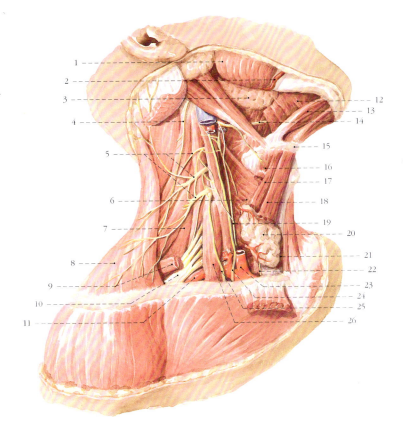

380. 颈部深层神经
Nerves of the deep layer of the neck

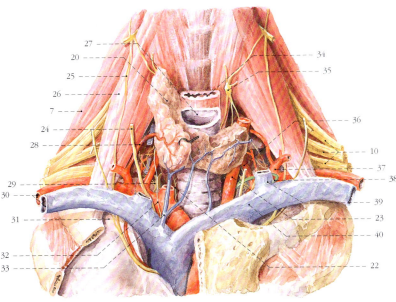

381. 臂丛及毗邻（1）
Brachial plexus and its relations (1)

1.咬肌 masseter
2.面动脉 facial artery
3.下颌下腺 submandibular gland
4.副神经 accessory nerve
5.颈丛 cervical plexus
6.咽下缩肌 inferior constrictor of pharynx
7.后斜角肌 scalenus posterior
8.斜方肌 trapezius
9.肩胛舌骨肌下腹 inferior belly of omohyoid
10.臂丛 brachial plexus
11.锁骨下动脉 subclavian artery
12.下颌舌骨肌 mylohyoid
13.二腹肌前腹 anterior belly of digastric muscle
14.舌下神经 hypoglossal nerve
15.舌骨 hyoid bone
16.甲状舌骨肌 thyrohyoid
17.肩胛舌骨肌上腹 superior belly of omohyoid
18.胸骨舌骨肌 sternohyoid
19.交感干 sympathetic trunk
20.甲状腺 thyroid gland
21.胸骨甲状肌 sternothyroid
22.喉返神经 recurrent laryngeal nerve
23.颈总动脉 common carotid artery
24.迷走神经 vagus nerve
25.膈神经 phrenic nerve
26.前斜角肌 scalenus anterior
27.气管 trachea
28.甲状腺下动脉 inferior thyroid artery
29.颈胸神经节 cervicothoracic ganglion
30.锁骨下动、静脉 subclavian artery and vein
31.胸膜顶 cupula of pleura
32.锁骨下袢 ansa subclavia
33.甲状腺下静脉 inferior thyroid vein
34.食管 esophagus
35.颈中神经节 middle cervical ganglion
36.椎动脉 vertebral artery
37.甲状颈干 thyrocervical trunk
38.胸导管 thoracic duct
39.颈内静脉 internal jugular vein
40.头臂静脉 brachiocephalic vein

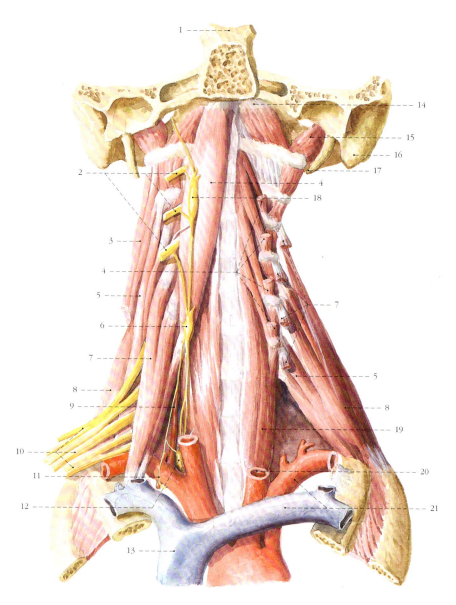

382. 臂丛及毗邻（2）

Brachial plexus and its relations (2)

1.枕骨基底部 basilar part of occipital bone
2.颈神经前支 anterior branches of cervical nerves
3.肩胛提肌 levator scapulae
4.头长肌 longus capitis
5.中斜角肌 scalenus medius
6.颈中神经节 middle cervical ganglion
7.前斜角肌 scalenus anterior

8.后斜角肌 scalenus posterior
9.椎动脉 vertebral artery
10.臂丛 brachial plexus
11.锁骨下袢 ansa subclavia
12.颈胸神经节 cervicothoracic ganglion
13.上腔静脉 superior vena cava
14.头前直肌 rectus capitis anterior
15.头外侧直肌 rectus capitis lateralis

16.乳突 mastoid process
17.茎突 styloid process
18.颈上神经节 superior cervical ganglion
19.颈长肌 longus collum
20.颈总动脉 common carotid artery
21.锁骨下动、静脉 subclavian artery and vein

1.臂外侧上皮神经 superior lateral brachial cutaneous nerve
2.臂外侧下皮神经 inferior lateral brachial cutaneous nerve
3.臂内侧皮神经 medial brachial cutaneous nerve
4.前臂后皮神经 posterior antebrachial cutaneous nerve
5.前臂外侧皮神经 lateral antebrachial cutaneous nerve
6.桡神经浅支 superficial branch of radial nerve
7.正中神经掌支 palmar branch of median nerve
8.指掌侧总神经 common palmar digital nerves
9.颈横神经 transverse nerve of neck
10.锁骨上神经 supraclavicular nerve
11.胸神经前支前皮支 anterior cutaneous branch of anterior branches of thoracic nerves
12.胸神经前支外侧皮支 lateral cutaneous branch of anterior branches of thoracic nerves

383. 上肢的皮神经（前面观）
Cutaneous nerves of upper limb (anterior aspect)

384. 上肢的皮神经（后面观）
Cutaneous nerves of upper limb (posterior aspect)

13.前臂内侧皮神经 medial antebrachial cutaneous nerve
14.胸神经后支外侧皮支 lateral cutaneous branch of posterior branches of thoracic nerves
15.尺神经手背支 dorsal branch of ulnar nerve
16.臂后皮神经 posterior brachial cutaneous nerve

191

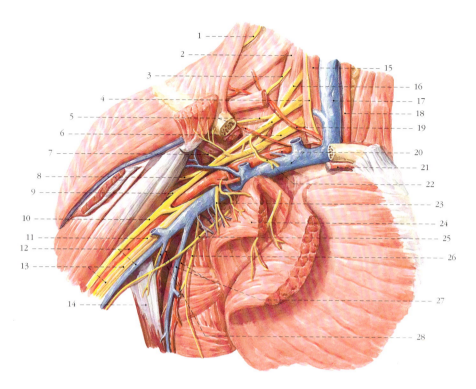

1.副神经 accessory nerve
2.中斜角肌 scalenus medius
3.肩胛背神经 dorsal scapular nerve
4.膈神经 phrenic nerve
5.肩胛上动脉、神经 suprascapular artery and nerve
6.臂丛干 brachial plexus trunks
7.肩胛下神经 subscapular nerve
8.腋神经 axillary nerve
9.肌皮神经 musculocutaneous nerve
10.正中神经 median nerve
11.尺神经 ulnar nerve
12.肱动、静脉 brachial artery and vein
13.前臂、臂内侧皮神经 medial antebrachial and medial brachial cutaneous nerves
14.背阔肌 latissimus dorsi
15.前斜角肌 scalenus anterior
16.臂丛根 brachial plexus roots
17.颈内静脉 internal jugular vein
18.颈总动脉 common carotid artery
19.颈横动脉 transverse cervical artery
20.锁骨下动、静脉 subclavian artery and vein
21.锁骨下肌 subclavius
22.胸外侧神经 lateral pectoral nerve
23.胸内侧神经 medial pectoral nerve
24.胸小肌 pectoralis minor
25.肋间臂神经 intercostobrachial nerves
26.胸长神经 long thoracic nerve
27.胸外侧动、静脉 lateral thoracic artery and vein
28.胸背动、静脉 thoracodorsal artery and vein
29.肩胛上神经 superascapular nerve
30.桡神经 radial nerve
31.前臂内侧神经 medial antebrachial nerve
32.臂内侧皮神经 medial brachial cutaneous nerve

385. 腋窝的神经及其毗邻（1）
Nerves of axillary fossa and their neighbours (1)

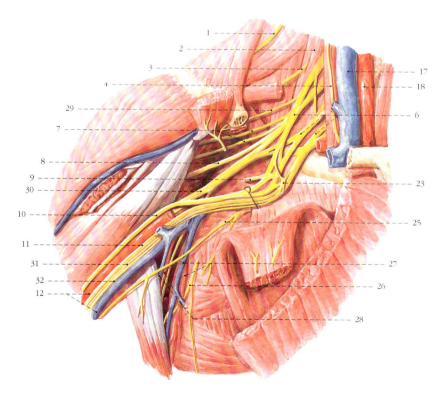

386. 腋窝的神经及其毗邻（2）
Nerves of axillary fossa and its neighbours (2)

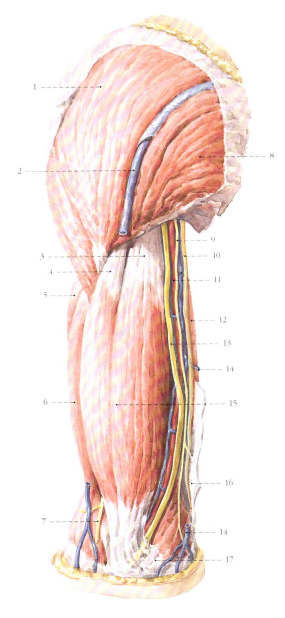

387. 臂部的神经（前面观）（1）
Nerves of the arm (anterior aspect) (1)

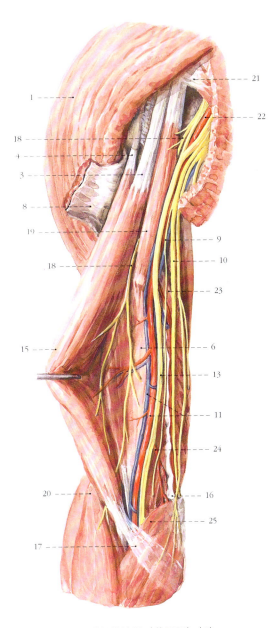

388. 臂部的神经（前面观）（2）
Nerves of the arm (anterior aspect) (2)

1.三角肌 deltoid
2.头静脉 cephalic vein
3.肱二头肌短头 short head of biceps brachii
4.肱二头肌长头 long head of biceps brachii
5.肱三头肌外侧头 lateral head of triceps brachii
6.肱肌 brachialis
7.前臂外侧皮神经 lateral antebrachial cutaneous nerve
8.胸大肌 pectoralis major
9.前臂内侧皮神经 medial autebrachial cutaneous nerve
10.尺神经 ulnar nerve
11.肱动、静脉 brachial artery and vein
12.肱三头肌内侧头 medial head of triceps brachii
13.正中神经 median nerve
14.贵要静脉 basilic vein
15.肱二头肌 biceps brachii
16.臂内侧肌间隔 medial brachial intermuscular septum
17.肱二头肌腱膜 bicipital aponeurosis
18.肌皮神经 musculocutaneous nerve
19.喙肱肌 coracobrachialis
20.肱桡肌 brachioradialis
21.胸小肌 pectoralis minor
22.腋动脉 brachial artery
23.尺侧上副动脉 superior ulnar collateral artery
24.尺侧下副动脉 inferior ulnar collateral artery
25.旋前圆肌 pronator teres

193

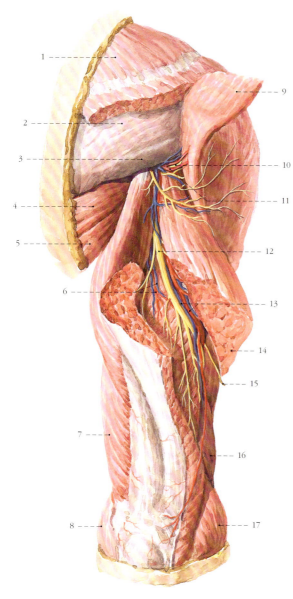

389. 臂部的神经（后面观）
Nerves of the arm (posterior aspect)

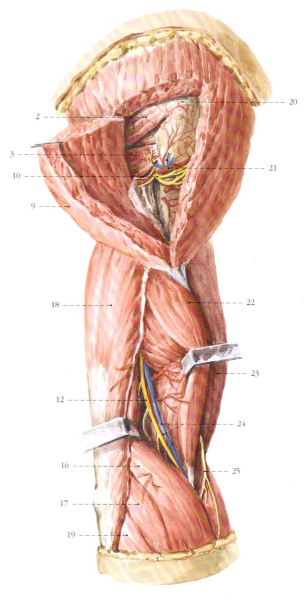

390. 臂部的神经（外侧面观）
Nerves of the arm (lateral aspect)

1.斜方肌 trapezius
2.冈下肌 infraspinatus
3.小圆肌 teres minor
4.大圆肌 teres major
5.背阔肌 latissimus dorsi
6.中副动、静脉 middle collateral artery and vein
7.肱三头肌内侧头 medial head of triceps brachii
8.尺侧腕屈肌 flexor carpi ulnaris
9.三角肌 deltoid
10.腋神经 axillary nerve
11.旋肱后动脉 posterior humeral circumflex artery
12.桡神经 radial nerve
13.肱深动、静脉 deep brachial artery and vein
14.肱三头肌外侧头 lateral head of triceps brachii
15.前臂后皮神经 posterior antebrachial cutaneous nerve
16.肱桡肌 brachioradialis
17.桡侧腕长伸肌 extensor carpi radialis longus
18.肱三头肌 triceps brachii
19.桡侧腕短伸肌 extensor carpi radialis brevis
20.大结节 greater tubercle
21.旋肱后动、静脉 posterior humeral circumflex artery and vein
22.肱肌 brachialis
23.肱二头肌 biceps brachii
24.桡侧副动、静脉 radial collateral artery and vein
25.前臂外侧皮神经 lateral antebrachial cutaneous nerve

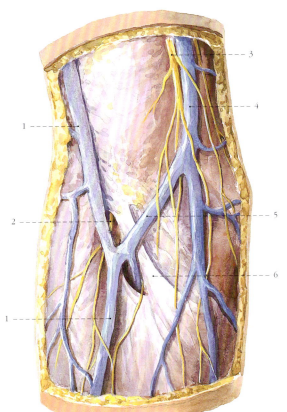

1.头静脉 cephalic vein
2.前臂外侧皮神经 lateral antebrachial cutaneous nerve
3.前臂内侧皮神经 medial antebrachial cutaneous nerve
4.贵要静脉 basilic vein
5.肘正中静脉 median cubital vein
6.肱二头肌腱膜 bicipital aponeurosis
7.肱肌 brachialis
8.肱二头肌 biceps brachii
9.肱桡肌 brachioradialis
10.正中神经 median nerve
11.肱动、静脉 brachial artery and vein
12.臂内侧肌间隔 medial brachial intermuscular septum
13.旋前圆肌 pronator teres
14.桡侧腕屈肌 flexor carpi radialis

391. 肘窝的神经（1）
Nerves of cubital fossa (1)

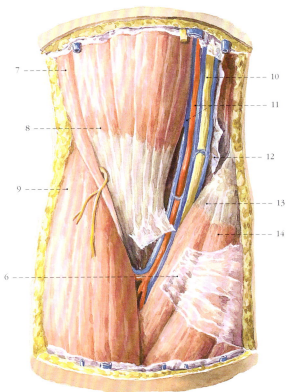

392. 肘窝的神经（2）
Nerves of cubital fossa (2)

195

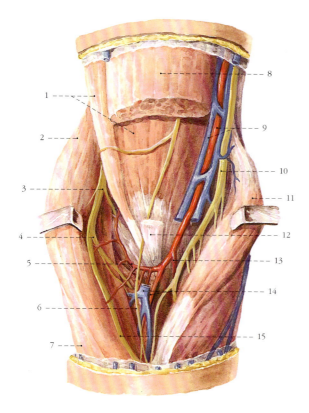

1.肱肌 brachialis
2.肱桡肌 brachioradialis
3.桡神经 radial nerve
4.桡神经深支 deep branch of radial nerve
5.桡侧返动脉 radial recurrent artery
6.前臂外侧皮神经 lateral antebrachial cutaneous nerve
7.桡侧腕长伸肌 extersor carpi radialis longus
8.肱二头肌 biceps brachii
9.肱动、静脉 brachial artery and vein
10.正中神经 median nerve
11.旋前圆肌 pronator teres
12.肱二头肌腱 bicipital tendon
13.尺动脉 ulnar artery
14.桡动、静脉 radial artery and vein
15.桡神经浅支 superficial branch of radial nerve
16.肱二头肌腱膜 bicipital aponeurosis
17.桡侧腕屈肌 flexor carpi radialis
18.掌长肌 palmaris longus
19.肱三头肌 triceps brachii
20.尺神经 ulnar nerve
21.内上髁 medial epicondyle
22.指深屈肌 flexor digitorum profundus
23.尺侧腕屈肌 flexor carpi ulnaris

393. 肘窝的神经（3）
Nerves of cubital fossa (3)

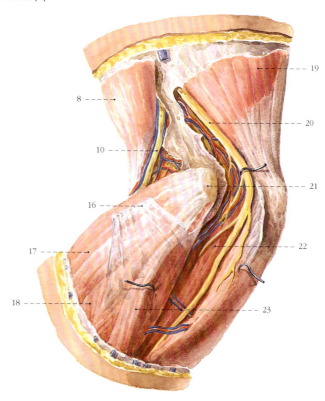

394. 肘窝的神经（内侧面观）
Nerves of cubital fossa (medial aspect)

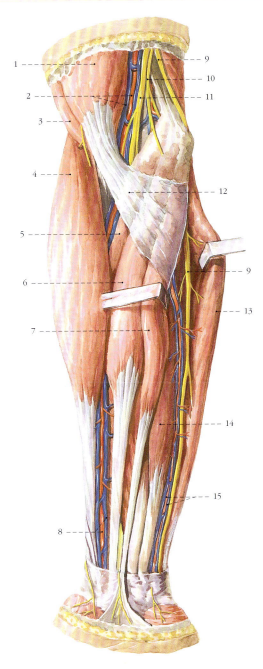

395. 前臂的神经（前面观）（1）
Nerves of the forearm (anterior aspect) (1)

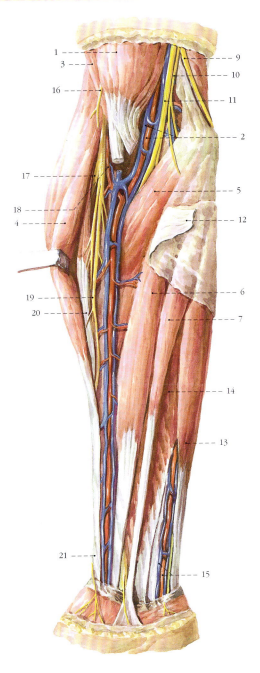

396. 前臂的神经（前面观）（2）
Nerves of the forearm (anterior aspect) (2)

1.肱二头肌 biceps brachii
2.肱动、静脉 brachial artery and vein
3.肱肌 brachialis
4.肱桡肌 brachioradialis
5.旋前圆肌 pronator teres
6.桡侧腕屈肌 flexor carpi radialis
7.掌长肌 palmaris longus
8.桡动、静脉 radial artery and vein

9.尺神经 ulnar nerve
10.前臂内侧皮神经 medial antebrachial cutaneous nerve
11.正中神经 median nerve
12.肱二头肌腱膜 bicipital aponeurosis
13.尺侧腕屈肌 flexor carpi ulnaris
14.指浅屈肌 flexor digitorum superficialis

15.尺动、静脉 ulnar artery and vein
16.前臂外侧皮神经 lateral antebrachial cutaneous nerve
17.桡神经深支 deep branch of radial nerve
18.桡神经返动脉 radial recurrent artery
19.桡神经浅支 superficial branch of radial nerve
20.桡侧腕长伸肌 extensor carpi radialis longus
21.拇长展肌 abductor pollicis longus

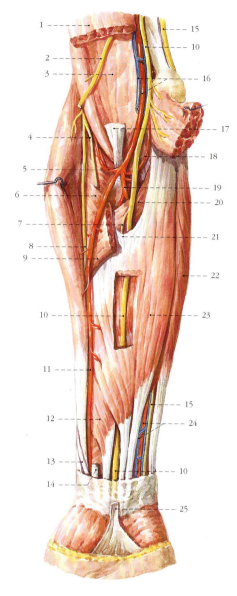

397. 前臂的神经（前面观）（3）
Nerves of the forearm (anterior aspect) (3)

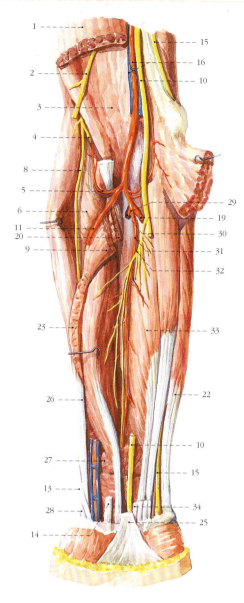

398. 前臂的神经（前面观）（4）
Nerves of the forearm (anterior aspect) (4)

1.肱二头肌 biceps brachii
2.肌皮神经 musculocutaneous nerve
3.肱肌 brachialis
4.桡神经深支 deep branch of radial nerve
5.桡侧返动脉 radial recurrent artery
6.旋后肌 supinator
7.骨间前神经 anterior interosseous nerve
8.桡神经浅支 superficial branch of radial nerve
9.旋前圆肌（肱头）humeral head of pronator teres
10.正中神经 median nerve
11.桡动脉 radial artery
12.拇长屈肌 flexor pollicis longus
13.拇长展肌腱 tendon of abductor pollicis longus
14.桡侧腕屈肌腱 tendon of flexor carpi radialis

15.尺神经 ulnar nerve
16.肱动、静脉 brachial artery and vein
17.肱二头肌腱 bicipital tendon
18.尺侧返动脉 ulnar recurrent artery
19.尺动脉 ulnar artery
20.旋前圆肌（尺头）ulnar head of pronator teres
21.指浅屈肌腱弓 tendinous arch of flexor digitorum superficialis
22.尺侧腕屈肌 flexor carpi ulnaris
23.指浅屈肌 flexor digitorum superficialis
24.尺动、静脉 ulnar artery and vein
25.掌长肌腱 tendon of palmaris longus
26.肱桡肌腱 tendon of brachioradialis

27.旋前方肌 pronator quadratus
28.拇短伸肌 extensor pollicis brevis
29.骨间总动脉 common interosseous artery
30.骨间后动脉 posterior interosseous artery
31.骨间前动脉 anterior interosseous artery
32.骨间前神经 anterior interosseous nerve
33.指深屈肌 flexor digitorum profundus
34.指浅屈肌腱 tendon of flexor digitorum superficialis

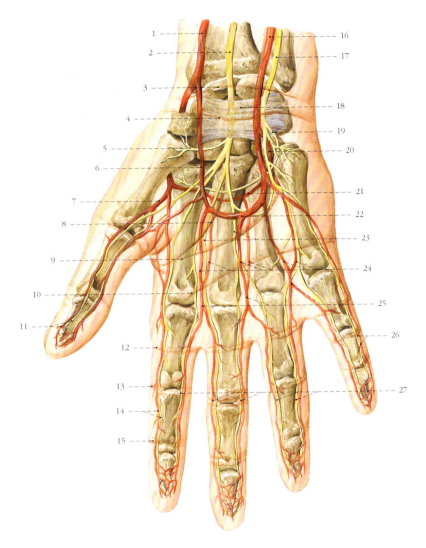

399. 手部神经及血管的体表投影

Surface projection of the nerves and blood vessels of
the hand

1.桡动脉 radial artery

2.正中神经 median nerve

3.腕横纹 carpal cross striation

4.腕远纹 carpal distal striation

5.正中神经返支 recurrent branch of median
nerve

6.桡动脉掌浅支 superficial palmar branch
of radial artery

7.拇主要动脉 principal artery of thumb

8.鱼际纹 thenar striation

9.掌中纹 plamar middle striation

10.掌远纹 palmar distal striation

11.拇掌侧固有动脉、神经 proper palmar
pollical arteries and nerves

12.近侧纹 proximal striation

13.中横纹 middle cross striation

14.示指桡掌侧固有动脉、神经 radial
proper palmar digital artery of index
finger and nerve

15.远横纹 distal cross striation

16.尺动脉 ulnar artery

17.尺神经 ulnar nerve

18.屈肌支持带 flexor retinaculum

19.尺神经深支 deep branch of ulnar
nerve

20.尺动脉掌深支 deep palmar branch
of ulnar artery

21.掌深弓 deep palmar arch

22.掌浅弓 superficial palmar
arch

23.指掌侧总神经 common
palmar digital nerve

24.掌心动脉 palmar metacarpal
arteries

25.指掌侧总动脉 common
palmar digital arteries

26.小指尺掌侧固有动脉、神经
proper palmar ulnar arteries
and nerves of little finger

27.指掌侧固有动脉、神经
proper palmar digital arteries
and nerves

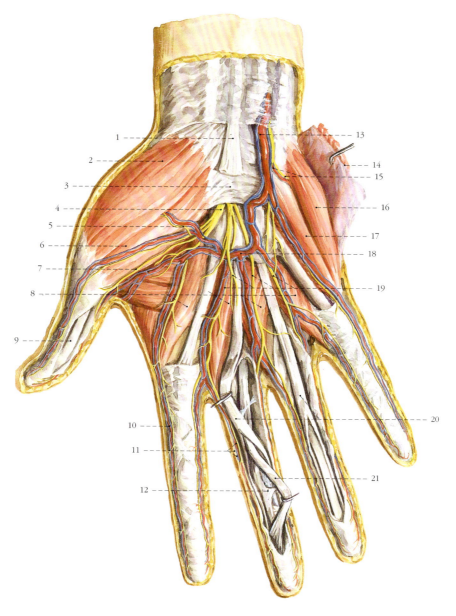

400. 手掌侧的神经及血管

Nerves and blood vessels of the palm of the hand

1.掌长肌腱 tendon of palmaris longus
2.拇短展肌 abductor pollicis brevis
3.屈肌支持带 flexor retinaculum
4.指掌侧总神经 common palmar digital nerves
5.正中神经返支 recurrent branch of median nerve
6.拇短屈肌 flexor pollicis brevis
7.指掌侧固有神经 proper palmar digital nerves
8.蚓状肌 lumbricales
9.拇长屈肌腱 flexor pollicis longus

10.示指桡掌侧固有动脉 radial proper palmar digital artery of index finger
11.指掌侧固有动、静脉、神经 proper palmar digital artery，veins and nerves
12.腱纽 vincula tendinum
13.尺动脉 ulnar artery
14.掌短肌 palmaris brevis
15.尺神经和动脉深支 deep branch of ulnar nerve and ulnar artery

16.小指展肌 abductor digiti minimi
17.小指短屈肌 flexor digiti minimi brevis
18.掌浅弓 superficial palmar arch
19.指掌侧总动脉、神经 common palmar digital arteries and nerves
20.指浅屈肌腱 flexor digitorum superficialis
21.指深屈肌腱 flexor digitorum profundus

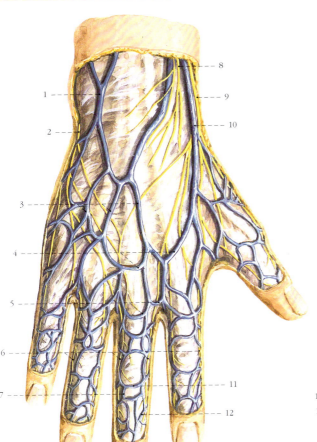

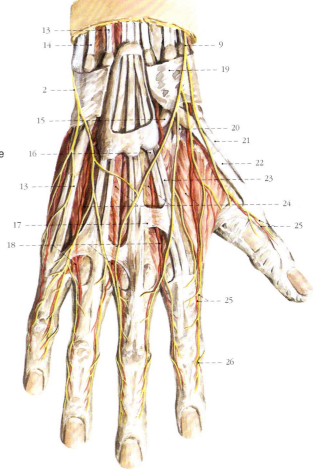

1.贵要静脉 basilic vein
2.尺神经手背支 dorsal branch of ulnar nerve
3.手背静脉网 dorsal venous rete of hand
4.掌背静脉 dorsal metacarpal veins
5.掌骨头间静脉 intercapital veins
6.指背神经 dorsal digital nerve
7.指尺侧静脉 digital ulnar vein
8.前臂外侧皮神经 lateral antebrachial cutaneous nerve
9.桡神经浅支 superficial branch of radial nerve
10.头静脉 cephalic vein
11.指静脉弓 digital venous arch
12.指桡侧静脉 digital radial vein

401. 手背部的神经及其毗邻结构（1）
The nerves and neighboring structures of the
dorsum of the hand (1)

13.小指伸肌腱 extensor digiti minimi
14.尺侧腕伸肌腱 extensor carpi ulnaris
15.桡侧腕短伸肌腱 extensor carpi radialis brevis
16.示指伸肌腱 extensor indicis
17.腱间结合 intertendinous connections
18.掌背动脉 dorsal metacarpal arteries
19.伸肌支持带 extensor retinaculum
20.桡侧腕长伸肌腱 extensor carpi radialis longus
21.拇短伸肌腱 extensor pollicis brevis
22.拇长伸肌腱 extensor pollicis longus
23.指伸肌腱 extensor digitorum
24.骨间背侧肌 doral interossei
25.指背动脉、神经 doral digital arteries and nerves
26.指掌侧固有神经 proper palmar digital nerves

402. 手背部的神经及其毗邻结构（2）
The nerves and adjacent structures of the dorsum of the hand (2)

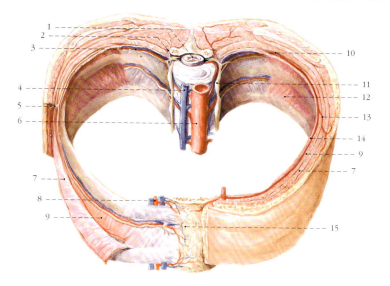

403. 肋间神经及其分布
Intercostal nerves and their distribution

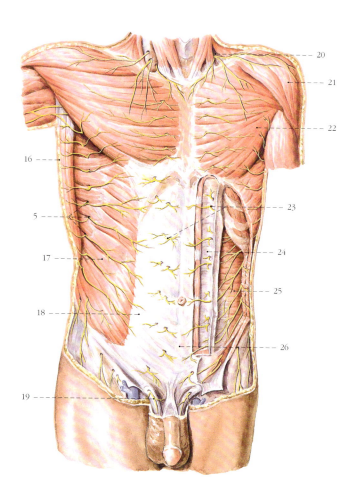

404. 胸神经前支的配布
Distribution of anterior branches of thoracic nerves

1.脊髓 spinal cord
2.胸神经后支 posterior branches of thoracic nerves
3.肋间后动、静脉，肋间神经 posterior intercostal arteries, veins, intercostal nerves
4.奇静脉 azygos vein
5.肋间神经外侧皮支 lateral cutaneous branch of intercostal nerves
6.胸主动脉 thoracic aorta
7.肋间外肌 intercostales externi
8.胸廓内动、静脉 internal thoracic artery and vein
9.肋间内肌 intercostales interni
10.肋间后动脉 posterior intercostal arteries
11.胸交感干 thoracic sympathetic trunk
12.肋间最内肌 intercostales intimi
13.肋间动脉前皮支 anterior cutaneous branch of intercostal artery
14.肋间动脉 intercostal arteries
15.胸骨 sternum
16.背阔肌 latissimus dorsi
17.腹外斜肌 obliquus externus abdominis
18.腹外斜肌腱膜 aponeurosis of obliquus externus abdominis
19.精索 spermatic cord
20.锁骨上神经 supraclavicular nerves
21.三角肌 deltoid
22.胸大肌 pectoralis major
23.肋间神经（前皮支）intercostal nerves (anterior cutaneous branch)
24.腹直肌鞘（后层）tendon sheath of rectus abdominis (posterior layer)
25.腹横肌 transversus abdominis
26.腹白线 linea alba abdominis

1.肋下神经外侧皮支 lateral cutaneous branch of subcostal nerve
2.生殖股神经股支 femoral branch of genitofemoral nerve
3.股外侧皮神经 lateral femoral cutaneous nerve
4.股神经前皮支 anterior cutaneous braches of femoral nerve
5.腓肠外侧皮神经 lateral sural cutaneous nerve
6.腓浅神经皮支 cutaneous branch of superficial peroneal nerve
7.足背中间皮神经 intermediate dorsal cutaneous nerve of foot
8.足背外侧皮神经 lateral dorsal cutaneous nerve of foot
9.髂腹下神经前皮支 anterior cutaneous branch of iliohypogastric nerve
10.髂腹股沟神经 ilioinguinal nerve
11.闭孔神经皮支 cutaneous branch of obturator nerve
12.隐神经髌下支 infrapatollar branch of saphenous nerve
13.隐神经 saphenous nerve
14.足背内侧皮神经 medial dorsal cutaneous nerve of foot

405. 下肢的皮神经和节段分布（前面观）
Cutaneous nerves and segmental distributions of the lower limb (anterior view)

15.腓深神经皮支 cutaneous branch of deep peroneal nerve
16.臀上皮神经 superior cluneal nerve
17.臀中皮神经 middle cluneal nerve
18.臀下皮神经 inf cluneal nerve
19.股后皮神经 posterior femoral cutaneous nerve
20.足底内侧神经足底皮支 plantar cutaneous branch of medial plantar nerve
21.髂腹下神经外侧皮支 lateral cutaneous branch of iliohypogastric nerve
22.腓肠内侧皮神经 medial sural cutaneous nerve
23.腓肠神经 sural nerve
24.足底外侧神经足底皮支 plantar cutaneous branch of lateral planar nerve

406. 下肢的皮神经和节段分布（后面观）
Cutaneous nerves and segmental distributions of the lower limb (posterior view)

203

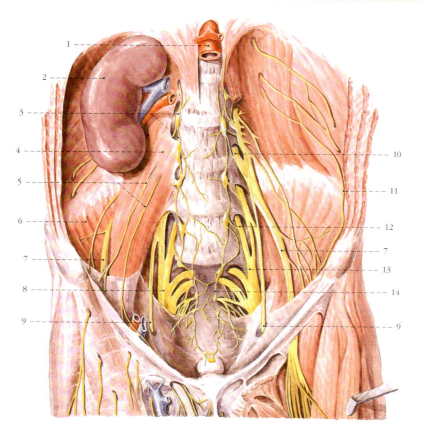

407. 腰丛和骶丛
Lumbar plexus and sacral plexus

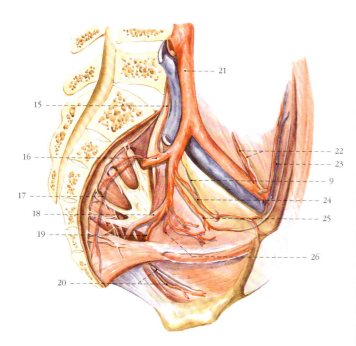

408. 骶尾丛及其毗邻结构
Sacrococcygeal plexus and its neighbours

1.腹主动脉 abdominal aorta
2.右肾 right kidney
3.腰交感神经节及干 lumbar sympathetic ganglion and trunk
4.腰大肌 psoas major
5.生殖股神经 genitofemoral nerve
6.髂肌 iliacus
7.股神经 femoral nerve
8.骶丛 sacral plexus
9.闭孔神经 obturator nerve
10.第3腰神经 third sacral nerve
11.髂腹股沟神经 ilioinguinal nerve
12.第5腰神经 fifth lumbar nerve
13.腰骶干 lumbosacral trunk
14.骶交感干 sacral sympathetic trunk
15.髂腰动脉 iliolumbar artery
16.臀上动脉 superior gluteal arteries
17.骶外侧动脉 lateral sacral arteris
18.臀下动脉 inferior gluteal artery
19.阴部内动脉 internal pudendal artery
20.阴部内动脉、神经 internal pudendal artery, nerve
21.左髂总动脉 left common iliac artery
22.旋髂深动脉 deep iliac circumflex artery
23.腹壁下动脉 inferior epigastric artery
24.闭孔动脉 obturator artery
25.脐动脉 umbilical artery
26.直肠下动脉 inferior rectal artery

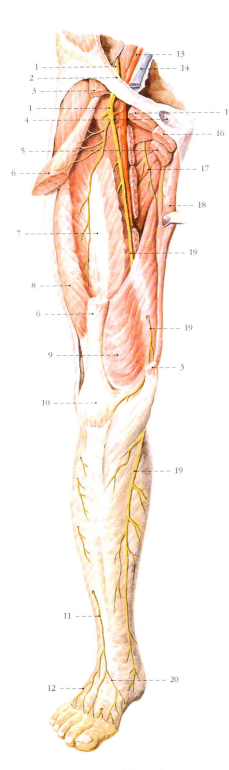

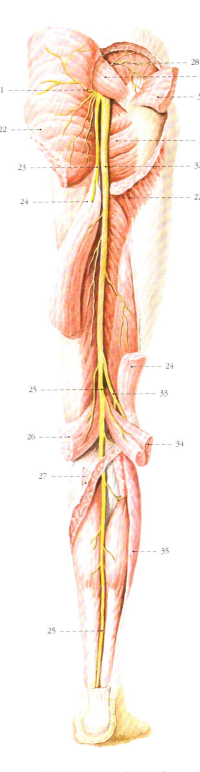

1.股神经 femoral nerve
2.腹股沟韧带 inguinal ligament
3.缝匠肌 sartorius
4.腹股沟管浅环 superficial inguinal ring
5.短收肌 adductor brevis
6.股直肌 rectus femoris
7.股中间肌 vastus intermedius
8.股外侧肌 vastus lateralis
9.股内侧肌 vastus medialis
10.髌骨 patella
11.腓浅神经 superficial peroneal nerve
12.足背外侧皮神经 lateral dorsal cutaneous nerve of foot
13.髂外动脉 external iliac artery
14.髂外静脉 external iliac vein
15.耻骨肌 pectineus
16.长收肌 adductor longus
17.闭孔神经后支 posterior branch of obturator nerve
18.股薄肌 gracilis
19.隐神经 saphenous nerve
20.足背内侧皮神经 medial dorsal cutaneous nerve of foot
21.臀下神经 inferior gluteal nerves
22.臀大肌 gluteus maximus
23.股后皮神经 posterior femoral cutaneous nerve
24.股二头肌长头 long head of biceps femoris
25.胫神经 tibial nerve
26.腓肠肌内侧头 medial head of gastrocnemius
27.腘肌 popliteus
28.臀上神经 superior gluteal nerves
29.梨状肌 piriformis
30.臀中肌 gluteus medius
31.股方肌 quadratus femoris
32.坐骨神经 sciatic nerve
33.腓总神经 common peroneal nerve
34.腓肠肌外侧头 lateral head of gastrocnemius
35.腓骨长肌 peroneus longus

409. 下肢的神经（前面观）
Nerves of the lower limb (anterior aspect)

410. 下肢的神经（后面观）
Nerves of the lower limb (posterior aspect)

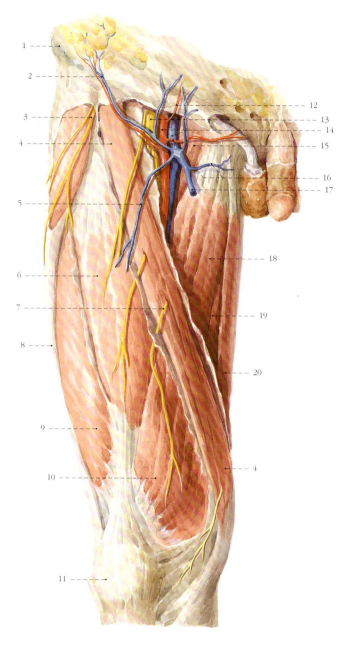

411. 股前部神经及其毗邻结构（1）

Nerves of the anterior aspect of the thigh and their adjacent
structures (1)

1.髂前上棘 anterior superior iliac spine

2.旋髂浅动、静脉 superficial iliac
circumflex artery and vein

3.股外侧皮神经 lateral femoral cutaneous
nerve

4.缝匠肌 sartorius

5.股外侧浅静脉 lateral femoral superficial
vein

6.股直肌 rectus femoris

7.股神经前皮支 anterior cutaneous
branch of femoral nerve

8.髂胫束 iliotibial tract

9.股外侧肌 vastus lateralis

10.股内侧肌 vastus medialis

11.髌骨 patella

12.腹壁浅动脉 superficial epigastric
artery

13.股神经 femoral nerve

14.股动、静脉 femoral artery and vein

15.耻骨肌 pectineus

16.阴部外动、静脉 external pudendal
artery and vein

17.大隐静脉 great saphenous vein

18.长收肌 adductor longus

19.大收肌 adductor magnus

20.股薄肌 gracilis

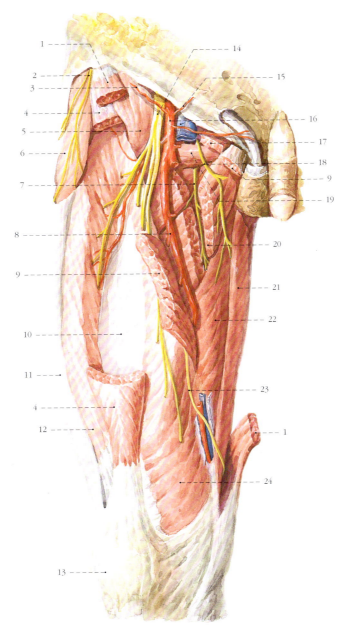

412. 股前部神经及其毗邻结构（2）

Nerves of the anterior aspect of the thigh and their adjacent
structures (2)

1.缝匠肌 sartorius

2.股外侧皮神经 lateral femoral cutaneous
　nerve

3.旋髂浅动脉 superficial iliac circumflex artery

4.股直肌 rectus femoris

5.髂腰肌 iliopsoas

6.阔筋膜张肌 tensor fasciae latae

7.闭孔神经后支 posterior branch of obturator
　neve

8.股深动脉 deep femoral artery

9.长收肌 adductor longus

10.股中间肌 vastus intermedius

11.髂胫束 iliotibial tract

12.股外侧肌 vastus lateralis

13.髌骨 patella

14.股神经 femoral nerve

15.腹壁浅动脉 superficial epigastric artery

16.股动、静脉 femoral artery and vein

17.耻骨肌 pectineus

18.闭孔神经前支 anterior branch of
　obturator nerve

19.闭孔外肌 obturator externus

20.短收肌 adductor brevis

21.股薄肌 gracilis

22.大收肌 adductor magnus

23.隐神经 saphenous nerve

24.股内侧肌 vastus medialis

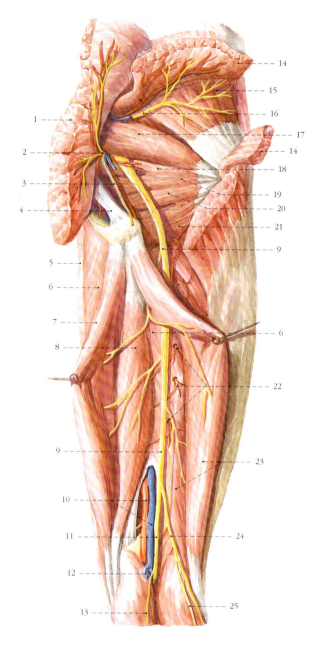

413. 臀部和股后部神经及其毗邻结构
The gluteal region and nerves of the posterior aspect of
the thigh and its adjacent structures

1.臀大肌 gluteus maximus
2.臀下动、静脉和神经 inferior gluteal artery，vein and nerve
3.股后皮神经 posterior femoral cutaneous nerve
4.骶结节韧带 sacrotuberous ligament
5.股薄肌 gracilis
6.大收肌 adductor magnus
7.半腱肌 semitendinosus
8.半膜肌 semimembranosus

9.坐骨神经 sciatic nerve
10.腘动、静脉 popliteal artery and vein
11.胫神经 tibial nerve
12.小隐静脉 small saphenous vein
13.腓肠内侧皮神经 medial sural cutaneous nerve
14.臀中肌 gluteus medius
15.臀小肌 gluteus minimus
16.臀上动、静脉和神经 superior gluteal artery, vein and nerve
17.梨状肌 piriformis

18.上孖肌 gemellus superior
19.闭孔内肌 obturator internus
20.下孖肌 gemellus inferior
21.股方肌 quadratus femoris
22.股深动脉穿支 perforating arteries of deep femoral artery
23.股二头肌长、短头 long head and short head of biceps femoris
24.腓总神经 common peroneal nerve
25.腓肠外侧皮神经 lateral sural cutaneous nerve

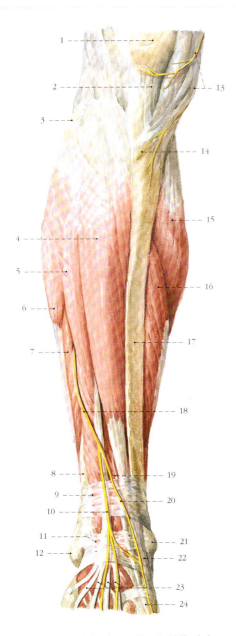

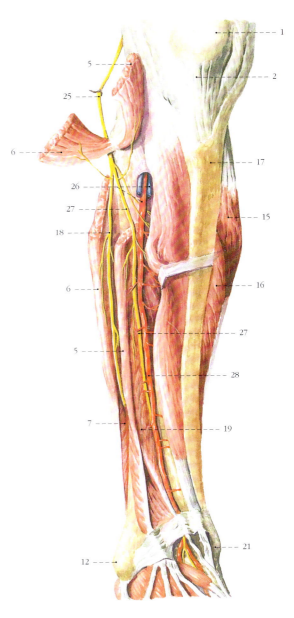

414. 小腿前部神经及其毗邻结构（1）
Nerves of the anterior aspect of the leg and their adjacent structures（1）

415. 小腿前部神经及其毗邻结构（2）
Nerves of the anterior aspect of the leg and their adjacent structures（2）

1.髌骨 patella

2.髌腱 patellar tendon

3.腓骨头 fibular head

4.胫骨前肌 tibialis anterior

5.趾长伸肌 extensor digitorum longus

6.腓骨长肌 peroneus longus

7.腓骨短肌 peroneus brevis

8.腓骨 fibula

9.伸肌上支持带 superior extensor retinaculum

10.足背中间皮神经 intermediate dorsal cutaneous nerve of foot

11.伸肌下支持带 inferior extensor retinaculum

12.外踝 lateral malleolus

13.隐神经髌下支 infrapatellar branch of saphenous nerve

14.胫骨粗隆 tibial tuberosity

15.腓肠肌 gastrocnemius

16.比目鱼肌 soleus

17.胫骨 tibia

18.腓浅神经 superficial peroneal nerve

19.踇长伸肌 extensor halluces longus

20.足背内侧皮神经 medial dorsal cutaneous nerve of foot

21.内踝 medial malleolus

22.胫骨前肌腱 tibialis anterior

23.趾长伸肌腱 extensor digitorum longus

24.踇长伸肌腱 extensor halluces longus

25.腓总神经 common peroneal nerve

26.胫前动、静脉 anterior tibial artery and vein

27.腓深神经 deep peroneal nerve

28.胫前动脉 anterior tibial artery

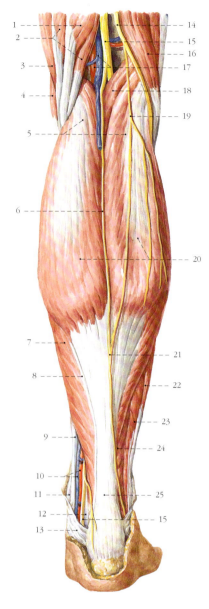

416. 小腿后部神经及其毗邻结构（1）

Nerves of the posterior aspect of the leg and their adjacent strucures（1）

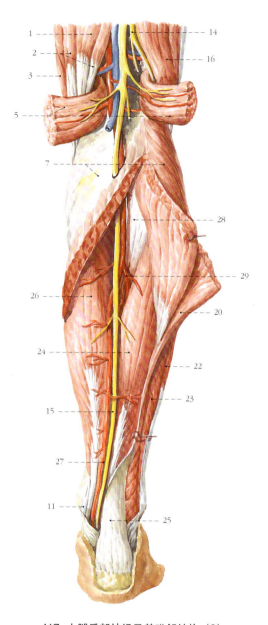

417. 小腿后部神经及其毗邻结构（2）

Nerves of the posterior aspect of the leg and their adjacent structures（2）

1.半腱肌 semitendinosus

2.半膜肌 semimembranosus

3.股薄肌 gracilis

4.缝匠肌 sartorius

5.腓肠肌内、外侧头 medial head and lateral head of gastrocnemius

6.腓肠内侧皮神经 medial sural cutaneous nerve

7.比目鱼肌 soleus

8.跖肌腱 tendon of plantaris

9.趾长屈肌腱 flexor digitorum longus

10.胫后动、静脉 posterior tibial artery and vein

11.胫骨后肌腱 tibialis posterior

12.踇长屈肌腱 flexor hallucis longus

13.屈肌支持带 flexor retinaculum

14.腓总神经 common peroneal nerve

15.胫神经 tibial nerve

16.股二头肌 biceps femoris

17.腘动、静脉 popliteal artery and vein

18.跖肌 plantaris

19.腓肠外侧皮神经 lateral sural cutaneous nerve

20.腓肠肌 gastrocnemius

21.腓肠神经 sural nerve

22.腓骨长肌 peroneus longus

23.腓骨短肌 peroneus brevis

24.踇长屈肌 flexor halluces longus

25.跟腱 tendo calcaneus

26.趾长屈肌 flexor digitorum longus

27.胫后动脉 posterior tibial artery

28.胫骨后肌 tibialis posterior

29.腓动脉 peroneal artery

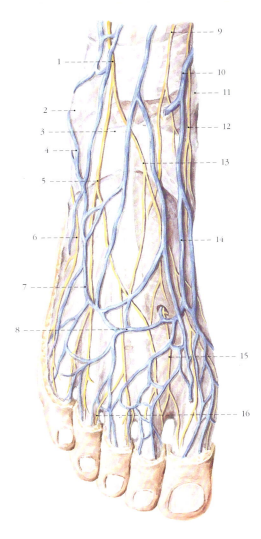

1.腓浅神经 superficial peroneal nerve
2.外踝 lateral malleolus
3.伸肌下支持带 inferior extensor retinaculum
4.小隐静脉 small saphenous vein
5.足背中间皮神经 intermediate dorsal cutaneous nerve of foot
6.足背外侧皮神经 lateral dorsal cutaneous nerve of foot
7.外侧缘静脉 lateral marginal vein
8.足背静脉弓 dorsal venous arch of foot
9.隐神经小腿内侧皮支 medial crural cutaneous branches of saphenous nerve
10.大隐静脉 great saphenous vein
11.内踝 medial malleolus
12.隐神经 saphenous nerve
13.足背内侧皮神经 medial dorsal cutaneous nerve of foot
14.内侧缘静脉 medial marginal vein
15.腓深神经皮支 cutaneous branches of deep peroneal nerve
16.趾背神经 dorsal digital nerves of foot
17.踇长伸肌 extensor halluces longus
18.趾长伸肌 extensor digitorum longus
19.腓动脉穿支 perforating branch of peroneal artery

418. 足背部的神经及静脉
Nerves and veins of the dorsum of the foot

20.外踝前动脉 lateral anterior malleolar artery
21.踇短伸肌、趾短伸肌 extensor halluces brevis，extensor digitorum brevis
22.第三腓骨肌腱 peroneus tertius
23.弓状动脉 arcuate artery
24.跖背动脉 dorsal metatarsal arteries
25.趾长伸肌腱 extensor digitorum longus
26.趾背动脉 dorsal digital arteries
27.胫骨前肌 tibialis anterior
28.胫前动脉 anterior tibial artery
29.腓深神经 deep peroneal nerve
30.内踝前动脉 medial anterior malleolar artery
31.腓深神经外侧支 lateral branch of deep fibular nerve
32.跗内侧动脉 medial tarsal arteries
33.跗外侧动脉 lateral tarsal artery
34.跖骨 metatarsal bones
35.骨间背侧肌 dorsal interossei
36.趾短伸肌腱 extensor digitorum brevis
37.踇短伸肌腱 extensor halluces brevis
38.趾背神经 dorsal digital nerve of foot

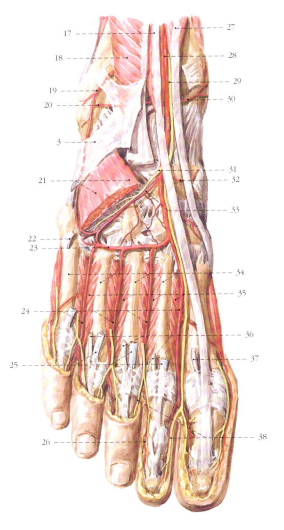

419. 足背部的神经及动脉
Nerves and arteries of the dorsum of the foot

1.蚓状肌 lumbricales

2.小趾短屈肌 flexor digiti minimi brevis

3.足底外侧动脉、神经 lateral plantar artery and nerve

4.小趾展肌 abductor digiti minimi

5.趾足底固有动脉、神经 proper plantar digital arteries，nerves

6.趾足底总动脉 common plantar digital arteries

7.踇短屈肌内、外侧头 medial head and lateral head of flexor halluces brevis

8.踇展肌 abductor halluces

9.趾短屈肌 flexor digitorum brevis

10.足底腱膜 plantar aponeurosis

11.跟骨结节 calcaneal tuberosity

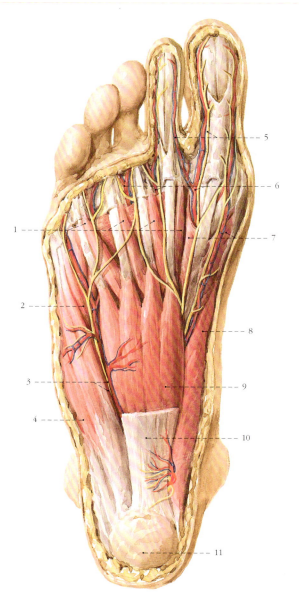

420. 足底部的神经及血管（1）
Nerves and blood vessels of the sole of the foot (1)

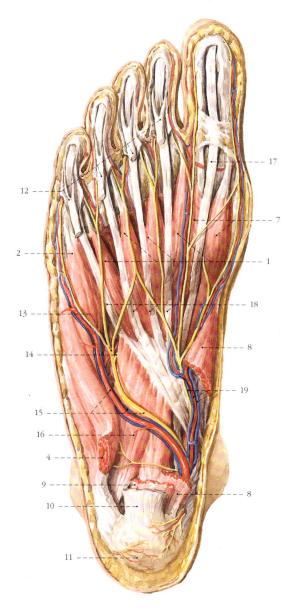

421. 足底部的神经及血管（2）
Nerves and blood vessels of the sole of the foot (2)

12.趾短屈肌腱 flexor digitorum brevis

13.浅支 superficial branch

14.深支 deep branch

15.足底外侧动、静脉和神经 lateral plantar artery，vein and nerve

16.足底方肌 quadratus plantae

17.踇长屈肌腱 flexor halluces longus

18.趾长屈肌腱 flexor digitorum longus

19.足底内侧动、静脉和神经 medial plantar artery，vein and nerve

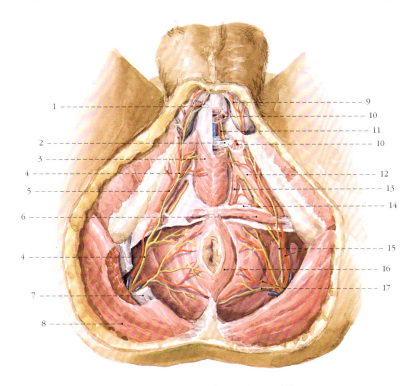

422. 男性会阴部的神经及其毗邻结构
Nerves in the male perineum and their adjacent structures

1. 阴囊后神经　posterior scrotal nerves
2. 会阴横韧带　transverse ligament of perineum
3. 球海绵体肌　bulbocavernosus
4. 会阴动脉、神经　perineal artery, nerve
5. 阴茎深动脉、阴茎背神经　deep artery of penis, dorsal nerve of penis
6. 会阴浅横肌　superficial transverse muscle of perineum
7. 骶结节韧带　sacrotuberous ligament
8. 臀大肌　gluteus maximus
9. 阴部内动脉阴囊后支　posterior scrotal branches of internal pudendal artery
10. 阴茎深动脉　deep artery of penis
11. 阴茎背动脉、神经　dorsal artery, nerve of penis
12. 坐骨海绵体肌　ischiocavernosus
13. 会阴深横肌　deep transverse muscle of perineum
14. 尿生殖膈下筋膜　inferior fascia of urogenital diaphragm
15. 阴部内动、静脉及阴部神经　internal pudendal artery, vein and pudendal nerve
16. 肛门外括约肌　sphincter ani externus
17. 肛动、静脉及神经　anal artery, vein and nerve
18. 前庭球　bulb of vestibule
19. 阴唇后神经　posterior labial nerve
20. 阴蒂深动脉、阴蒂背神经　deep artery of clitoris, dorsal nerve of clitoris
21. 前庭大腺　great vestibular gland
22. 阴唇后支、阴唇后神经　posterior labial branches and posterior labial nerve

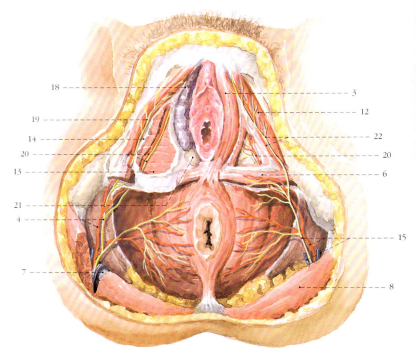

423. 女性会阴部的神经及其毗邻结构
Nerves in the female perineum and their adjacent structures

1.头静脉 cephalic vein
2.胸大肌 pectoralis major
3.肱二头肌长头 long head of biceps brachii
4.肱二头肌短头 short head of biceps brachii
5.肌皮神经 musculocutaneous nerve
6.肱骨 humerus
7.肱三头肌 triceps brachii
8.三角肌 deltoid
9.臂筋膜 brachial fascia
10.喙肱肌 coracobrachialis
11.大圆肌 teres major
12.正中神经 median nerve
13.前臂内侧皮神经 medial antebrachial cutaneous nerve
14.肱静脉 brachial veins
15.尺神经 ulnar nerve
16.肱深动脉 deep brachial artery
17.臂内侧皮神经 medial brachial cutaneous nerve
18.桡神经 radial nerve
19.肱动脉 brachial artery
20.背阔肌腱 tendon of latissimus dorsi
21.肱二头肌 biceps brachii
22.肱肌 brachialis
23.前臂后皮神经 posterior antebrachial cutaneous nerve
24.桡侧副动脉 radial collateral artery
25.外侧肌间隔 lateral brachial intermuscular septum
26.中副动脉 middle collateral artery
27.内侧肌间隔 medial brachial intermuscular septum
28.肱动、静脉 brachial artery, vein
29.尺侧上副动、静脉 superior ulnar collateral artery, vein
30.前臂外侧皮神经 lateral antebrachial cutaneous nerve
31.肱桡肌 brachioradialis
32.桡侧腕长伸肌 extensor carpi radialis longus

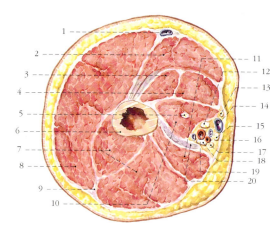

424. 右臂近侧 1/3 横切面（A）
The transverse section through the porximal
1/3 of the right arm (A)

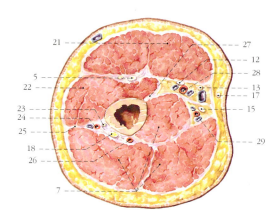

425. 右臂中 1/3 横切面（B）
The transverse section through the
middle 1/3 of the right arm (B)

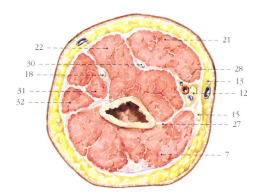

426. 右臂远侧 1/3 横切面（C）
The transverse section through the distal 1/3 of the
right arm (C)

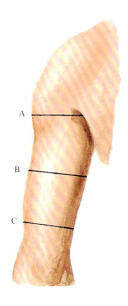

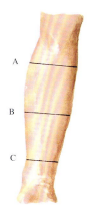

1.桡动脉、桡神经浅支 radial artery and superficial branch of radial nerve

2.肱桡肌 brachioradialis

3.桡侧腕长伸肌 extensor carpi radialis longus

4.旋后肌 supinator

5.指浅屈肌 flexor digitorum superficialis

6.拇长屈肌 flexor pollicis longus

7.桡神经深支 deep branch of radial nerve

8.桡侧腕短伸肌 extensor carpi radialis brevis

9.指伸肌 extensor digitorum

10.小指伸肌 extensor digiti minimi

11.肘肌 anconeus

12.桡骨 radius

13.旋前圆肌 pronator teres

14.掌长肌 palmaris longus

15.指浅屈肌 flexor digitorum superficialis

16.桡侧腕屈肌 flexor carpi radialis

17.尺侧腕屈肌 flexor carpi ulnaris

18.尺神经 ulnar nerve

19.尺动脉、正中神经 ulnar artery，median nerve

20.骨间总动脉 common interosseous artery

21.尺骨 ulna

22.指深屈肌 flexor digitorum profundus

23.尺侧腕伸肌 extensor carpi ulnaris

24.骨间前动脉、神经 anterior interosseous artery，nerve

25.骨间后动脉、神经 posterior interosseous artery，nerve

26.正中神经 median nerve

27.尺动脉、神经 ulnar artery，nerve

28.拇长伸肌 extensor pollicis longus

29.掌长肌腱 tendon of palmaris longus

30.桡侧腕屈肌腱 tendon of flexor carpi ulnaris

31.桡动脉 radial artery

32.肱桡肌腱 tendon of brachioradialis

33.桡神经浅支 superficial branch of radial nerve

34.拇长、短展肌腱 tendon of abductor pollicis longus and brevis

35.桡侧腕长伸肌腱 tendon of extensor carpi radialis longus

36.桡侧腕短伸肌腱 tendon of extensor carpi radialis brevis

37.拇长伸肌腱 tendon of extensor pollicis longus

38.指伸肌腱 tendon of extensor digitorum

39.指浅屈肌腱 tendon of flexor digitorum superficialis

40.指深屈肌腱 tendon of flexor digitorum profundus

41.旋前方肌 pronator quadratus

42.示指伸肌腱 extensor indicis

43.桡神经背支 dorsal branch of radial nerve

44.尺侧腕伸肌腱 tendon of extensor carpi ulnaris

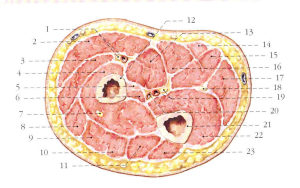

427. 右前臂近侧 1/3 横切面（A）
The transverse section through the proximal
1/3 of right forearm (A)

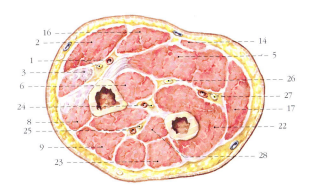

428. 右前臂中 1/3 横切面（B）
The transverse section through the
middle 1/3 of right forearm (B)

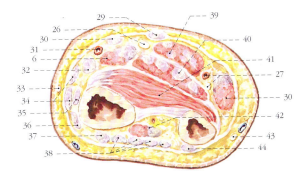

429. 右前臂远侧 1/3 横切面（C）
The transverse section through the distal
1/3 of right forearm (C)

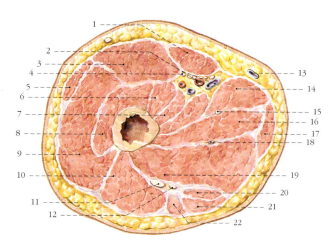

430. 右大腿近侧 1/3 横切面（A）

The transverse section through the proximal 1/3 of
the right thigh (A)

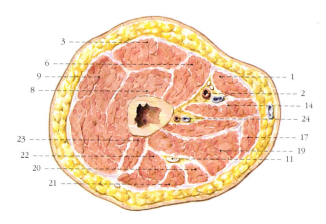

431. 右大腿中 1/3 横切面（B）

The transverse section through the middle 1/3 of the
right thigh (B)

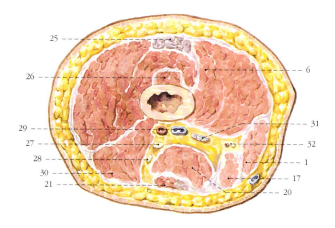

432. 右大腿远侧 1/3 横切面（C）

The transverse section through the distal 1/3 of the
right thigh (C)

1.缝匠肌 sartorius
2.股动、静脉 femoral artery，vein
3.股直肌 rectus femoris
4.股神经 femoral nerve
5.阔筋膜张肌 tensor fasciae latae
6.股内侧肌 vastus medialis
7.髂腰肌 iliopsoas
8.股中间肌 vastus intermedius
9.股外侧肌 vastus lateralis
10.臀大肌 gluteus maximus
11.坐骨神经 sciatic nerve
12.股后皮神经 posterior femoral cutaneous nerve
13.大隐静脉 great saphenous vein
14.长收肌 adductor longus
15.闭孔神经前支 anterior branch of obturator nerve
16.短收肌 adductor brevis
17.股薄肌 gracilis
18.闭孔神经后支 posterior branch of obturator nerve
19.大收肌 adductor magnus
20.半膜肌 semimembranosus
21.半腱肌 semitendinosus
22.股二头肌长头 long head of biceps femoris
23.股二头肌短头 short head of biceps femoris
24.股深动、静脉 deep femoral artery，vein
25.股四头肌腱 tendon of quadriceps femoris
26.膝关节肌 articularis genus
27.胫神经 tibial nerve
28.腓总神经 common peroneal nerve
29.腘动、静脉 popliteal artery，vein
30.股二头肌 biceps femoris
31.大收肌腱 adductor magnus
32.隐神经 saphenous nerve

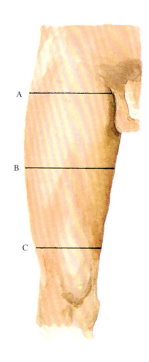

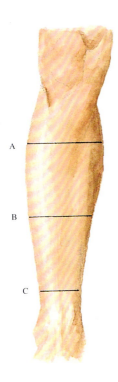

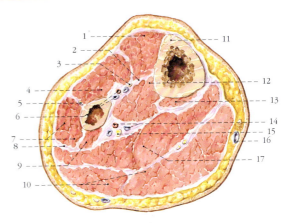

433. 右小腿近侧 1/3 横切面（A）
The transverse section through the proximal 1/3 of the right leg (A)

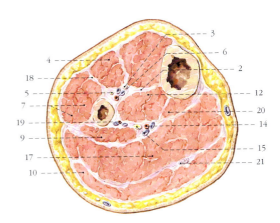

434. 右小腿中 1/3 横切面（B）
The transverse section through the middle 1/3 of the right leg (B)

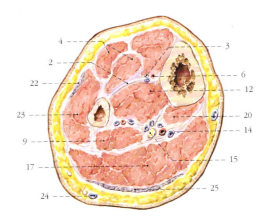

435. 右小腿远侧 1/3 横切面（C）
The transverse section through the distal 1/3 of the right leg (C)

1. 胫骨前肌 tibialis anterior
2. 小腿骨间膜 interosseous membrane of leg
3. 腓深神经 deep peroneal nerve
4. 趾长、踇长伸肌 extensor digitorum longus, extensor hallucis longus
5. 腓浅神经 superficial peroneal nerve
6. 胫前动、静脉 anterior tibial artery, vein
7. 腓骨长、短肌 peroneus longus and brevis
8. 小腿后肌间隔 posterior crural intermuscular septum
9. 踇长屈肌 flexor hallucis longus
10. 腓肠肌 gastrocnemius
11. 胫骨 tibia
12. 胫骨后肌 tibialis posterior
13. 腘肌 popliteus
14. 胫后动、静脉 posterior tibial artery
15. 胫神经 tibial nerve
16. 大隐静脉 great saphenous vein
17. 比目鱼肌 soleus
18. 小腿前肌间隔 anterior crural intermuscular septum
19. 腓动、静脉 peroneal artery, vein
20. 趾长屈肌 flexor digitorum longus
21. 跖肌 plantaris
22. 腓骨长肌 peroneus longus
23. 腓骨短肌 peroneus brevis
24. 小隐静脉 small saphenous vein
25. 腓肠肌腱 tendon of gastrocnemius

217

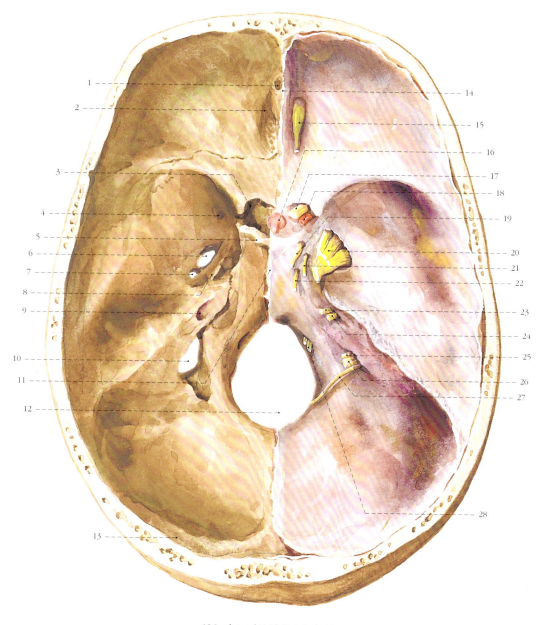

436. 十二对脑神经出颅部位

The inlet and exit points of the 12 pairs of cranial nerves

1.盲孔 foramen cecum

2.筛板 cribriform plate

3.视神经管 optic canal

4.圆孔 foramen rotundum

5.鞍背 dorsum sellae

6.卵圆孔 foramen ovale

7.棘孔 foramen spinosum

8.破裂孔 foramen lacerum

9.内耳门 internal acoustic pore

10.颈静脉孔 jugular foramen

11.斜坡 clivus

12.枕骨大孔 foramen magnum of occipital bone

13.横窦沟 sulcus for transverse sinus

14.鸡冠 crista galli

15.嗅球 olfactory bulb

16.垂体 hypophysis

17.视神经 optic nerve

18.眼动脉 ophthalmic artery

19.动眼神经 oculomotor nerve

20.三叉神经节 trigeminal ganglion

21.滑车神经 trochlear nerve

22.展神经 abducent nerve

23.面神经 facial nerve

24.前庭蜗神经 vestibulocochlear nerve

25.舌咽神经 glossopharyngeal nerve

26.迷走神经 vagus nerve

27.副神经 accessory nerve

28.舌下神经 hypoglossal nerve

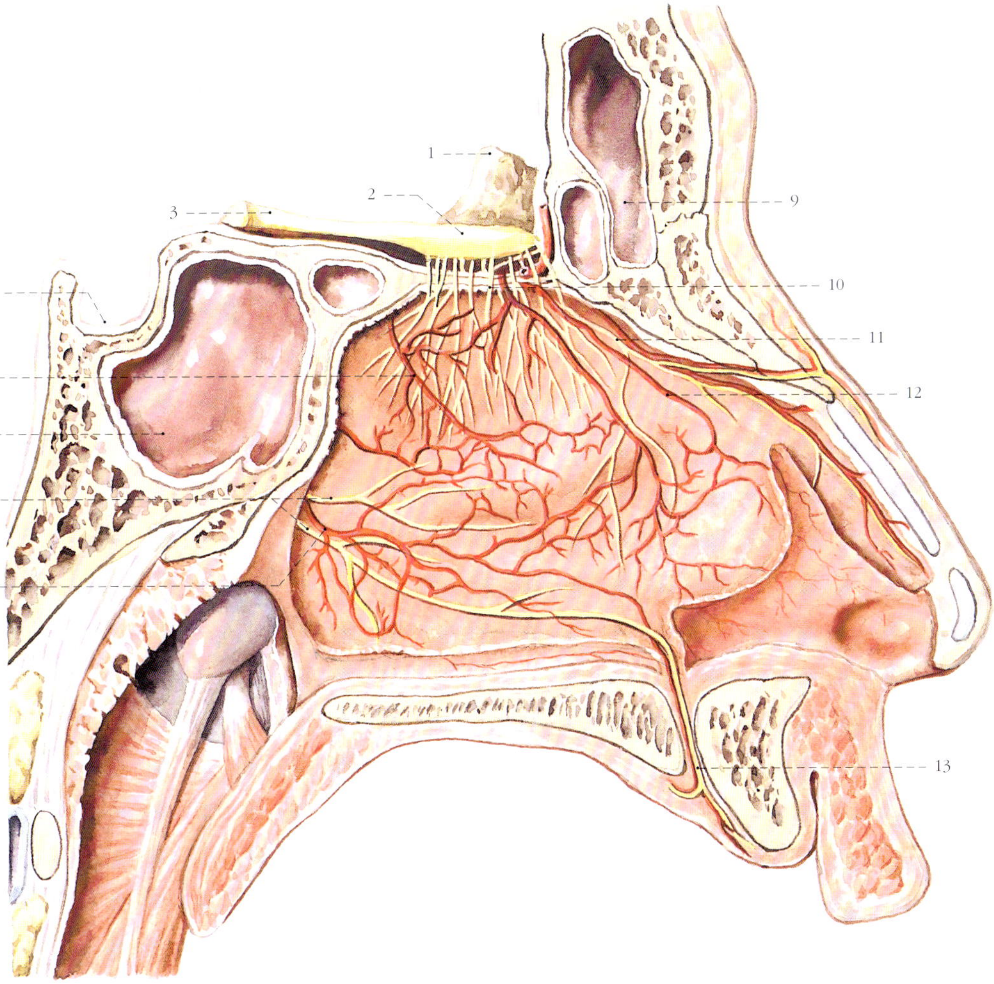

437. 鼻腔内的神经

Nerves in the nasal cavity

1.鸡冠 crista galli

2.嗅球 olfactory bulb

3.嗅束 olfactory tract

4.垂体窝 hypophysial fossa

5.筛后动脉 posterior ethmoidal artery

6.蝶窦 sphenoid sinus

7.鼻后支 posterior nasal branches

8.蝶腭动脉 sphenopalatine artery

9.额窦 frontal sinus

10.嗅神经 olfactory nerves

11.筛前神经（鼻支）anterior ethmoidal nerve（nasal branch）

12.筛前动脉 anterior ethmoidal artery

13.鼻腭神经 nasopalatine nerves

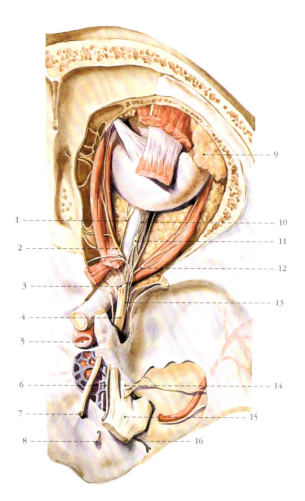

1. 睫状长神经 long ciliary nerve
2. 鼻睫神经 nasociliary nerve
3. 额神经 frontal nerve
4. 眼神经 ophthalmic nerve
5. 眼动脉 ophthalmic artery
6. 滑车神经 trochlear nerve
7. 动眼神经 oculomotor nerve
8. 展神经 abducent nerve
9. 泪腺 lacrimal gland
10. 睫状短神经 short ciliary nerve
11. 睫状神经节 ciliary ganglion
12. 展神经 abducent nerve
13. 泪腺神经 lacrimal nerve
14. 上颌神经 maxillary nerve
15. 三叉神经节 trigeminal ganglion
16. 三叉神经 trigeminal nerve
17. 上斜肌 superior obliquus
18. 外直肌 lateral rectus
19. 下颌神经 mandibular nerve
20. 眶上神经 superior orbital nerve
21. 滑车上神经 superior trochlear nerve
22. 上睑提肌 levator palpebrae superioris
23. 上直肌 superior rectus
24. 上睑 upper eyelid
25. 下睑 lower eyelid
26. 下斜肌 inferior obliquus

438. 眶腔内的神经（上面观）
Nerves in the orbit (superior aspect)

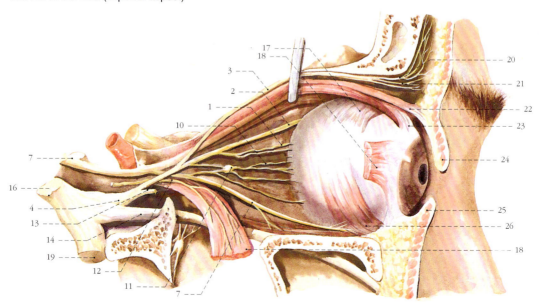

439. 眶腔内的神经（外侧面观）
Nerves in the orbit（lateral aspect）

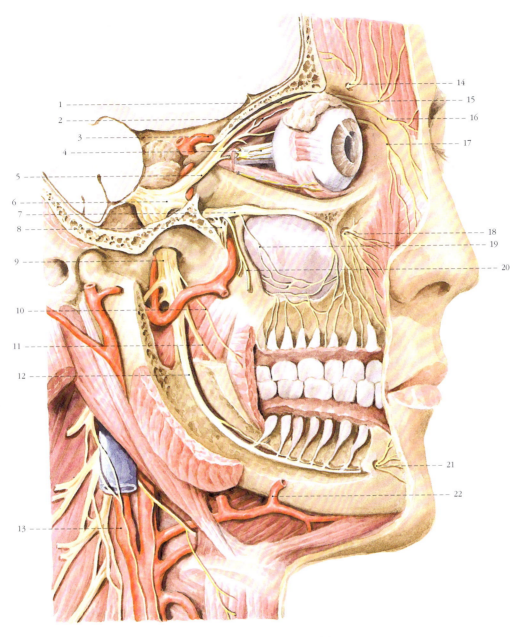

440. 三叉神经及其分支（1）
The trigeminal nerve and its branches (1)

1.额神经 frontal nerve
2.泪腺神经 lacrimal nerve
3.眼动脉 ophthalmic artery
4.视神经 optic nerve
5.眼神经 ophthalmic nerve
6.三叉神经节 trigeminal ganglion
7.上颌神经 maxillary nerve
8.翼腭神经节 pterygopalatine ganglion

9.下颌神经 mandibular nerve
10.颊神经 buccal nerve
11.舌神经 lingual nerve
12.下牙槽神经 inferior alveolar nerve
13.颈内动脉 internal carotid artery
14.眶上神经 supraorbital nerve
15.滑车上神经 supratrochlear nerve
16.滑车下神经 infratrochlear nerve

17.筛前神经 anterior ethmoidal nerve
18.眶下神经 infraorbital nerve
19.上牙槽前支 anterior superior alveolar branches
20.上牙槽后支 posterior superior alveolar branches
21.颏神经 mental nerve
22.面动脉 facial artery

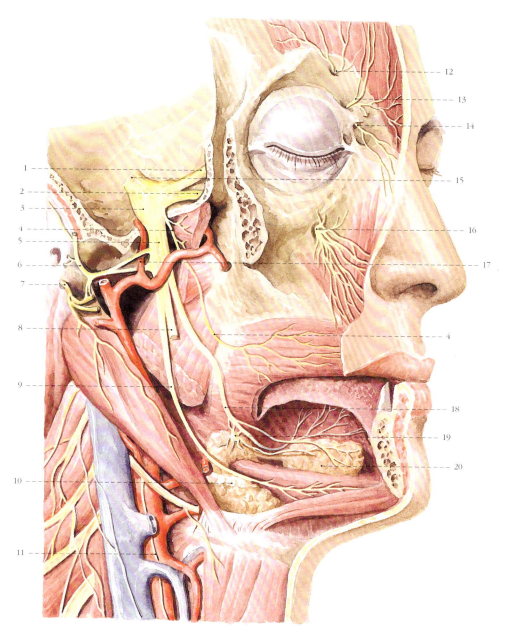

441. 三叉神经及其分支（2）

The trigeminal nerve and its branches (2)

1.眼神经 ophthalmic nerve
2.上颌神经 maxillary nerve
3.三叉神经节 trigeminal ganglion
4.颊神经 buccal nerve
5.下颌神经 mandibular nerve
6.耳颞神经 auriculotemporal nerve
7.面神经 facial nerve

8.下牙槽神经 inferior alveolar nerve
9.下颌舌骨肌神经 mylohyoid nerve
10.下颌下腺 submandibular gland
11.舌下神经降支 descending branch
　　of sublingual nerve
12.眶上神经 supraorbital nerve
13.滑车上神经 supratrochlear nerve

14.筛前神经 anterior ethmoidal nerve
15.三叉神经 trigeminal nerve
16.眶下神经 infraorbital nerve
17.脑膜中动脉 middle meningeal artery
18.舌神经 lingual nerve
19.下颌下神经节 submandibular ganglion
20.舌下腺 sublingual gland

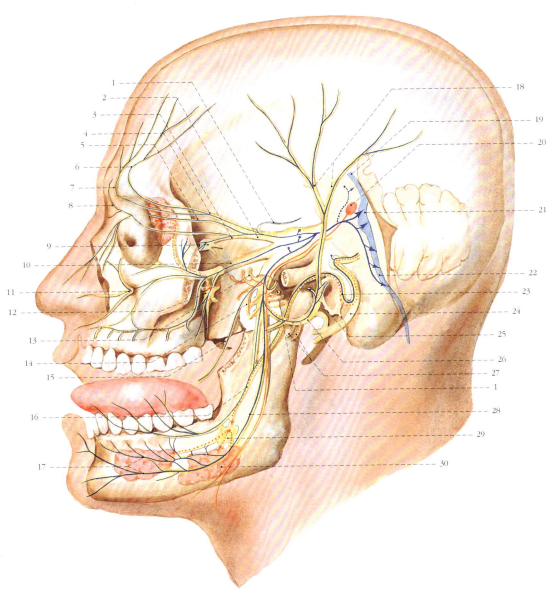

442. 三叉神经的纤维成分及其分布（模式图）

Fiber compositions and distribution of the trigeminal nerve (diagram)

1.脑膜支 meningeal branch

2.眼神经 ophthalmic nerve

3.鼻睫神经 nasociliary nerve

4.额神经 frontal nerve

5.泪腺神经 lacrimal nerve

6.眶上神经 supraorbital nerve

7.滑车上神经 supratrochlear nerve

8.滑车下神经 infratrochlear nerve

9.睫状神经节 ciliary ganglion

10.上颌神经 maxillary nerve

11.眶下神经 infraorbital nerve

12.翼腭神经节 pterygopalatine ganglion

13.颞深神经 deep temporal nerves

14.咀嚼肌神经 nerves of masticatory muscles

15.颊神经 buccal nerve

16.舌神经 lingual nerve

17.下牙丛 inferior dental plexus

18.颞浅支 superficial temporal branch

19.三叉神经中脑核 mesencephalic nucleus of trigeminal nerve

20.三叉神经运动核 motor nucleus of trigeminal nerve

21.三叉神经脑桥核 pontine nucleus of trigeminal nerve

22.三叉神经脊束核 spinal tract nucleus of trigeminal nerve

23.鼓索 chorda tympani

24.面神经 facial nerve

25.耳支 auricular branch

26.耳颞神经 auriculotemporal nerve

27.腮腺支 parotid branches

28.下牙槽神经 inferior alveolar nerve

29.下颌下神经节 submandibular ganglion

30.下颌下腺 submandibular gland

223

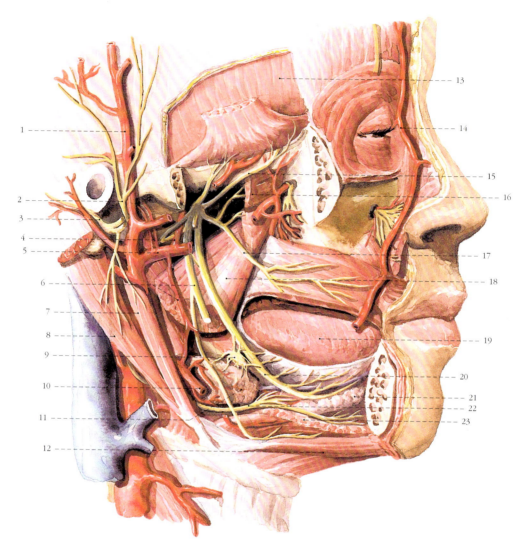

443. 下颌神经的分支和下颌下神经节
Branches of mandibular nerue and submandibular gonglion

1.颞浅动脉 superficial temporal artery
2.耳颞神经 auriculotemporal nerve
3.面神经 facial nerve
4.脑膜中动脉 middle meningeal artery
5.上颌动脉 maxillary artery
6.下牙槽动脉、神经 inferior alveolar artery, nerve
7.茎突舌骨肌 stylohyoid

8.二腹肌（后腹）posterior belly of digastric
9.下颌下神经节 submandibular ganglion
10.面动脉 facial artery
11.下颌下腺 submandibular gland
12.二腹肌（前腹）anterior belly of digastric
13.颞肌 temporalis
14.内眦动脉 angular artery
15.颞深神经 deep temporal nerve

16.翼外肌 lateral pterygoid
17.颊神经 buccal nerve
18.翼内肌 medial pterygoid
19.舌 tongue
20.舌神经 lingual nerve
21.舌下腺 sublingual gland
22.舌下神经 hypoglossal nerve
23.下颌舌骨肌 mylohyoid

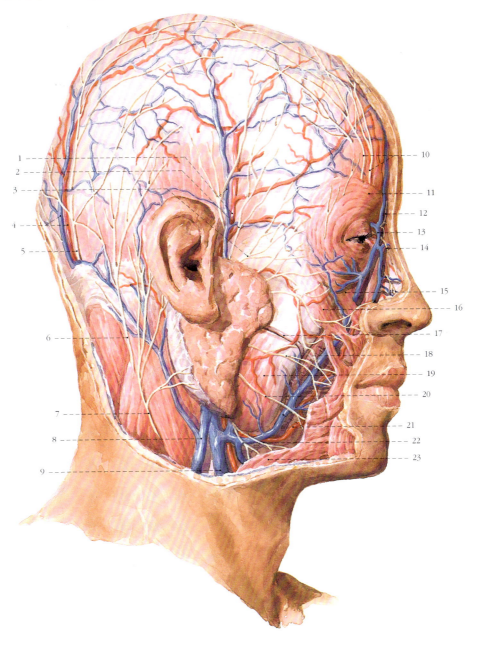

444. 面神经的分支及其毗邻结构

Branches and adjacent structures of the facial nerve

1.颞浅动、静脉 superficial temporal artery，vein

2.面神经颞支 temporal branches of facial nerve

3.面神经颧支 zygomatic branches of facial nerve

4.枕动、静脉 occipital artery，vein

5.枕大神经 greater occipital nerve

6.枕小神经 lesser occipital nerve

7.耳大神经 great auricular nerve

8.颈外静脉 external carotid artery

9.颈内静脉 retromandibular vein

10.额神经内、外侧支 lateral and medial branches of frontal nerve

11.眼轮匝肌 orbicularis oculi

12.滑车上神经 supratrochlear nerve

13.内眦静脉 angular vein

14.滑车下神经 infratrochlear nerve

15.颧小肌 zygomaticus minor

16.颧大肌 zygomaticus major

17.腮腺管 parotid duct

18.面神经颊支 buccal branches of facial nerve

19.咬肌 masseter

20.面神经下颌缘支 marginal mandibular branch of facial nerve

21.面动、静脉 facial artery，vein

22.面神经颈支 cervical branch of facial nerve

23.颈阔肌 platysma

225

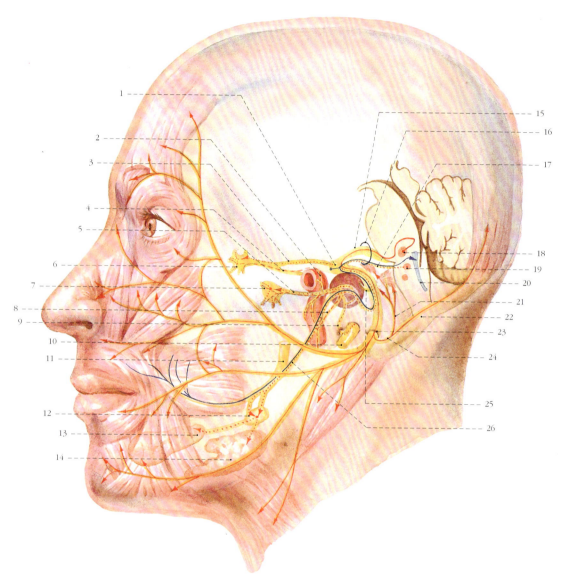

445. 面神经的纤维成分及其分布（模式图）
Fiber compositions and distribution of the facial nerve (diagram)

1.膝神经节 geniculate ganglion
2.颈内动脉及神经丛 internal carotid artery and nerve plexus
3.岩大神经 greater petrosal nerve
4.岩深神经 deep petrosal nerve
5.岩小神经 lesser petrosal nerve
6.翼腭神经节 pterygopalatine ganglion
7.耳神经节 otic ganglion
8.颈鼓神经 caroticotympanic nerves
9.鼓室神经 tympanic nerve

10.舌咽神经 glossopharyngeal nerve
11.舌神经 lingual nerve
12.下颌下神经节 submandibular ganglion
13.舌下腺 sublingual gland
14.下颌下腺 submandibular gland
15.面神经 facial nerve
16.内听道 internal acoustic meatus
17.中间神经 intermediate nerve
18.面神经核 nucleus of facial nerve
19.上涎核 superior salivary nucleus

20.孤束核 solitary tract nucleus
21.耳后神经耳肌支 auriculomuscular branch of posterior auricular nerve
22.耳后神经枕支 occipital branch of posterior auricular nerve
23.茎乳孔 stylomastoid foramen
24.耳后神经 posterior auricular nerve
25.镫骨肌支 stapedial nerve
26.鼓索 chorda tympani

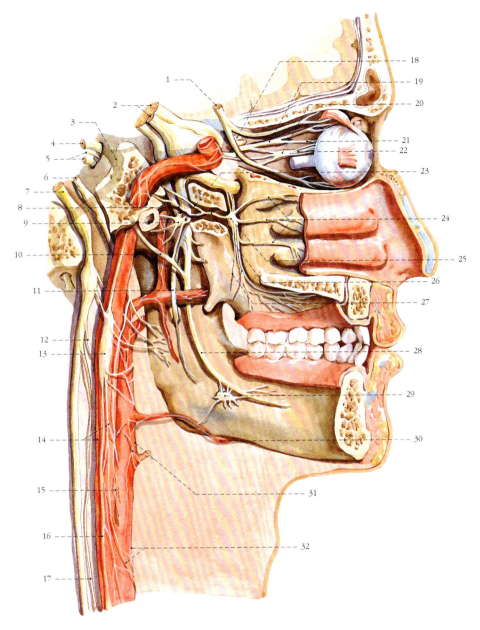

446. 睫状神经节、翼腭神经节、耳神经节及下颌下神经节和脑神经

Ciliary ganglion，pterygopalatine ganglion，otic ganglion，submandibular ganglion and cranial nerves

1.动眼神经 oculomotor nerve

2.三叉神经 trigeminal nerve

3.膝神经节 geniculate ganglion

4.面神经 facial nerve

5.前庭蜗神经 vestibulocochlear nerve

6.舌咽神经 glossopharyngeal nerve

7.迷走神经 vagus nerve

8.岩深神经 deep petrosal nerve

9.耳神经节 otic ganglion

10.鼓索 chorda tympani

11.下牙槽神经 inferior alveolar nerve

12.喉上神经 superior laryngeal nerve

13.颈上节 superior cervical ganglion

14.颈内动脉及神经丛 internal carotid artery and nerve plexus

15.舌咽神经颈动脉窦支 carotid sinus branch of glossopharyngeal nerve

16.颈交感干 cervical sympathetic trunk

17.迷走神经心上支 superior cardiac branch of vagus nerve

18.眼神经 ophthalmic nerve

19.鼻睫神经 nasociliary nerve

20.睫状神经节 ciliary ganglion

21.睫状长神经 long ciliary nerve

22.睫状短神经 short ciliary nerve

23.岩大神经 greater petrosal nerve

24.后外侧鼻神经 posterior lateral nasal nerve

25.翼腭神经节 pterygopalatine ganglion

26.翼管神经 nerve of pterygoid canal

27.腭大、小神经 greater and lesser palatine nerves

28.舌神经 lingual nerve

29.下颌下神经节 submandibular ganglion

30.面动脉及神经丛 facial artery and nerve plexus

31.颈外动脉及神经丛 external carotid artery and nerve plexus

32.颈总动脉及神经丛 common carotid artery and nerve plexus

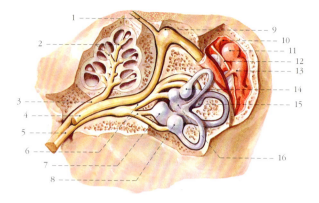

447. 前庭蜗神经和面神经（模式图）
Vestibulocochlear nerve and facial nerve (diagram)

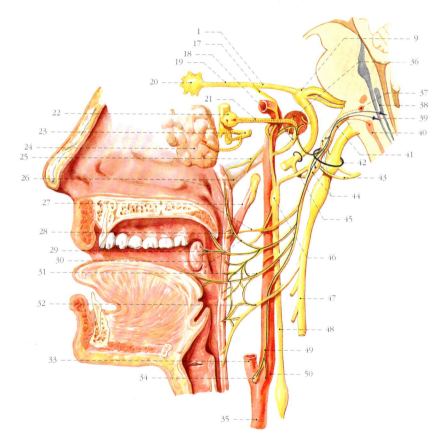

448. 舌咽神经的纤维成分及其分布
Fiber composition and distribution of the glossopharyngeal nerve

14.上半规管壶腹 ampulla of superior semicircular canal
15.外半规管壶腹 ampulla of lateral semicircular canal
16.椭圆囊 utricle
17.岩深神经 deep petrosal nerve
18.颈鼓神经 caroticotympanic nerves
19.翼管神经 nerve of pterygoid canal
20.翼腭神经节 pterygopalatine ganglion
21.岩小神经 lesser petrosal nerve
22.耳神经节 otic ganglion
23.耳颞神经 auriculotemporal nerve
24.腮腺 parotid gland
25.鼓室丛咽鼓管支 tubal branch of tympamic plexus
26.咽鼓管及咽口 eustachian tube and pharyngeal ostium
27.茎突咽肌及神经支 stylopharyngeal muscle and nerve branch
28.咽丛 pharyngeal plexus
29.扁桃体支 tonsil branches
30.咽支 pharyngeal branches
31.舌支 lingual branches
32.迷走神经咽支 pharyngeal branches of vagus nerve
33.颈外动脉 external carotid artery
34.颈动脉体 carotid body
35.颈总动脉 common carotid artery
36.鼓室神经 tympanic nerve
37.下涎核 inferior salivary nucleus
38.孤束核 solitary tract nucleus
39.三叉神经脊束核 spinal nucleus of trigeminal nerve
40.疑核 nucleus ambiguus
41.舌咽神经 glossopharyngeal nerve
42.颈静脉孔 jugular foramen
43.迷走神经耳支 auricular branch of vagus nerve
44.舌咽神经上、下节 superior and inferior ganglions of glossopharyngeal nerve
45.面神经的交通支 communicating branches to facial nerve
46.颈上节 superior cervical ganglion
47.迷走神经 vagus nerve
48.交感干 sympathetic trunk
49.颈动脉窦支 carotid sinus branch
50.颈动脉窦 carotid sinus

1.岩大神经 greater petrosal nerve
2.螺旋神经节 spiral ganglion
3.蜗神经 cochlear nerve
4.面神经 facial nerve
5.前庭神经 vestibular nerve
6.前庭 vestibule
7.球囊 saccule
8.后半规管壶腹 ampulla of posterior semicircular canal
9.面神经膝节 genu of facial nerve
10.鼓室 tympanic carity
11.锤骨头 head of malleus
12.鼓索 chorda tympani
13.砧骨 incus

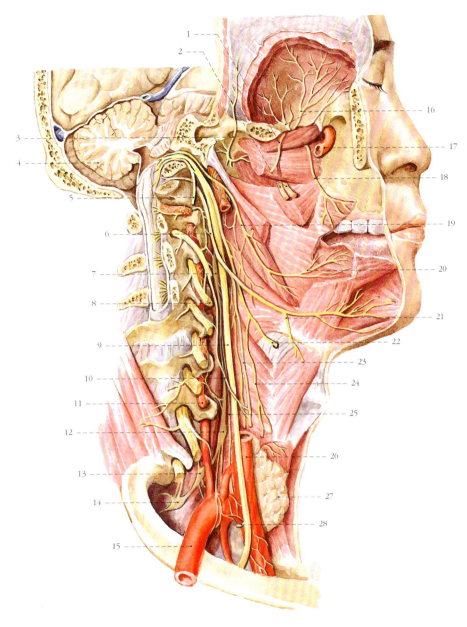

449. 舌咽神经、迷走神经、副神经和舌下神经
Glossopharyngeal nerve, vagus nerve, accessory nerve and hypoglossal nerve

1.咬肌神经 masseter nerve

2.下牙槽神经和舌神经 inferior alveolar nerve and lingual nerve

3.耳颞神经 auriculotemporal nerve

4.小脑 cerebellum

5.副神经 accessory nerve

6.舌下神经 hypoglossal nerve

7.颈上神经节 superior cervical ganglion

8.第三颈神经前支 anterior branch of third cervical nerve

9.迷走神经 vagus nerve

10.颈袢 ansa cervicalis

11.椎动脉 vertebral artery

12.颈中神经节 middle cervical ganglion

13.颈下神经节 inferior cervical ganglion

14.第一胸神经节 first thoracic ganglion

15.锁骨下动脉 subclavian artery

16.颞深神经 deep temporal nerve

17.上颌动脉 maxillary artery

18.颊神经 buccal nerve

19.舌咽神经 glossopharyngeal nerve

20.舌咽神经舌支 lingual branch of glossopharygeal nerve

21.舌下神经肌支 muscular branch of hypoglossal nerve

22.喉上神经（内支）superior laryngeal nerve（internal branch）

23.颈袢上根 superior root of ansa cervicalis

24.喉上神经（外支）superior laryngeal nerve（external branch）

25.迷走神经心上支 superior cardiac branch of vagus nerve

26.颈总动脉 common carotid artery

27.甲状腺 thyroid gland

28.右喉返神经 right recurrent laryngeal nerve

229

1.迷走神经下神经节 inferior ganglion of vagus nerve
2.舌咽神经 glossopharyngeal nerve
3.腭垂 uvula
4.左喉上神经 left superior laryngeal nerve
5.喉口 aperture of larynx
6.左迷走神经 left vagus nerve
7.甲状腺 thyroid gland
8.甲状腺下动脉 inferior thyroid artery
9.喉下神经 inferior laryngeal nerve
10.气管 trachea
11.主动脉弓 aortic arch
12.左喉返神经 left recurrent laryngeal nerve
13.左主支气管 left main bronchus
14.左肺静脉 left pulmonary vein
15.心脏 heart
16.胸主动脉 thoracic aorta
17.左肺 left lung
18.颈上神经节 superior cervical ganglion
19.咽丛 pharyngeal plexus
20.咽后壁 posterior pharyngeal wall
21.交感干 sympathetic trunk
22.右迷走神经 right vagus nerve
23.颈中神经节 middle cervical ganglion
24.食管 esophagus
25.颈胸神经节 cervicothoracic ganglion
26.右喉返神经 right recurrent laryngeal nerve
27.气管杈 bifurcation of trachea
28.右主支气管 right main bronchus
29.右肺静脉 right pulmonary vein
30.食管后丛 posterior esophagus plexus
31.下腔静脉 inferior vena cava
32.膈 diaphragm

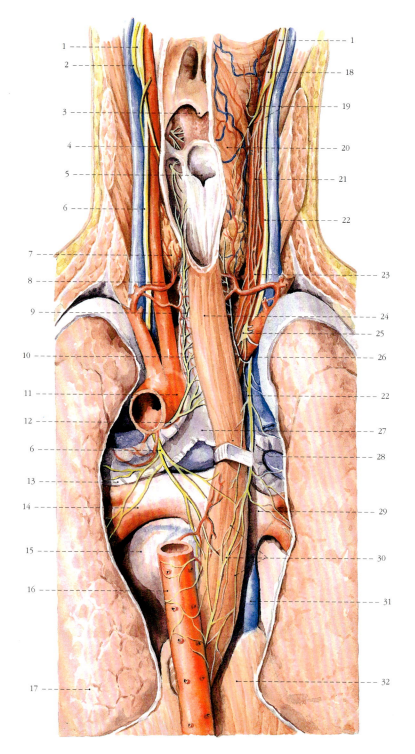

450. 左、右迷走神经颈胸部的分支（后面观）
Cervicothoracic branches of left and right vagus nerves
(posterior aspect)

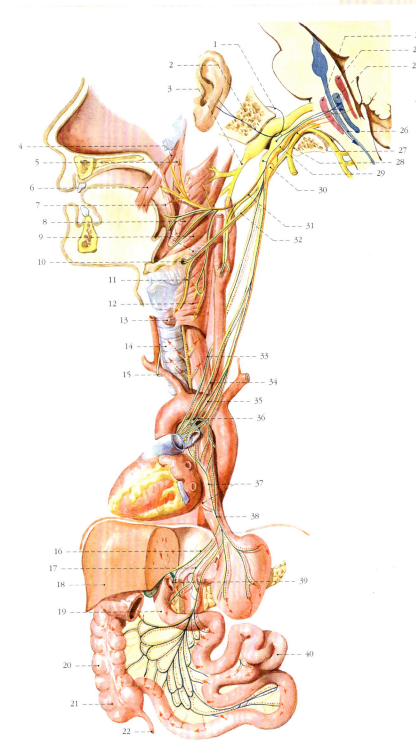

1.脑膜支 meningeal branch
2.耳支 auricular branch
3.舌咽神经 glossopharyngeal nerve
4.腭帆提肌 levator veli palatini
5.咽鼓管咽肌 salpingopharyngeus
6.腭舌肌 palatoglossus
7.腭咽肌 palatopharyngeus
8.咽上缩肌 superior constrictor of pharynx
9.咽中缩肌 middle constrictor of pharynx
10.喉上神经（内支）internal branch of superior laryngeal nerve
11.喉上神经（外支）external branch of superior laryngeal nerve
12.咽下缩肌 inferior constrictor of pharynx
13.环甲肌 cricothyroid
14.气管 trachea
15.右喉返神经 right recurrent laryngeal nerve
16.迷走神经前干肝支 hepatic branches of anterior vagal trunk
17.迷走神经后干腹腔支 celiac branches of posterior vagal trunk
18.肝 liver
19.十二指肠 duodenum
20.升结肠 ascending colon
21.盲肠 cecum
22.阑尾 vermiform appendix
23.疑核 nucleus ambiguus
24.迷走神经背核 dorsal nucleus of the vagus nerve
25.孤束核 solitary tract nucleus
26.三叉神经脊束与脊束核 spinal tract and spinal nucleus of trigeminal nerve
27.迷走神经 vagus nerve
28.颈静脉孔 jugular foramen
29.迷走神经上节 superior ganglion of vagus nerve
30.迷走神经下节 inferior ganglion of vagus nerve
31.迷走神经咽支 pharyngeal branch of vagus nerve
32.喉上神经 superior lanyngeal nerve
33.迷走神经心上支 superior cardiac branch of vagus nerve
34.迷走神经心下支 inferior cardiac branch of vagus nerve
35.迷走神经胸心支 thoracic cardiac branches of vagus nerve
36.左喉返神经 left recurrent laryngeal nerve
37.食管丛 esophageal plexus
38.迷走神经前干 anterior vagal trunk
39.肝丛幽门支 pyloric branch of hepatic plexus
40.小肠 small intestine

451. 迷走神经的纤维成分及其分布（模式图）
Fiber compositions and distribution of the vagus nerve (diagram)

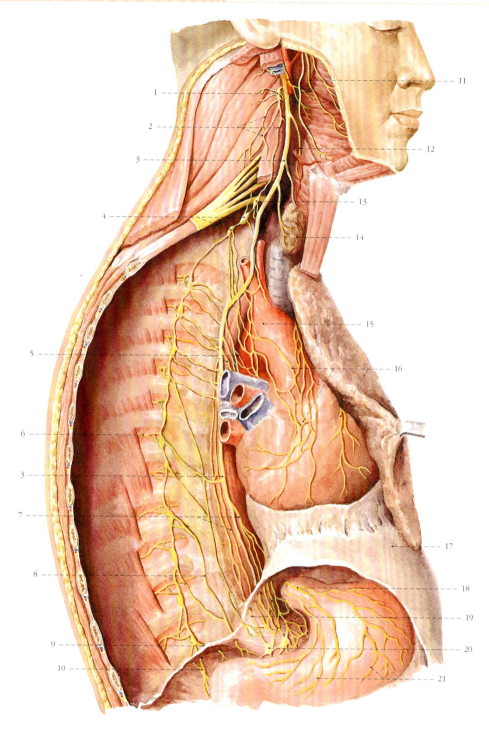

452. 胸部自主神经
Autonomic nerves of the thorax

1.颈上神经节 superior cervical ganglion
2.颈丛 cervical plexus
3.迷走神经 vagus nerve
4.颈胸神经节 cervicothoracic ganglion
5.肺丛 pulmonary plexus
6.肋间神经 intercostal nerves
7.食管丛 esophageal plexus

8.内脏大神经 greater splanchnic nerve
9.内脏小神经 lesser splanchnic nerve
10.腰神经节 lumbar ganglion
11.舌咽神经 glossopharyngeal nerve
12.喉上神经 superior laryngeal nerve
13.颈中神经节 middle cervical ganglion
14.甲状腺 thyroid gland

15.主动脉弓 aortic arch
16.心丛 cardiac plexus
17.膈 diaphragm
18.迷走神经前干 anterior vagal trunk
19.腹腔丛 celiac plexus
20.腹腔神经节 celiac ganglion
21.胃丛 gastric plexuses

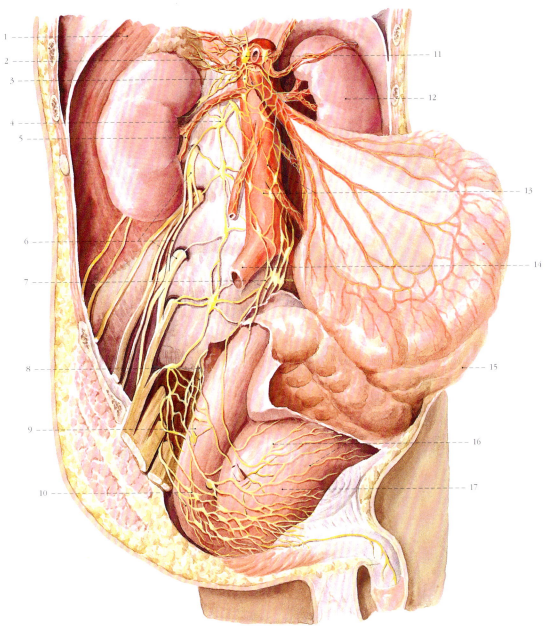

453. 腹、盆部的自主神经丛和节
Plexuses and ganglia of autonomic nerves in
abdomen and pelvis

1.膈 diaphragm
2.肾上腺丛 suprarenal plexus
3.肠系膜上神经节 superior mesenteric ganglion
4.腰神经节 lumbar ganglion
5.肾丛 renal plexus
6.腰丛 lumbar plexus
7.上腹下丛 superior hypogastric plexus
8.下腹下丛 inferior hypogastric plexus
9.直肠 rectum

10.直肠中丛 middle rectal plexus
11.腹腔神经节 celiac ganglia
12.肾 kidney
13.腹主动脉丛 abdominal aortic
   plexus
14.髂总动脉 common iliac artery
15.小肠 small intestine
16.膀胱丛 vesical plexus
17.膀胱 urinary bladder

233

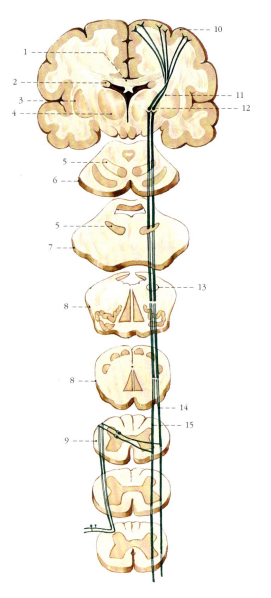

454. 躯干、四肢痛、温、触觉传导路

The pain, thalpotic and pselaphesic conductive
pathways of the trunk and limbs

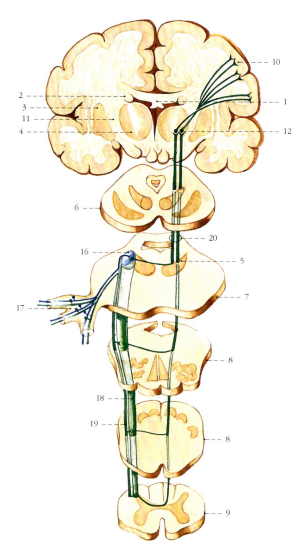

455. 头面部痛、温、触觉传导路

Pathways of pain, thalposis, tactile sensation of
head and face

1.胼胝体 corpus callosum
2.尾状核 caudate nucleus
3.豆状核 lentiform nucleus
4.背侧丘脑 dorsal thalamus
5.内侧丘系 medial lemniscus
6.中脑 midbrain
7.桥脑 pons

8.延髓 medulla oblongata
9.脊髓 spinal cord
10.中央后回 postcentral gyrus
11.内囊 internal capsule
12.腹后外侧核 ventral posterolateral nucleus
13.脊髓丘脑束 spinothalamic tract
14.脊髓丘脑侧束 lateral spinothalamic tract

15.脊髓丘脑前束 anterior spinothalamic tract
16.三叉神经脑桥核 pontine nucleus of trigeminal nerve
17.三叉神经节 trigeminal ganglion
18.三叉神经脊束核 spinal nucleus of trigeminal nerve
19.三叉神经脊束 spinal tract of trigeminal nerve
20.三叉丘系 trigeminal lemniscus

1.豆状核 lenticular nucleus
2.内囊 internal capsule
3.背侧丘脑 dorsal thalamus
4.中脑 midbrain
5.延髓 medulla oblongata
6.薄束核 gracile nucleus
7.楔束核 cuneate nucleus
8.内侧丘系交叉 decussation of medial lemniscus
9.楔束 fasciculus cuneatus
10.薄束 fasciculus gracilis
11.中央后回 postcentral gyrus
12.腹后外侧核 ventral posterolateral nucleus
13.脑桥 pons
14.脊髓 spinal cord
15.脊髓小脑前束 anterior spinocerebellar tract
16.旧小脑皮质 paleocerebellar cortex
17.脊髓小脑后束 posterior spinocerebellar tract

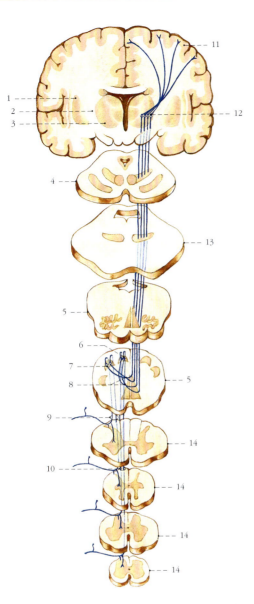

456. 躯干、四肢本体感觉和精细触觉传导路
The proprioception and refined tactile sensation
pathway of trunk and limbs

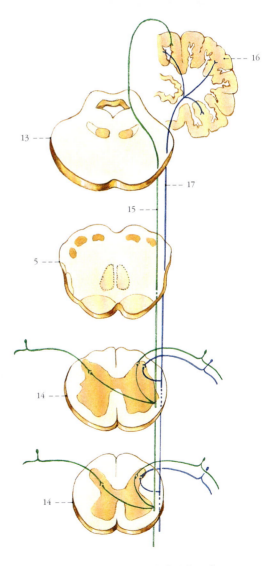

457. 传向小脑的本体感觉传导路
Pathway of the proprioceptive sensibility
conducting to the cerebellum

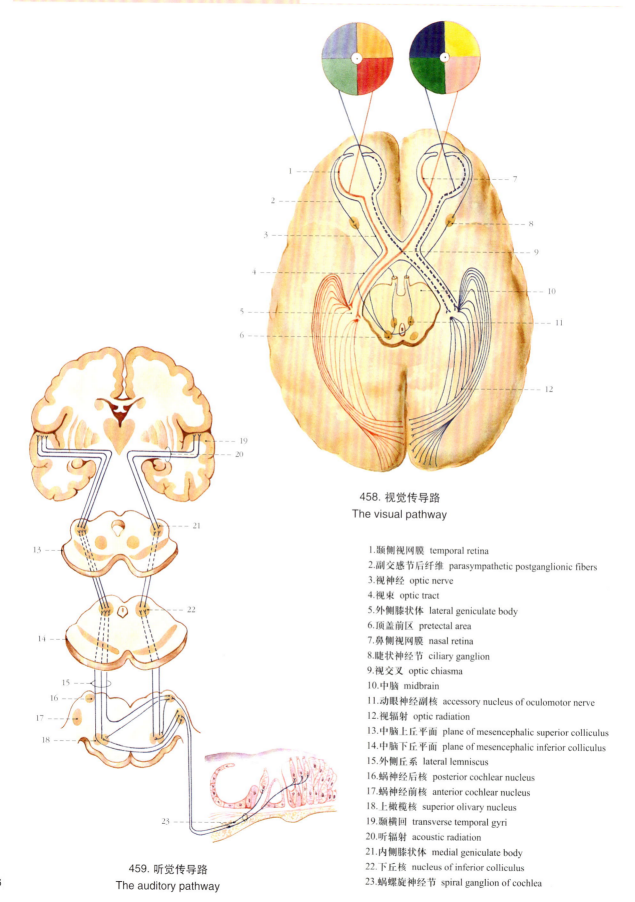

458. 视觉传导路
The visual pathway

459. 听觉传导路
The auditory pathway

1.颞侧视网膜 temporal retina
2.副交感节后纤维 parasympathetic postganglionic fibers
3.视神经 optic nerve
4.视束 optic tract
5.外侧膝状体 lateral geniculate body
6.顶盖前区 pretectal area
7.鼻侧视网膜 nasal retina
8.睫状神经节 ciliary ganglion
9.视交叉 optic chiasma
10.中脑 midbrain
11.动眼神经副核 accessory nucleus of oculomotor nerve
12.视辐射 optic radiation
13.中脑上丘平面 plane of mesencephalic superior colliculus
14.中脑下丘平面 plane of mesencephalic inferior colliculus
15.外侧丘系 lateral lemniscus
16.蜗神经后核 posterior cochlear nucleus
17.蜗神经前核 anterior cochlear nucleus
18.上橄榄核 superior olivary nucleus
19.颞横回 transverse temporal gyri
20.听辐射 acoustic radiation
21.内侧膝状体 medial geniculate body
22.下丘核 nucleus of inferior colliculus
23.蜗螺旋神经节 spiral ganglion of cochlea

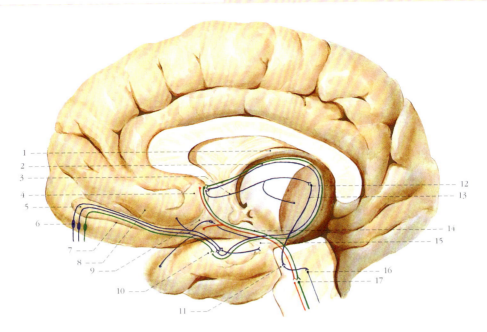

460. 嗅觉传导路
The olfactory pathway

1.穹窿 fornix

2.终纹 terminal stria

3.丘脑髓纹 thalamic medullary stria

4.隔区 septal area

5.嗅球 olfactory bulb

6.嗅细胞 olfactory cells

7.嗅束 olfactory tract

8.眶回 orbital gyri

9.前穿质 anterior perforated substance

10.梨状区 piriform area

11.脚间核 interpeduncular nucleus

12.缰核 habenular nucleus

13.缰核脚间束 habenulointerpeduncular tract

14.前脑内侧束 medial forebrain bundle

15.海马 hippocampus

16.被盖核 tegmental nucleus

17.网状核 reticular nucleus

18.大脑皮质 cerebral cortex

19.背侧丘脑 dorsal thalamus

20.展神经核 nucleus of abducent nerve

21.前庭神经上核 superior vestibular nucleus

22.球状核 globose nucleus

23.前庭神经外侧核 lateral vestibular nucleus

24.前庭神经下核 inferior vestibular nucleus

25.前庭神经内侧核 medial vestibular nucleus

26.网状结构 reticular formation

27.疑核 nucleus ambiguus

28.前庭脊髓束 vestibulospinal tract

29.副神经核 accessory nucleus

30.后连合核 nucleus of posterior commissure

31.Cajal 中介核 Cajal intercalatus nucleus

32.红核 red nucleus

33.动眼神经核 nucleus of oculomotor nerve

34.滑车神经核 nucleus of trochlear nerve

35.前庭神经节细胞 cells of vestibular ganglion

36.内侧纵束 medial longitudinal fasciculus

37.脊髓前角运动细胞 motor neuron of anterior
   horn of the spinal cord

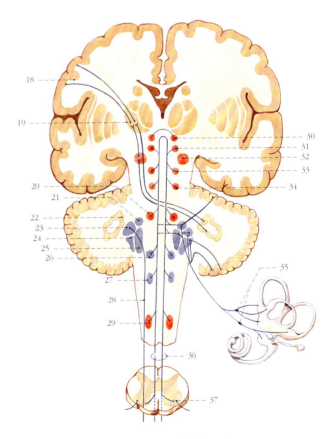

461. 平衡觉传导路
The pathway of the equilibrium sense

237

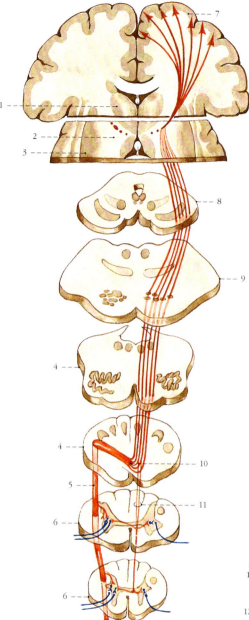

1. 背侧丘脑 dorsal thalamus
2. 内囊 internal capsule
3. 豆状核 lenticular nucleus
4. 延髓 medulla oblongata
5. 皮质脊髓侧束 lateral corticospinal tract
6. 脊髓 spinal cord
7. 中央前回 precentral gyrus
8. 中脑 midbrain
9. 脑桥 pons
10. 锥体交叉 decussation of pyramid
11. 皮质脊髓前束 anterior corticospinal tract
12. 动眼神经核 nucleus of oculomotor nerve
13. 三叉神经运动核 motor nucleus of trigeminal nerve
14. 展神经核 nucleus of abducent nerve
15. 疑核 ambiguous nucleus (nucleus ambiguus)
16. 副神经核 nucleus of accessory nerve
17. 皮质核束 corticobulbar tract
18. 滑车神经核 nucleus of trochlear nerve
19. 面神经核 nucleus of facial nerve
20. 舌下神经核 nucleus of hypoglossal nerve

462. 锥体系（皮质脊髓束）
The pyramidal system（corticospinal tract）

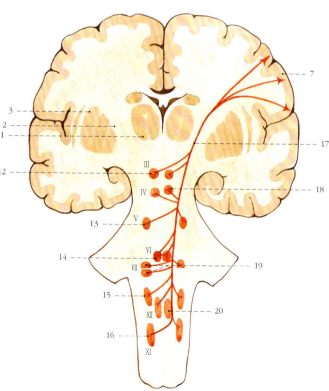

463. 锥体系（皮质核束）
The pyramidal system（corticobulbar tract）

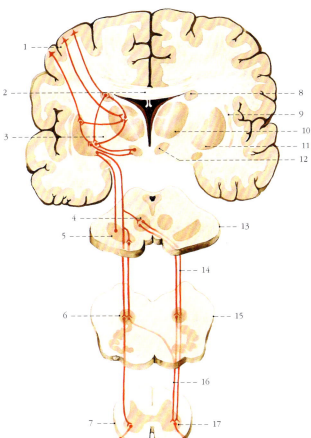

1.大脑皮质 cerebral cortex
2.胼胝体 corpus callosum
3.内囊 internal capsule
4.红核 red nucleus
5.黑质 substantia nigra
6.网状结构 reticular formation
7.脊髓 spinal cord
8.尾状核 caudate nucleus
9.屏状核 claustrum
10.背侧丘脑 dorsal thalamus
11.豆状核 lentiform nucleus
12.底丘脑核 subthalamic nucleus
13.中脑 midbrain
14.红核脊髓束 rubrospinal tract
15.延髓 medulla oblongata
16.网状脊髓束 reticulospinal tract
17.前角 anterior horn
18.皮质核束 corticobulbar tract
19.脑桥核 pontine nucleus
20.齿状核 dentate nucleus
21.齿状丘脑束 dentatothalamic tract
22.齿状红核束 dentatorubral tract
23.脑桥小脑束 pontocerebellar tract
24.脊髓小脑后（背侧）束 posterior dorsal spinocerebellar tract

464. 锥体外系（纹状体—苍白球系）
Extrapyramidal system
(corpus striatum-globus pallidus)

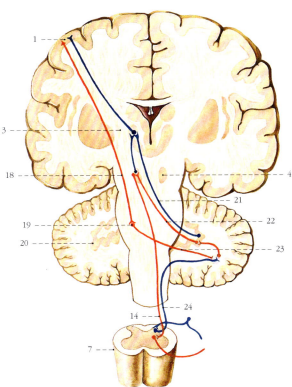

465. 锥体外系（皮质—脑桥—小脑系）
The extrapyramidal system (cortex-pons-cerebellum system)

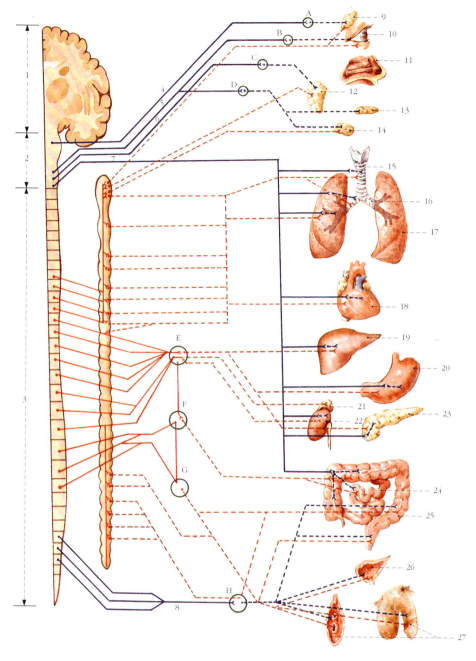

466. 自主神经系概观

General view of autonomic nervous system

1.大脑 cerebrum
2.脑干 brain stem
3.脊髓 spinal cord
4.动眼神经 oculomoter nerve
5.面神经 facial nerve
6.舌咽神经 glossopharyngeal nerve
7.迷走神经 vagus nerve
8.盆内脏神经 pelvic splanchnic nerves
9.泪腺 lacrimal gland

10.眼 eye
11.鼻 nose
12.腮腺 parotid gland
13.舌下腺 sublingual gland
14.下颌下腺 submandibular gland
15.气管 trachea
16.主支气管 main bronchus
17.肺 lung
18.心 heart
19.肝 liver

20.胃 stomach
21.肾上腺 adrenal gland
22.肾 kidney
23.胰 pancreas
24.小肠 small intestine
25.大肠 large intestine
26.膀胱 urinary bladder
27.男、女生殖器 male and female genital organs
A.睫状神经节 ciliary ganglion
B.翼腭神经节 pterygopalatine

ganglion
C.耳神经节 otic ganglion
D.下颌下神经节 submandibular ganglion
E.腹腔神经节 celiac ganglion
F.肠系膜上神经节 superior mesenteric ganglion
G.肠系膜下神经节 inferior mesenteric ganglion
H.盆神经节 pelvic ganglion

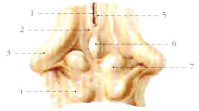

467. 松果体
Pineal body

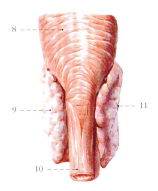

468. 甲状腺和甲状旁腺
Thyroid gland and parathyroid gland

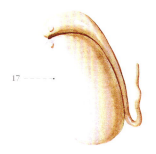

469. 睾丸
Testis

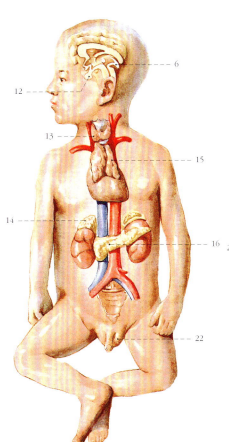

470. 内分泌腺概观
General view of endocrine glands

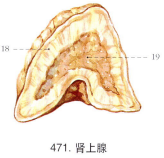

471. 肾上腺
Suprarenal gland

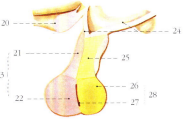

472. 垂体的分部
Divisions of the hypophysis

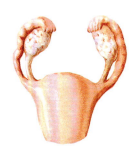

473. 卵巢
Ovary

1.第三脑室 third ventricle
2.缰连合 habenular commissure
3.背侧丘脑 dorsal thalamus
4.下丘 inferior colliculus
5.缰三角 habenular trigone
6.松果体 pineal body
7.上丘 superior colliculus
8.咽 pharynx
9.甲状腺侧叶 lateral lobe of thyroid gland
10.食管 esophagus
11.甲状旁腺 parathyroid gland
12.脑垂体 hypophysis
13.甲状腺 thyroid gland
14.肾上腺 suprarenal gland
15.胸腺 thymus
16.胰 pancreas

17.睾丸 testis
18.肾上腺皮质 cortex of suprarenal gland
19.肾上腺髓质 medulla of suprarenal gland
20.视交叉 optic chiasma
21.结节部 tuberal part
22.远部 distal part
23.前叶（腺垂体）anterior lobe
   (adenohypo physis)
24.正中隆起 median eminence
25.漏斗干核 infundbular nucleus
26.神经部 posterior lobe
27.正中部 median part
28.后叶（神经垂体）posterior lobe (neu-
   rohypophysis)
29.卵巢 ovary